New York Journal
Volume 1 (1

Various

Alpha Editions

This edition published in 2022

ISBN: 9789356784840

Design and Setting By

Alpha Editions

www.alphaedis.com

Email - info@alphaedis.com

Contents

NEW YORK JOURNAL OF PHARMACY. JANUARY, 1852.

TO OUR READERS.

The College of Pharmacy was founded with a view to the elevation of the professional standing and scientific attainments of Apothecaries, as well as to guard their material interests by raising a barrier against ignorance and imposture. What they have accomplished and how far they have been successful it does not become the Board of Trustees to state; if the results have not, in all respects, been what might be desired, it has not arisen from want of earnest effort and honest intention on their part. As a further means of benefiting their profession, of keeping its members acquainted with the progress it is making at home and abroad, and of inspiring among them a spirit of scientific inquiry, they believe that the establishment of a Journal, devoted to the pursuits and the interests of Apothecaries, would be of the highest utility.

By far the wealthiest and most populous city in the Union, New York, with its environs, contains several hundred Apothecaries, among whom are many of great experience and eminent ability; it contains numerous Laboratories where chemicals are manufactured on a large scale, and where the appliances and refinements of modern science are compelled into the service of commerce; it contains within itself all the means of scientific progress, and yet these means lie, for the most part, waste and idle; the observations that are made and the processes that are invented profit only the observer and the inventor. Both they and their consequences—for even apparently trivial observations may contain in themselves the germ of important discoveries, and no man can tell what fruit they may produce in the minds of others—are lost to the world.

New York is the commercial centre of the Union, the point to which our products are brought for exportation, and from which various goods, obtained from abroad, are distributed to the remainder of the United States. It is the chief drug mart of the Union; the source from which the largest part of our country draws its supplies of all medicines that are not the products of their own immediate vicinities. It is thus connected more intimately with the Druggists of a large portion of our country than any other city;

many visit it annually or oftener; most have business relations with it. Is the spirit of trade incompatible with that of science? Is money-getting to absorb all our faculties to the exclusion of anything nobler or higher? Are we ever to remain merely the commercial metropolis of our Union, but to permit science and art to centre in more congenial and less busy abodes? Shall we not rather attempt to profit by our many advantages, to use the facilities thrown in our way by the channels of trade for the diffusion of scientific knowledge, and in return avail ourselves of the information which may flow into us from the interior?

But it is not alone, we hope, by the information it would impart that a Journal such as is contemplated would be useful. A higher and no less useful object would be that it would excite a spirit of inquiry and emulation among the profession itself; it would encourage observation and experiment; it would train our young men to more exact habits of scientific inquiry. In diffusing information it would create it, and would be doubly happy in being the means of making discoveries it was intended to promulgate.

Such are the views which have determined the Trustees of the College to publish a Journal of Pharmacy. It will appear on the first day of every month, each number containing thirty-two octavo pages. It will be devoted exclusively to the interests and pursuits of the Druggist and Apothecary. While it is hoped that its pages will present everything that is important relating to the scientific progress of Pharmacy, it is intended to be mainly practical in its character, subserving the daily wants of the Apothecary, and presenting, as far as possible, that kind of information which can be turned to immediate account, whether it relates to new drugs and formulæ, or improved processes, manipulations, and apparatus. Such are the aims and ends of the New York Journal of Pharmacy; and the Druggists of New York are more particularly appealed to to sustain it, not only by their subscriptions, but by contributions from their pens. This last, indeed, is urgently pressed upon them; for, unless it receives such aid, however successful otherwise, it will fail in one great object for which it was originated. When special information is wanted on any particular subject, the conductors of the Journal, if in their power, will always be happy to afford it.

It is no part of the intention of the College to derive an income from the Journal. As soon as the state of the subscription list warrants it, it is intended to increase its size so that each number shall contain forty-eight instead of thirty-two pages.

REPORT OF COMMITTEE OF COLLEGE OF PHARMACY AS AMENDED.

The Committee to whom was referred the subject of the establishment of a Journal of Pharmacy in the city of New York, have given their attention to the subject, and beg leave to report as follows:

1. That in their opinion it is all important that a Journal of Pharmacy should be established in this city as soon as practicable, for reasons well known, and therefore unnecessary here to enumerate.

2. They recommend that the first number of a Journal of thirty-two octavo pages be issued on the 1st day of January next, and one number each month thereafter, to be called the New York Journal of Pharmacy.

3. The general control of the Journal shall be vested in a committee of five, which shall review every article intended for publication, four of whom shall be elected annually by the Board of Trustees at the first stated meeting succeeding the annual election of officers; and a committee of the same number shall be now elected, who shall act until the next annual election, to be denominated the Publishing Committee. The President of the College of Pharmacy shall be "ex officio" a member of this Committee, and the whole number of this Committee shall be five, two of whom may act.

4. That an Editor be appointed by the Publishing Committee who shall attend to all the duties of its publication, and cause to be prepared all articles for the Journal, and to have the entire management of it under the control and direction of the Publishing Committee.

5. The compensation for the services of the Editor, together with all financial matters connected with the Journal, shall be subject to the control of the Publishing Committee.

6. The matter to be published in the Journal shall be original communications, extracts from foreign and domestic journals, and editorials. No matter shall be published except what may relate directly or indirectly to the subject of Pharmacy, and the legitimate

business of Druggists and Apothecaries. No advertisements of nostrums shall be admitted.

7. The subscription list shall be kept in the hands of the Publishers, subject to the disposal of the Publishing Committee.

(Signed) T. B. MERRICK,
Chairman.

The Board then balloted for members of the Publishing Committee, when the following were found to be elected.

MESSRS. JNO. H. CURRIE,
THOS. B. MERRICK,
C. B. GUTHRIE,
EUGENE DUPUY,
with Ex Officio, GEO. D. COGGESHALL,
President of the College.

<hr size=0 width="100%" align=center>

ON TWO VARIETIES OF FALSE JALAP.

BY JOHN H. CURRIE.

Two different roots have for some time back been brought to the New York market, for the purpose of adulterating or counterfeiting the various preparations of Jalap. They differ materially from the Mechoacan and other varieties of false Jalap which formerly existed in our markets, as described by Wood and Bache in the United States Dispensatory, while some of the pieces bear no slight resemblance to the true root. The specimens I have been able to procure are so imperfect, and so altered by the process of drying, that the botanists I have consulted are unable to give any information even as to the order to which they belong. I have not been able either to trace their commercial history, nor do I know how, under the present able administration of the law for the inspection of drugs, they have obtained admission to our port. The article or articles, since there are at least two of them, come done up in bales like those of the true Jalap, and are probably brought from the same port, Vera Cruz.

No. 1 appears to be the rhizome or underground stem of an exogenous perennial herb, throwing up at one end each year one or more shoots, which after flowering die down to the ground. It comes in pieces varying in length from two to five inches, and in thickness from the third of an inch to three inches. In some of the pieces the root has apparently been split or cut lengthwise; in others, particularly in the large pieces, it has been sliced transversely like Colombo root. The pieces are somewhat twisted or contorted, corrugated longitudinally and externally, varying in color from a yellowish to a dark brown. The transverse sections appear as if the rhizome may have been broken in pieces at nodes from two to four inches distant from each other, and at which the stem was enlarged. Or the same appearance may have been caused by the rhizome having been cut into sections of various length; and the resinous juice exuding on the cut surfaces, has hindered them from contracting to the same extent as the intervening part of the root. On the cut or broken surfaces are seen concentric circles of woody fibres, the intervening parenchyma being contracted and depressed. The fresh broken surfaces of these pieces exhibit in a marked manner the concentric layers of woody fibres. The pieces that are cut longitudinally, on the other hand, are heavier than those just described, though their specific gravity is still not near so great as that of genuine Jalap. Their fracture is more uniform, of a greyish brown color, and highly resinous.

This variety of false Jalap, when exhausted with alcohol, the tincture thus obtained evaporated, and the residuum washed with water, yielded from 9½ to 15½ per cent. of resin, the average of ten experiments being 13 per cent. Its appearance was strikingly like that of Jalap resin. It had a slightly sweetish mucilaginous taste, leaving a little acridity, and the odor was faintly jalapine. It resembled Jalap resin in being slowly soluble in concentrated sulphuric acid, but unlike Jalap resin it was wholly soluble in ether. In a dose of ten grains it proved feebly purgative, causing two or three moderate liquid stools. Its operation was unattended with griping or other unpleasant effect, except a slight feeling of nausea felt about half an hour after the extract had been swallowed, and continuing for some time.

This variety of false Jalap is probably used, when ground, for the purpose of mixing with and adulterating the powder of true Jalap, or is sold for it, or for the purpose of obtaining from it its resin or extract, which is sold as genuine resin or extract of Jalap. The powder strikingly resembles that of true Jalap, has a faint odor of Jalap, but is destitute, to a great extent, of its flavor. The dust, too, arising from it, is much less irritating to the air passages.

The second variety is a tuber possibly of an orchidate plant, a good deal resembling in shape, color and size, a butternut, (Juglans cinerea.) Externally it is black or nearly so, in some places shining as if varnished by some resinous exudation, but generally dull, marked by deep longitudinal cuts extending almost to the centre of the tubers; internally it is yellow or yellowish white, having a somewhat horny fracture, and marked in its transverse sections with dots as if from sparse, delicate fibres. When first imported the root is comparatively soft, but becomes dry and brittle by keeping. Its odor resembles that of Jalap, and its taste is nauseous, sweetish, and mucilaginous.

This root contains no resin whatever. Treated with boiling water it yields a large amount (75 per cent.) of extract. This is soluble, to a great extent, likewise in alcohol. With iodine no blue color is produced.

The extract obtained from this drug appears, in ordinary doses, perfectly inert, five or ten grains producing, when swallowed, no effect whatever. Is this root employed for the purpose of obtaining its extract, and is this latter sold as genuine extract of Jalap?

Of the effect which frauds of this kind cannot fail to have on the practice of medicine it does not fall within my province to speak, but commercially its working is sufficiently obvious. One hundred pounds of Jalap at the market price, 60 cents per pound, will cost $60. In extracting this there will be employed about $5 worth of alcohol, making in all $65. There will be obtained forty pounds of extract, costing thus $1 62½ per pound.

One hundred pounds of false Jalap, No. 1, may be obtained for $20; admitting the alcohol to cost $5, it will make in all $25. This will produce thirty-six pounds of extract, costing rather less than 70 cents per pound.

One hundred pounds of variety No. 2 may be had for $20, and no alcohol is necessary in obtaining the extract. The yield being seventy-five pounds, the extract will cost rather less than twenty-seven cents per pound.

VIRGIN SCAMMONY,

WITH SOME REMARKS UPON THE CHARACTERISTICS OF SCAMMONY RESIN. BY B. W. BULL.

The more extended use in medicine which this substance has acquired within a few years, and its consequent greater consumption, render the knowledge of its peculiarities and the modes of ascertaining its purity doubly important to the druggist and apothecary.

An instance occurred a few weeks since, showing the necessity of careful and thorough examination of every parcel of this drug, and possessing some interest, from the fact that no description of any similar attempt at falsification has, I believe, been before published.

The commercial house with which I am connected, purchased a parcel of what purported to be virgin scammony from the importer, who obtained it direct from Smyrna. A sample of it was examined and found to contain seventy per cent. of resinous matter, but when the whole lot was received, it was found to consist evidently of two different grades of the article.

The whole of it was composed of amorphous pieces, possessing externally a similar appearance. Upon breaking them, however, a manifest difference was observable. Some of the pieces possessed the resinous fracture, and the other characteristics of virgin scammony, while the remainder, which constituted about five eighths of the whole, exposed a dull, non-resinous surface when freshly broken.

I selected two samples, each possessing in the highest degree the characteristics of the two varieties, and subjected them to the action of sulphuric ether with the following results, designating the resinous or best No. 1, and the other specimen No. 2:—

	No. 1.	No. 2.
Specific gravity	1,143	1,3935
	Per cent.	Per cent.
Resinous matter and water	94.35	49.86

Vegetable substance insoluble in ether	3.20	45.16
Inorganic matter	2.45	4.98
	100.00	100.00

The vegetable substance in No. 2 was principally, if not entirely, farinaceous or starchy matter, of which the other contained not a trace. The result shows that this parcel of scammony was composed partly of true virgin scammony mixed with that of an inferior quality; and also indicates the necessity of examining the whole of every parcel, and of not trusting to the favorable result of the examination of a mere sample.

The powder in the two specimens was very similar in shade, and they possessed in about the same degree the odor peculiar to the substance, showing the fallacy of relying upon this as a means of judging of the comparative goodness of different samples. This fact may appear anomalous, but on different occasions the powder of No. 2 was selected as having the most decided scammony odor.

Since examining the above, I have had an opportunity of experimenting upon a portion of scammony imported from Trieste as the true Aleppo scammony, of which there are exported from Aleppo not more than from two hundred and fifty to three hundred pounds annually.

The parcel consisted of a sample of one pound only, which was obtained from a druggist of respectability in that place by one of my partners, who was assured that the sample in question was from the above source, and the kind above alluded to. This scammony was in somewhat flattish pieces, covered externally with a thin coating of chalk in which it had been rolled, the structure was uniformly compact, the color of the fracture greenish, and it possessed in a high degree the caseous odor.

The fracture was unusually sensitive to the action of moisture. By merely breathing upon a freshly exposed surface, a film resembling the bloom upon fruit was at once perceived. Its specific gravity was 1,209, which, it will be observed, approximates with unusual accuracy to that given by Pereira as the specific gravity of true scammony, viz. 1,210. It contained

Resinous matter and water	89.53 per cent.
Vegetable substance insoluble in ether	7.55 per cent.
Inorganic matter	2.92 per cent.

There was no starchy matter present in the portion examined.

The mode of deciding upon the value or goodness of different samples of scammony, by ascertaining the amount of matter soluble in sulphuric ether, has seemed to me productive of a negative result in showing how much non-resinous matter was present, rather than a certain method of ascertaining the actual amount of scammony resin present; but some experiments upon the resinous residuum lead to a more favorable conclusion.

The results of the analyses made by Johnston, who seems to be the only chemist who has paid any attention to its ultimate composition, show that it varies in composition materially from many other resins.

According to his analyses, as contained in Löwig, it has the formula $\begin{array}{c} C_{40} H_{33} \\ O_8 \end{array}$

While that of Guaiac resin is $\begin{array}{c} C_{40} H_{23} \\ O_{10} \end{array}$

Of Colophony $\begin{array}{c} C_{40} H_{30} \\ O_4 \end{array}$

Or expressed in per cents:—

	Scammony.	Guaiac.	Colophony.
Carbon	56.08	70.37	79.81
Hydrogen	7.93	6.60	9.77
Oxygen	35.99	23.03	10.42
	100.00	100.00	100.00

The resin analysed by Johnston was obtained by evaporating the alcoholic solution, and he describes it as opaque, pale yellow, hard, and brittle; when obtained, however, by evaporating the ethereal solution I have found it transparent.

It might be inferred that, with a composition so different from that of the substances above adduced, its behavior with re-agents would be different from theirs; and its action with strong acids confirms the supposition, as may be seen by reference to the appended papers from a late number of the Paris Journal of Pharmacy.

The Edinburgh Pharmacopœia has an extract of scammony among its officinal preparations, prepared by treating scammony with proof spirit, and evaporating the solution. It is described as of a dirty greenish brown color. This color, however, is not a necessary accompaniment, but is owing either to some coloring matter being dissolved in the menstruum or to the partial oxydation of the dissolved substance under the influence of the air and the heat of the operation.

The ethereal solution of scammony resin, when gradually evaporated, and without exposure to heat, leaves a colorless or amber-colored resin, perfectly transparent and soluble in alcohol; when heated, however, during the operation, more or less insoluble matter of a dark color is found. Sometimes the ethereal solution, when spontaneously evaporated, leaves a dark residuum, but a second solution and evaporation leave it as above described.

This product, obtained from several different parcels of virgin scammony, I have considered free from admixture with any of the substances with which scammony is said to be adulterated, and from the similarity of their behavior, and, as the circumstances under which the sample from Trieste above alluded to was obtained are such as to make its genuineness very certain, feel warranted in so doing.

Sulphuric acid does not immediately decompose it, but produces the effect described by M. Thorel.

Nitric acid produces no discoloration, nor does hydrochloric acid immediately.

If scammony should be adulterated with colophony, sulphuric acid would be a very ready method of detection, though it would seem that this substance would hardly be resorted to, unless an entirely new mode of sophisticating the article should be adopted abroad.

The introduction of farinaceous substances and chalk is effected while the scammony is in a soft condition, in which state it would be difficult to incorporate colophony completely with the mass.

An admixture of resin of guaiac is also detected by the same agent, a fact which seems to have escaped observation.

When brought in contact with sulphuric acid, resin of guaiac immediately assumes a deep crimson hue, and this reaction is so distinct that a proportion of not more than four or five per cent. is readily detected.

The deep red mixture of sulphuric acid with resin of guaiac becomes green when diluted with water, a remarkable change, which adds to the efficacy of the test. Scammony resin, on the contrary, suffers no alteration by dilution.

In addition, nitric acid affords a ready mode of ascertaining the presence of resin of guaiac. It is well known that nitric acid, when mixed with an alcoholic solution of guaiac, causes a deep green color, which soon passes into brown, or if the solution is dilute, into yellow.

This reaction is manifest when scammony resin is mixed with guaiac resin in the proportion above mentioned, though the greenish blue tinge is then very transient, and sometimes not readily perceived.

Chloride of soda is a delicate test for the presence of guaiac resin. Added to an alcoholic solution, a beautiful green color appears, while it produces no effect on scammony resin. This reaction is very evident, though transient, when a very small proportion of guaiac is present. Nitrate of silver causes a blue color in a solution of guaiac resin, as does also sesqui-chloride of iron, neither of which agents affects the color of a solution of scammony resin. In fact, the evidences of the presence of guaiac are so numerous and distinct that there can be no possibility of an undetected adulteration with this substance.

The high price of resin of jalap would seem to be sufficient to prevent its being resorted to as a means of sophisticating scammony; but in case this substance should be made use of, the method proposed for detecting it by means of ether is defective, since, according to authorities, resin of jalap is partially soluble in that substance.

It becomes of interest to know whether in the preparation of scammony the juice of the plant from which it is obtained is ever mixed with that of other plants of similar properties, or with that of plants destitute of efficacy. This information can, of course, only be furnished by those familiar with the localities and with the mode of its preparation.

1"In advancing the opinion that scammony should only be employed for therapeutic purposes in the state of resin, I mean that this resin should only be prepared by the apothecary himself. When, however, it is impossible for the apothecary to do so, and the commercial article is in consequence resorted to, there arises a liability to deception. We must then be enabled to recognise its purity.

To avoid detection of the fraud, the admixture must either be in small quantity, or it must possess nearly the same action. In this latter case, resin of jalap would be employed as being less in price and nearly as active.

The method I propose for detecting an adulteration of this nature, in case it should be attempted, is based on the one side upon the entire insolubility of resin of jalap in rectified sulphuric ether, and on the other, upon the solubility of scammony resin in this liquid. Nothing is easier than the detection of a mixture of these two resins, since eight grammes of ether dissolve completely ten centigrammes of scammony resin.

Thus by agitating for a short time a mixture of twenty centigrammes of suspected resin with sixteen grammes of sulphuric ether, we shall be certain of the presence of resin of jalap, provided there is no other admixture, if a portion remains undissolved. This undissolved portion, dried and weighed, gives the proportion of the two resins.

Other more culpable sophistications may be attempted, either by the addition of resin of guaiac, or by that of colophony or other substances.

The resin of guaiac may easily be detected by means of the solution of gum, which I have specified as one of the most certain re-agents (Repertoire du Pharmacien, vol. iv., 1848), or by the means of nitrous gas, or bichloride of mercury.

Many re-agents disclose the presence of common resin or of pitch in the resin of scammony. First, spirits of turpentine, which dissolves the common resin at the ordinary temperature, and which leaves scammony resin almost untouched. The most certain re-agent, however, in my opinion, is sulphuric acid. This acid possesses the property of dissolving many resins—modifying their composition more or less.

Thus, if a small quantity is poured on common resin, an intense red color is produced by contact; poured on scammony resin, on the contrary, it does not produce an immediate change; only after some minutes, and with exposure to the air, does it become colored, and then but feebly, with the production of a color resembling the lees of wine, while in the first case the color is a very deep scarlet.

By this method one twentieth part of colophony may be detected in scammony resin. It is sufficient to pour upon twenty-five or thirty centigrammes of resin, placed in a glass or porcelain mortar, four or five grammes of commercial sulphuric acid, and to give one or two turns of the pestle; if colophony is present, the mixture will redden immediately upon contact; if, on the contrary, it is pure, the liquid will only become colored after the lapse of some time.

Colophony being more soluble in sulphuric acid is acted upon with more rapidity."

2"Scammony resin obtained by alcohol of 86 degrees occurs in form of powder or in thin transparent scales, if the alcoholic solution has been evaporated on a stove upon plates, or upon sheets of tin.

It is characterized by the peculiar odor of the substance from which it is obtained, the *odeur de brioche*, or of rancid butter.

If scammony resin has been mixed with one twentieth of common resin, trituration in a mortar develops the odor of the latter to a sufficient degree to cause detection of the fraud. Heated in a tube, a peculiar odor manifests itself with sufficient distinctness to indicate its purity.

This pure resin is soluble in all proportions in ether of 56 degrees (·752). This property affords a means of purifying it, by means of which it is obtained in thin flakes, by exposure to the air on plates.

Solution of ammonia at 24 degrees (·910) dissolves scammony resin completely. The solution has a more or less green color. These different properties, which the resin of scammony, obtained by alcohol, possesses, are sufficiently distinct to assist in distinguishing it from other resins or to establish its purity."

December, 1851.

---

1 Methods for detecting Resin of Jalap, Resin of Guaiac, and Colophony, in Resin of Scammony. By MR. THOREL.—*From the Journal de Pharmacie et de Chimie, for Nov. 1851.*

---

2 Note by MR. DUBLANC.—*From the Journal de Pharmacie et de Chimie, Nov. 1851.*

ON THE PREPARATION OF STRAMONIUM OINTMENT.

BY EUGENE DUPUY, PHARMACEUTIST, NEW YORK CITY.

The powerful narcotic and sedative properties of the Datura stramonium; added to the fact of its luxuriant growth in the vacant grounds of the inhabited districts of the United States, has made its use popular with most of our practising physicians. Besides its use smoked as tobacco in asthmatic cases, its properties analogous to those of hyosciamus and belladonna, have enabled practitioners to use it with success for producing dilatation of the pupil and in anodyne fomentations. In fact, the consequence of its demonstrated efficient activity as a remedial agent, has prompted its adoption in the United States Pharmacopœia, where the leaves and seeds are recognised, and the Tincture, Extract, and Ointment are officinal. According to our Pharmacopœia, last edition, to prepare the ointment, one drachm of the extract of stramonium is mixed to the proportion of one ounce of lard. Such a mixture, though possibly as effectual as need be, lacks the green color and homogeneity to which both patients and physicians have been accustomed. To remedy these objections, I have found the following process to give a good preparation both in quality and appearance. I am inclined to think that the objections which have been made to the former officinal ointment are chiefly ascribable to the difficulty of obtaining readily an ointment which would keep one year, that is free from water of vegetation or not impaired by a too protracted ebullition, and consequent decomposition, which deprives it of its properties, spoiling its appearance, and giving it an unpleasant pyrogenous odor, which shows the extent of the alteration it has undergone, making of it an irritating rather than a soothing unguent. In the process I now submit to the opinion of the profession, I had in view, 1st. To obtain at all seasons an ointment fulfilling the reasonable expectations of practitioners; 2d. Which could be easily prepared by competent Pharmaceutists throughout the United States. It is as follows:

Stramonium Leaves,   half a pound.

Alcohol at 95°,   a sufficient quantity.

Prepared lard,   fourteen ounces.

Moisten the leaves, previously reduced to a coarse powder, with sufficient alcohol, in a tight vessel having a suitable cover; melt the lard in a pan three times in capacity to the bulk of the lard, and stir in it gradually the prepared stramonium; keep the mixture in a warm place for five hours, stirring occasionally, till the alcohol has disappeared from the ointment, which may be ascertained by placing a lighted match on the surface of the warm ointment just stirred. Filter the mixture through flannel, in an appropriate vessel. The stramonium ointment thus prepared is a reliable preparation, possessed of a handsome green color, a rather pleasant herbaceous odor, and forms a homogeneous mass containing all the valuable constituents of the Datura stramonium, if the leaves have been gathered while the plant is in bud, and properly preserved. For the warm days of summer the substitution of two ounces of beeswax for the same quantity of lard gives it the consistence which it has at the low temperature of the remaining seasons.

COMPOUND FLUID EXTRACT OF SENNA AND DANDELION.

BY EUGENE DUPUY, PHARMACEUTIST, NEW YORK CITY.

Senna (officinal),	two pounds.
Torrefied Dandelion Root,	one pound.
Chamomile,	quarter of a pound.
Sugar,	twenty ounces.
Carbonate of Potash or Soda,	one ounce.
Oil of Gaultheria,	half a drachm.
Alcohol,	two ounces.
Water,	half a gallon.

Mix the dry plants, previously reduced to a coarse powder, with the water holding the alkaline carbonate in solution; let the mixture stand twelve hours; introduce it in a percolator, and gradually pour in water until a gallon of liquid shall have passed; evaporate it to twenty ounces by means of a water bath, then add the sugar, filter, and make the addition of the alcoholic solution of gaultheria when cold. By following this process, I believe that a kind of saponification takes place, which allows of the more ready solution of the active principle of the senna in the aqueous vehicle, probably because chlorophylle being united to a dried essential oil, participating in the properties of resins, is rendered soluble, and the extractive portion being denuded of its resinoid covering, is more readily extracted by the percolating liquid. I make use of a percolator possessed of a convenient hydraulic power; it has rendered readily, within thirty hours, a highly saturated liquid, containing in a gallon all the soluble principles of this extract. Ordinary percolators will answer also; but the ingredients needing to be more loosely packed, do not yield so fully or so readily. The addition of torrefied dandelion root is intended to give to this fluid extract some greater value on account of its peculiar action on the hepatic system. I employ in preference the German chamomile (Camomila vulgaris3), because of its pleasant aroma and its carminative properties, joined to a bitter principle, which seems to increase the purgative effect of the senna.

This extract has become a favorite anti-bilious purgative with many of our practitioners, who, some of them at least, have used it with success with children, who can take it readily, as well as for adults, where an anti-bilious purgative is desirable, seldom producing pain or nausea, and not liable to induce constipation.

---

3 Matricaria.

ACCIDENTS CAUSED BY A VERY SMALL DOSE OF SANTONINE GIVEN TO A CHILD.

Santonine, being a tasteless vermifuge, is easily given to children, consequently its employment becomes daily more and more frequent; we therefore think it useful to expose the accidents which may follow the use of this medicine, when given in too large a dose. We refer to a case given in the Bulletin de Thérapeutique, by Dr. Spengler (d'Herborn). The patient, a child of four years old, who had been suffering for several months from intestinal worms, had taken at different times, and with success, a dose of a grain and a half. One day they gave him three grains in two doses; after the first dose he became troubled with pains in the epigastrium, colic, and vomiting. He had frequent stools, in which were found a number of ascarides. Notwithstanding these numerous evacuations, the bad symptoms continued to increase; his body became cold, his face livid, his eyes had a blue circle round them, a cold sweat broke out, his respiration became embarrassed, and his extremities convulsed. Besides these symptoms, M. Spengler mentions that there were dilatation of the pupils and great pain in the abdomen (not, however, increased by pressure). He prescribed milk in abundance, and after several evacuations, the potion of Rivière in an oily emulsion. The little patient was placed in a very warm bed; during the night he was much disturbed; the following day he took some doses of calomel, after which several worms were evacuated, and from that time he became convalescent. We have related this fact as a caution against the accidents which may result from the use of santonine, although the severity of the symptoms and the smallness of the dose may make us doubt whether the santonine was pure, or whether some other cause might not have produced the terrible results attributed to it.—*Journal de Pharmacie et Chimie.*

ON POISONING BY NICOTINE.

READ BEFORE THE NATIONAL ACADEMY OF MEDICINE.
BY M. ORFILA.

GENTLEMEN,—In laying before the Academy a memoir on Nicotine, on the 20th of last month, I stated that I did not think I ought to read it, fearing that it might exercise some influence on the proceedings which were to take place at Mons, eight days afterwards. My scruples are now entirely removed, because I was present at the three first sittings of the Court of Assizes at Hainault, and have heard the examination of the accused persons, and the depositions of some of the witnesses. My memoir, supposing it to be published to-morrow, and consequently much before the sentence will have been pronounced, will not aggravate the situation of the accused, nor increase the power of the ministers of justice. You will see, in fact, that after describing nicotine, I came to the conclusion, that it may be easily detected in the digestive canal, the liver, the lungs, and all those organs into which it has been carried after its absorption. Now, M. de Bocarmé confesses that he prepared some nicotine, that Gustave Fougnies took an appreciable dose of it, and died very shortly afterwards. Consequently, he cannot dispute the fact of M. Stas having found this alkaloid in the body of his brother-in-law. It is of little importance to us that Madame de Bocarmé accuses her husband of being the author of the crime, whilst he, on the other hand, attributes the death of Gustave to a mistake of his wife's, who might inadvertently have poured the nicotine into a glass instead of wine. It will be for the jury to decide what truth there is in these assertions; as scientific men, we ought to confine ourselves in this case to the solution of the chemical and medical problems relating to this subject.

I think I ought to read to the Academy the textual memoir, without the preamble, which I composed a fortnight ago, when the principal circumstances, which have since been developed, were but imperfectly known.

The principal object of this paper is to show:—

1. That we may characterize pure nicotine as easily as we can a poison derived from the mineral kingdom.

2. That we may detect this alkali in the digestive canal, and assert its existence there, although it is present only to the extent of a few drops.

3. That it is sufficiently easy to prove its presence in the liver and the other organs, after it has been absorbed.

1. *Pure Nicotine may be characterised as easily as a Poison derived from the Mineral Kingdom.*—Nicotine, discovered in 1809 by the illustrious Vauquelin, was studied in 1828 by Messrs. Posselt and Reimann, who found it in different species of nicotiana, in macrophylla rustica, and glutinosa. Messrs. Boutron, Charlard, and Henry described some of its properties in 1836. Havanna tobacco contains two per cent., that of Maryland 2·3, that of Virginia 6·9, that of Alsace 3·2, that of Pas-de-Calais 4·9, that of the Nord 6·6, and that of Lot 8. It is classed among the *natural volatile* vegetable alkalies, which are only three in number, namely, *conicine*, *theobromine*, and *nicotine*. This last is entirely composed of hydrogen, carbon, and nitrogen. It may be represented as a compound of one equivalent of ammonia (H_3N), and of one of a hydro-carbon containing four equivalents of hydrogen and ten of carbon (H_4C_{10}). It is now obtained by a much more simple process than was formerly adopted, which consists in passing the vapor of tobacco into water acidulated with sulphuric acid. Sulphate of nicotine is thus speedily produced, and this has to be decomposed by a strong alkali. It is then only necessary to apply sufficient heat to volatilize the nicotine. This mode of preparation indicates that smokers in respiring the smoke of tobacco introduce into their bodies a certain quantity of the vapor of nicotine.

Characters of pure Nicotine.—It is in the form of an oleaginous, transparent, colorless, tolerably fluid, anhydrous liquid, of the density of 1·048, becoming slightly yellow with keeping, and tending to become brown and thick from contact with the air from which it absorbs oxygen; its acrid odor resembles but slightly that of tobacco; its taste is very burning. It volatilizes at 77° F., and leaves a carbonaceous residue. The vapor which rises presents such a powerful smell of tobacco, and is so irritating, that it is difficult to breathe in a room in which one drop of it has been spilt. If this vapor be approached with a lighted taper, it burns with a white smoky flame, and leaves a carbonaceous residue as an essential oil would do. It *strongly blues* reddened litmus paper. *It is very soluble in water*, in alcohols, and in fat oils, as also in *ether*, which easily separates it from an aqueous solution. The great solubility of nicotine in both water and ether forms an important fact in its chemical history, as the greater number of vegetable alkalies, not to say all, if they dissolve easily in one of these liquids, are not readily soluble in the other.

Nicotine combines directly with acids, disengaging heat. Concentrated pure sulphuric acid, without heat, produces with it a wine-red color; on the application of heat to this it becomes thick, and acquires the color of the dregs of wine; if it be boiled it blackens and disengages sulphurous acid. With cold hydrochloric acid it disengages white vapors as ammonia does; if the mixture be heated it acquires a violet color, the intensity of which increases with prolonged ebullition. Nitric acid, aided with a little heat, imparts to it an orange-yellow color, and white vapors of nitric acid are first given off, then red vapors of hyponitrous acid. If it be further heated the liquor becomes yellow, and by ebullition it acquires a red color resembling that of chloride of platinum. Prolonged ebullition gives a black mass. Heated with stearic acid it dissolves and forms a soap, which congeals on cooling, and is slightly soluble in water, and very soluble in heated ether. The simple salts of nicotine are deliquescent, and difficultly crystallizable. The double salts which it yields with the different metallic oxides crystallize better.

The aqueous solution of nicotine is colorless, transparent, and strongly alkaline. It acts like ammonia on several reagents; thus, it gives a white precipitate with bichloride of mercury, acetate of lead, protochloride and bichloride of tin; a canary yellow precipitate with chloride of platinum, which precipitate is soluble in water; a white precipitate with salts of zinc, which is soluble in excess of nicotine; a blue precipitate with acetate of copper. This precipitate is gelatinous and soluble in excess of nicotine, forming a blue double acetate, similar to that formed by ammonia with the same salt. It gives an ochre-yellow precipitate with salts of the sesqui-oxide of iron, insoluble in excess of nicotine. With sulphate of protoxide of manganese it gives a white precipitate of oxide, which speedily becomes brown by contact with the oxygen of the air. It separates the green sesqui-oxide from the salts of chromium. The red permanganate of potash is instantly decolorized by nicotine, as by ammonia, although this latter alkali acts more slowly and must be used in larger proportion.

The following reactions may serve to distinguish the aqueous solutions of nicotine from ammonia Chloride of gold yields a reddish-yellow precipitate, *very soluble in an excess of nicotine*. Chloride of cobalt yields a blue precipitate, which changes to green; the oxide thus formed does not readily dissolve in excess of nicotine, whilst ammonia dissolves the green precipitate and forms a red solution. Aqueous solution of iodine gives a yellow precipitate with solution of nicotine, as chloride of platinum would do; with an excess of nicotine it acquires a straw color, and it is decolorized by the action of heat. Ammonia, on the contrary, immediately decolorizes the aqueous solution of iodine without rendering it turbid. Pure tannic acid gives with nicotine an abundant white precipitate. Ammonia gives no precipitate, but imparts a red color.[4]

---

4 It is interesting to compare the physical and chemical properties of nicotine with those of conicine.

Conicine is yellow; *its smell resembles that of the urine of the mouse*, and differs entirely from that of nicotine; it strongly blues reddened litmus paper. Added to water and shaken with it, it floats on the surface and is not readily dissolved. Ether dissolves it easily. When heated in a capsule it forms white vapors, *having a strong smell of celery mixed with that of the urine of the mouse*. Weak tincture of the iodine yields a white precipitate, which acquires an olive color with excess of the tincture. Pure and concentrated sulphuric acid *does not alter it*; when the mixture is heated it acquires a greenish brown color, and if the heat be continued it becomes blood-red and afterwards black. Nitric acid imparts to it a *topaz color*, which is not changed by the action of heat. Hydrochloric acid yields white vapors as ammonia does, and renders it violet, especially when heated. Tannic acid gives a white precipitate, and chloride of platinum a yellow precipitate. The red permanganate of potash is immediately decolorized. Corrosive sublimate yields a white precipitate. Acetate of copper gives a gelatinous blue precipitate, less soluble in an excess of conicine than is that formed with nicotine. Chloride of cobalt behaves with it as it does with nicotine. Chloride of gold gives a light yellow precipitate. *Neutral acetate of lead does not give any precipitate*; neither does the subacetate. Chloride of zinc gives a white gelatinous precipitate soluble in excess of the conicine. Sulphate of sesquioxide of iron gives a yellow precipitate. The words in italics indicate the means of distinguishing conicine from nicotine.

If to these chemical characters which permit one so easily to distinguish nicotine, we add those resulting from the action which it exercises on the animal economy, it will no longer be possible to confound it with any other body. The following are the results of the experiments I undertook in 1842 on this alkali, and which I published in 1843. (See the 4th edition of my work on Toxicology.)

First Experiment.—I applied three drops of nicotine on the tongue of a small but sufficiently robust dog; immediately afterwards, the animal became giddy, and voided urine; at the end of a minute, its breathing was quick and panting. This state lasted for forty seconds, and then the animal fell on its right side, and appeared intoxicated. Far from showing any stiffness or convulsions, it was feeble and flabby, although the fore paws slightly trembled. Five minutes after the administration of the poison, he uttered plaintive cries, and slightly stiffened his neck, carrying his head slightly backwards. The pupils were excessively dilated; the respiration was calm, and in no way accelerated. This state lasted ten minutes, during which the animal was not able to stand. From this time the effects appeared to diminish, and soon after it might have been predicted that they would speedily disappear entirely. Next day, the animal was quite well. The nicotine I used was evidently not anhydrous.

Second Experiment.—I repeated the experiment with five drops of nicotine on a dog of the same description. The animal showed the same effects, and died at the end of ten minutes, although during four minutes he showed slight convulsive movements.

Opening of the Body the day following.—The membranes of the brain were slightly injected, and the superficial vessels were gorged with blood; this injection was especially observed on the left side, and in the lower part of the brain. The brain itself of the ordinary consistence, had the two substances of which it is composed, slightly disintegrated, the striated substance was much injected, as well as the *pons varolii*. The membranes which envelope the cerebellum were still more injected than the other parts. Between the first and second cervical vertebræ on the right side, that is, on the side on which the animal fell, there was a rather considerable effusion of blood. The lungs appeared to be in their natural state. The heart, the vessels of which were gorged with blood, was greatly distended, especially on the right side, with clots of blood; the auricles and the right ventricle containing much, and the left ventricle none. The superior and inferior *vena cava*, and the aorta, were equally distended with clots of semi-fluid blood. The tongue was corroded along the middle line, and towards the posterior part, where the epithelium separated with facility. In the interior of the stomach there were found a black pitchy matter and a bloody liquid, which appeared to have resulted from an exudation of blood. The duodenum was inflamed in patches; the rest of the intestinal canal appeared in a healthy state.

Since the above period I have made the following experiments, which I have frequently repeated with the same results, only that in some cases I have found the blood contained in the cavities of the heart in a fluid state, even when proceeding to dissection immediately after death; nevertheless the blood speedily coagulated.

Third Experiment.—At eleven o'clock I administered, to a dog of moderate size, twelve drops of nicotine. A few instants afterwards giddiness came on, and *he fell on the right side;* he soon manifested convulsive movements, slightly at first, then sufficiently strong to constitute a tetanic fit with opisthotonos; he was in a remarkable state of drowsiness, and uttered no cry. His pupils were dilated; there was no action of the bowels, nor vomiting. He died at two minutes after eleven. The body was immediately opened. The abdomen and thorax, on being cut open, *sometimes* emitted a very decided smell of tobacco. The heart contained a considerable quantity of *black coagulated* blood. There was more in the right auricle and ventricle than in the left. The lungs appeared in a normal state. The stomach contained about forty grammes of a thick, yellow, slimy liquid; and here and there parts of the mucous membrane were inflamed. The œsophagus, the intestines, the liver, the spleen, and the kidneys, were in a normal state. The epithelium was easily detached from the tongue; the base of this organ was red and slightly excoriated. The brain was more injected than its enveloping membranes; the *pons varolii* was the same as in the second experiment.

Fourth Experiment.—I applied on the eye of a dog of moderate size one drop of nicotine; the animal instantly became giddy and weak in its limbs; a minute afterwards he fell on his right side and manifested convulsive fits, which became more and more powerful; the head was thrown back. At the end of two minutes the convulsions ceased, and extreme weakness ensued. Five minutes afterwards the animal could stand, but was unable to walk. Ten minutes later he was in the same state without having vomited or had any action of the bowels. Urged to walk, he made a few undecided steps, then vomited about one hundred grammes of a greyish alimentary paste. At the end of half an hour he was in the same state. It was evident that he was recovering. The conjunctiva was sensibly inflamed, and the transparent cornea was, to a great extent, opaque.

2. *We may detect nicotine in the digestive canal, and affirm its existence there, although it may be only present to the extent of a few drops.* I would call the particular attention of the Academy to this paragraph; I have never, in the course of my numerous experiments, seen animals whose death has been almost instantaneous, either vomit or have any action of the bowels.5 If it be the same with man, as everything tends to prove it is, the Chemist will, under such circumstances, be in the most favorable condition for detecting the poison, as there will most frequently be a sufficient quantity in the canal to determine its presence.

---

5 If life is prolonged the animals vomit.

Before describing the two processes to which I had recourse for the determining the existence of nicotine in the stomach and intestines, as well as in the œsophagus, it may be observed that I acted separately on the liquid and solid matters contained in these organs, and on the organs themselves.

First Process.—The contents of the stomach and intestines, or the organs themselves, are placed in a considerable proportion of sulphuric ether; after twelve hours of maceration, it is to be filtered; the ether passes through, holding nicotine in solution; most frequently when the matters on which the ether has acted are fatty, the ether holds in solution a soap composed of nicotine and one or several fatty acids; it may also happen that it contains non-saponified nicotine. The ethereal liquid is evaporated almost to dryness by very gentle heat. The greasy and soapy product obtained rarely shows any alkaline reaction. It is to be agitated, without heat, with caustic soda dissolved in water, to decompose the soap and set free the nicotine. The whole is then to be put into a retort furnished with a receiver plunged in cold water, and heat applied to the retort until no more liquid remains in it. The liquid condensed in the receiver contains either all, or at least a large proportion of the nicotine. It is well to know that, 1st, when heat is applied to the retort, the matter froths, augments in volume, and would certainly pass into the receiver, if the retort was not very large in relation to the quantity of liquid operated upon; 2ndly, even at a temperature of 212° Fahr., the vapor of water carries with it a certain quantity of nicotine, therefore the operation should be carried on as much as possible in close vessels. If these precautions be observed, the distilled liquid will be limpid and colorless; it suffices then to concentrate it over a water-bath, to about a ninth of its volume, to obtain with it all the reactions of nicotine.

Second Process.—The method of which I am now going to speak is evidently superior to the preceding. The matters contained in the stomach and intestines, or the organs themselves, as well as the œsophagus, are macerated in water acidulated by pure and concentrated sulphuric acid, taking, for instance, four or five drops of acid to one hundred and fifty or two hundred grammes of water. At the end of twelve hours it is to be filtered; the liquid, which is generally of a yellow color, contains sulphate of nicotine and a certain quantity of organic matter. It is then to be evaporated almost to dryness in close vessels over a water-bath; then treated with a few grammes of distilled water which dissolves the sulphate of nicotine, leaving the greater part of the organic matter undissolved; it is now to be filtered; the filtered liquor is to be saturated with a little pure hydrate of soda or potash, in order to take the sulphuric acid, and set free the nicotine. The mixture of nicotine and of sulphate of soda or potash is to be put into a retort, and heated as described in the first process; the distilled liquid is to be evaporated over a water-bath in order to concentrate the solution of nicotine.

Instead of distilling the liquor by heat, I have often treated it with ether; this latter decanted and submitted to spontaneous evaporation leaves the nicotine.

Everything tends to show that nicotine may be detected by other processes. Thus by treating the digestive canal with absolute alcohol, with the addition of a little soda, it would be dissolved, and by the reaction of the soda, a soap would be formed with the fatty matter, which would set free the nicotine; it would then only remain to distil it by heat, after having evaporated to dryness. Perhaps, also, it might be separated by acting on the tissues with pure soda or potash, then evaporating to dryness and heating it in closed vessels.

3. *It is sufficiently easy to prove the presence of nicotine in the liver and other organs after it has been absorbed.*—In 1839 when I had shown that poisons after having been absorbed might be extracted from the organs where they had been carried with the blood, I insisted so strongly on the necessity of examining these organs with a view to the detection of poisons, that it has now become the custom to proceed in this way. How often does it happen, that, in consequence of repeated vomiting and action of the bowels, and also from complete absorption having taken place, there remains

no trace of the poison in the digestive canal? Moreover, it is evident, that, in getting the poison from the organs to which it has been carried by absorption, we obtain, in reality, that portion of the poison which has been the cause of death, unless it be shown that it was carried to those organs after death by absorption. M. Stas has conformed, most wisely, to this precept. For my part, I could not, in my researches, neglect this important branch of the investigation. The livers of those animals which I had poisoned with twelve or fifteen drops of nicotine, when submitted to one or other of the processes I have described, furnished me with appreciable quantities of this alkali. I scarcely obtained any from the blood contained in the heart, but I had only operated upon a few grammes. Moreover, experience teaches that a great number of poisons absorbed rapidly pass from the blood into the organs, and most especially into the liver.

It may be readily conceived that the research for absorbed nicotine might be fruitless in those cases where death was occasioned by only a few drops of this body; but then the presence of the alkali may be detected in the digestive canal.

Gentlemen, after results such as those obtained by M. Stas and myself, society may feel satisfied. Without doubt intelligent and skilful criminals, intent on puzzling the Chemists, will sometimes have recourse to very active poisons, but little known to the community at large, and difficult to detect; but science is on the alert to surmount all difficulties. Penetrating to the recesses of our organs, she extracts evidence of the crime, and furnishes one of the great elements of conviction against the guilty. Do we not know that at the present time poisonings by morphine, brucine, strychnine, nicotine, conicine, hydrocyanic acid, and many other vegetable substances which were formerly believed to be inaccessible to our means of investigation, may be discovered and recognised in a manner to be perfectly characteristic?

During my stay at Mons, and consequently since the deposit of this memoir, I have had at my disposal the complete and remarkable Report of M. Stas, and I have satisfied myself:—

1st. That this Chemist has obtained nicotine from the tongue, from the stomach, and liquids contained in it, and also from the liver and lungs of Gustave Fougnies.

2ndly. That he also obtained nicotine by properly treating the boards of the dining-room where Gustave died, although these boards had been washed with warm water, with oil, and with soap.—*Repertoire de Pharmacie.*

The Count Hippolyte Visarte de Bocarmé confessed his guilt, and was executed at Mons.

ON THE ESTIMATION OF THE STRENGTH OF MEDICINAL HYDROCYANIC ACID, OF BITTER ALMOND WATER, AND OF CHERRY LAUREL WATER.

BY J. LIEBIG.

Liquids which contain prussic acid, and are mixed with caustic potash ley until they have a strong alkaline reaction, yield, on the gradual addition of a diluted solution of nitrate of silver, a precipitate, which, on being shaken, disappears to a certain extent. Alkaline liquids containing prussic acid, may also be mixed with a few drops of a solution of common salt without the production of any permanent precipitate, until at last, on an increased addition, chloride of silver falls down.

This phenomenon depends on the fact that oxide of silver and chloride of silver are soluble in the generated cyanide of potassium, until there is found a double salt, composed of equal equivalents of cyanide of potassium and cyanide of silver, which is not decomposed by an excess of alkali. Liebig's method of estimating the prussic acid consists in determining the quantity of silver which must be added to an alkaline liquid, containing prussic acid, until a precipitate appears. Each equivalent of silver corresponds to two equivalents of prussic acid. Having caused several experiments to be made, which prove the efficacy of this method; and having carefully observed that the presence of formic acid and muriatic acid in the prussic acid, does not interfere with the correctness of this method, the author gives the following directions for examining different liquids containing prussic acid:—The *aqua amygdalarum amarum* being turbid, must be clarified by the addition of a known quantity of water: 63 grs. of fused nitrate of silver are dissolved in 5937 grs. of water; 300 grs. of this liquid corresponds to 1 gr. of anhydrous prussic acid. Before applying the test, the vessel with the solution of silver is to be weighed, and of the latter so much is added to a weighed quantity (*e.g.* 60 grs.) of prussic acid, mixed with a small portion of potash ley and a few drops of a solution of common salt, shaking it in a common white medicine glass until a perceptible turbidness takes place, and does not disappear on shaking. The solution of silver is now again to be weighed; and supposing 360 grs. are found to have been employed for the test, the 60 grs. of the tested prussic acid contain 1,20 grs. anhydrous prussic acid, or 100 grs. contain two grains.

Aqua laurocerasi, which the author examined, contained in one litre, one decigram, and the same quantity of *aqua amygdal. amar.* 7·5 decigrammes of anhydrous prussic acid.—(In Pharmaceutical Journal, from *Ann. de Chem. U. Pharm. Bd.* lxxvii.)

THE PHARMACOPŒIA OF THE UNITED STATES OF AMERICA.

By authority of the National Convention, held at Washington A. D. 1850. Philadelphia: Lippincott, Grambo & Co. 1851.

The appearance of a new edition of the Pharmacopœia is to the apothecary always a matter of high interest; to it he looks for the recognized improvements in the various processes which he has constantly to perform; by it essentially he is to be guided in all the officinal preparations which he makes; and from it he learns what new articles, by their intrinsic merits and through the vogue they have obtained, are deemed of sufficient importance to be recognized officinally as additions to the materia medica. The general arrangement of the new Pharmacopœia is the same as that of 1840. Owing to the wise principles which governed the earlier framers of the Pharmacopœia—though, from the progress of botanical science, the scientific names of the plants to which many of the articles of the vegetable materia medics are referred, have been changed, and with improvements in chemistry, the nomenclature of several salts has been altered—this has led to little alteration in the designations employed in the Pharmacopœia. Assafœtida is now referred to Narthex Assafetida, instead of Ferula A.; Diosma is, after the Edinburgh Pharmacopœia, termed Barosma; Camphor to Camphora officinarum; Cardamom to Elettaria Cardamomum; Cinchona flava to C. calisaya; Cinchona pallida to C. condaminea and C. micrantha, while the source of Cinchona rubra is not yet indicated. Colocynth is now termed the fruit of Citrullus colocynthis; kino is said to be the inspissated juice of Pterocarpus marsupium, and of other plants; quassia is referred to Simaruba excelsa, and uva ursi to Artostaphylos uva-ursi.

Of the names of the articles of the materia medica, as was before stated, very few are changed. Myroxylon, of the old Pharmacopœia, is now Balsamum Peruvianum, Tolutanum, Balsamum Tolutanum; Diosma, after the Edinburgh Pharmacopœia, is now Buchu; Zinci carbonas is changed to the old name, calamina; iodinum, following the British Pharmacopœias, is iodinium, and brominum, brominium. Port wine has been introduced, and consequently, instead of the Vinum of 1840, we have now Vinum Album, Sherry, and Vinum Rubrum, Port Wine.

The secondary list of the materia medica, a peculiarity of our national pharmacopœia, is still retained, to what good purpose it is hard to understand. The framers of the book state that "it has the advantage of permitting a discrimination between medicines of acknowledged value and others of less estimation, which, however, may still have claims to notice." The advantage is not a very evident one. The distinction that is attempted is very difficult to make satisfactorily; it will vary with individuals, and, we fancy, too, with the place at which it is made. Certainly few in New York would put Angostura bark with Horsemint (Monarda), and Queen's root (Stillingia) in the primary list; while Apocynum cannabinum, one of the most active of our diuretics, and Malefern, in tape-worm, one of the most certain anthelmintics, are exiled to the secondary. If popular, instead of professional reputation, is to be the criterion, are not Arnica, and Matricaria, and Benne leaves, and horehound, quite as well entitled to a place in the primary list as many of the articles that now figure there? And are there not twenty simples in use among the old women of the country that deserve a place in the national Pharmacopœia as well as may weed, and frost wort, and fever root? Though, too, new articles should not readily be admitted until time has fixed their value, we should like to have seen some notice of Matico and of the salts of Valerianic acid. We are sorry, too, to see the old definition of rhubarb still adhered to; "the root of Rheum palmatum and of other species of Rheum;" that of the Edinburgh Pharmacopœia, "the root of an unknown species of Rheum," thus rendering the Russian or Chinese rhubarb alone officinal, is very much preferable.

Of the substances introduced into the Materia Medica, the chief are Aconite root (aconiti radix), Extractum cannabis (extract of hemp), Oleum morrhuæ (cod liver oil), Oleum amygdalæ amaræ (oil of bitter almonds), and Potassæ chloras (chlorate of potassa). By Arnica in the last Pharmacopœia was understood the root and herb of Arnica montana; for these, in the present—the name remaining unchanged—the flowers are substituted. The additions to the Materia Medica have been made with judgment, and certainly nothing has been admitted with the exception perhaps of Helianthemum (Frostwort), of doubtful utility, or that has not for some time been submitted to the test of experience.

The preparations introduced are all familiar to the pharmaceutist, and have for a long time been kept in most good shops. It is singular that in the last Pharmacopœia, by nitrate of silver was understood the fused nitrate. This oversight has been corrected, and by Argenti nitras now is understood the salt in crystals, while the common lunar caustic is Argenti nitras fusa. Among the new preparations are the active principles of Aconitum Napellus (Aconitia), Oxide of Silver, Iodide of Arsenic, Chloroform, Collodion, a number of fluid extracts, Citrate of Iron, Glycerine, Solution of Citrate of Magnesia, the oils of Copaiba, Tobacco, and Valerian, Iodide of Lead, Potassa cum calce, Bromide of Potassium, Syrup of Wild Cherry bark—of gum—and Tinctures of Aconite root, Kino, and Nux Vomica, and compound tincture of Cardamom.

The Iron by hydrogen, as it has been sometimes rather awkwardly termed, the Fer réduit of the French, after the British Pharmacopœias, is termed Ferri pulvis, powder of iron. Soubeiran's formula for the preparation of Donovan's Liquor (Liquor Arsenici et Hydrargyri Iodidi) is given as much simpler and of easier preparation than the original formula of Donovan; there is, too, a good formula for the extemporaneous preparations of pills of iodide of iron. The solution of the Persesquinitrate of Iron, as it has been sometimes termed, appears as solution of Nitrate of Iron; it is a preparation that soon becomes altered by keeping. Tincture of Aconite root is directed to be made by macerating a pound of bruised Aconite root for fourteen days with two pints of alcohol, expressing and filtering. A process by percolation is also given. This is weaker than the tincture of either of the British Pharmacopœias, and weaker, we believe, than the tincture ordinarily employed here. As an external application, for which it is chiefly used, this is a great disadvantage, and when administered internally, the varying strength of a medicine so powerful will be attended with serious evils.

The old formulæ for the preparation of the alcoholic extract of aconite and of the extractum aconiti (expressed juice), are retained, both being made from the leaves. The extracts when thus made, even when properly prepared, are for the most part inert. No formula is given for the preparation of an alcoholic extract from the root.

There are three new preparations among the ointments:— Unguentum Belladonnæ, Potassii Iodidi, and Sulphuris Iodidi. The ointment of Iodide of Potassium is directed to be made by dissolving a drachm of the iodide in a drachm of boiling water, and afterwards incorporating the solution with the lard.

On the whole, there is much more to praise than to find fault with in the Pharmacopœia. Upon some of the preparations we will hereafter find further occasion perhaps to comment.

PHARMACEUTICAL CONVENTION.

In pursuance of a call issued by the College of Pharmacy of the City of New York, a Committee of Delegates from the different Colleges of Pharmacy in the United States assembled at the College Rooms in New York at 5 o'clock P. M. on Wednesday, the 15th of October.

Delegates from Philadelphia and Boston were in attendance. The Maryland College (at Baltimore) and the Cincinnati College were not represented, although Delegates from each had been previously reported to the Committee of Arrangements in New York. A communication of some length was received from the Cincinnati Delegation.

The Convention was organized by the appointment of Mr. Charles Ellis of Philadelphia as Chairman, and Dr. Samuel R. Philbrick of Boston as Secretary, pro tem. A Committee was then appointed by the nomination of each delegation, consisting of Messrs. Samuel M. Colcord of Boston, Alfred B. Taylor of Philadelphia, and George D. Coggeshall of New York, to examine credentials and nominate officers for the Convention. The Committee retired, and on their return reported the credentials satisfactory, and proposed Dr. B. Guthrie of New York as President, and Mr. Alfred B. Taylor of Philadelphia as Secretary, who were unanimously confirmed.

Dr. Guthrie, on taking the chair, made a few remarks expressive of his sense of the honor conferred by appointing him presiding officer of the first Convention of the kind ever held in the United States, and explanatory of the objects of the Convention, which were in accordance with the growing feeling amongst druggists and pharmaceutists of its necessity to establish standards of the qualities of imported Drugs and Medicines for the government of the United States Inspectors at the different ports, and in addition to act upon such matters of general interest to the Profession as may be presented to the consideration of the Convention.

Reports were presented by the majority (Messrs. Guthrie and Coggeshall) and the minority (Mr. Merrick) of the New York delegates, embodying their views upon the subject of standards, and also in regard to false drugs which should be excluded.

A communication from the Cincinnati Delegates was read, and Mr. Restieaux of Boston read an interesting statement of the working of the Drug Law in that city.

A general discussion ensued upon various topics connected with the business of the Convention, and resulted in the appointment of a committee, consisting of Messrs. Proctor of Philadelphia, Restieaux of Boston, and Coggeshall of New York, to consider the several communications, and to arrange the general plan of business, and report at the next sitting.

The Convention then adjourned to Thursday, at 12 o'clock.

Second sitting, Oct. 16th.—The Convention met at 12 o'clock. The Committee appointed yesterday made a report, reviewing the numerous propositions presented by the different Colleges, and submitting a general system for regulating standards, which, in their judgment, should prevail uniformly at the ports of entry, with numerous specifications of prominent articles to which their attention was called by their importance, and the difficulty that has been sometimes found in deciding upon them.

The report was considered in sections in a lengthy and very interesting discussion, in which the members generally participated. With some amendments it was adopted.

The Committee also offered the following preamble and resolutions, which were adopted, viz.

WHEREAS, The advancement of the true interests of the great body of Pharmaceutical practitioners in all sections of our country is a subject worthy earnest consideration; and whereas Pharmaceutists, in their intercourse among themselves, with physicians and the public, should be governed by a code of ethics calculated to elevate the standard and improve the practice of their art; and whereas, the means of a regular pharmaceutical education should be offered to the rising Pharmaceutists by the establishment of Schools of Pharmacy in suitable locations; and whereas, it is greatly to be desired that the united action of the profession should be directed to the accomplishment of these objects; therefore,

Resolved, That, in the opinion of this Convention, much good will result from a more extended intercourse between the Pharmaceutists of the several sections of the Union, by which their customs and practice may be assimilated; that Pharmaceutists would promote their individual interests and advance their professional standing by forming associations for mutual protection, and the education of their assistants, when such associations have become sufficiently matured; and that, in view of these important ends, it is further

Resolved, That a Convention be called, consisting of three delegates each from incorporated and unincorporated Pharmaceutical Societies, to meet at Philadelphia on the first Wednesday in October, 1852, when all the important questions bearing on the profession may be considered, and measures adopted for the organization of a National Association, to meet every year.

On motion, it was resolved that the New York Delegation be appointed a Committee to lay the proceedings of this Convention before the Secretary of the Treasury of the United States, and afterwards have them published in pamphlet form.

Dr. Philbrick of Boston offered the following preamble and resolution, which were adopted:—

Whereas, to secure the full benefits of the prohibition of sophisticated drugs and chemicals from abroad, it is necessary to prevent home adulteration; therefore,

Resolved, that this convention recommend to the several colleges to adopt such measures as in their respective states may be best calculated to secure that object.

On motion of mr. Colcord of boston, it was

Resolved, that a committee of three be appointed by this convention to act as a standing committee to collect and receive such information as may be valuable, and memorials and suggestions from any medical and pharmaceutical association, to be presented at the next convention.

The president appointed g. D. Coggeshall of new york, s. M. Colcord of boston, and w. Proctor, jr., of philadelphia, as the committee.

A vote of thanks to the officers was passed, and then the convention adjourned, to meet in philadelphia on the first wednesday in october, 1852,

The following circular letter has since been issued by the president of the convention, and addressed to the leading pharmaceutists throughout the union:—

New york, november 25, 1851.

Sir:—at a meeting of delegates from the colleges of pharmacy of the united states, held in this city on the 15th of october, 1851, the following preamble and resolutions, explanatory of themselves, was offered, and, after a free and full discussion, unanimously adopted:—

[here follow the preamble and resolutions introduced by messrs. Proctor, restieaux, and coggeshall.]

The objects set forth in the above, i trust, will meet the hearty approbation of yourself and the apothecaries of your place, and lead to the formation (if not already in existence) of such an association as will co-operate in the furtherance of the proposed association.

Our medical brethren have, as you are doubtless aware, an organization, similar in character, holding its sessions annually, in which all matters pertaining to their profession are fully discussed—the beneficial effects of which are already apparent, though the association has been in existence but a few years.

They cannot give to the subject of pharmacy the attention it requires and deserves, neither is it a matter legitimately falling under their cognizance, but belongs to pharmaceutists themselves.

The medical profession and the community at large rightfully look to us for the correction of any existing abuses, the advancement of the science, and the elevation of the business of an apothecary to the dignity and standing of a profession.

To this end we invite you to the formation of such associations, in view of the convention, to be held in philadelphia, on the first wednesday of october, 1852.

Communications intended for said convention may be addressed to william proctor, jr., philadelphia, george d. Coggeshall, new york, or s. M. Colcord, boston.

Any communication touching the subject of the above letter will be cheerfully responded to by the president of the convention.

G. B. Guthrie, m. D.,
president convention of colleges of pharmacy.

NEW YORK JOURNAL OF PHARMACY. FEBRUARY, 1852.

ON THE PREPARATION OF PURE HYDRATE OF POTASH AND CARBONATE OF POTASH.

BY HENRY WURTZ, A. M.

In preparing pure potash compounds, it is highly necessary, especially in order to avoid the possibility of the presence of soda, to select, as a starting point, some compound of potash which differs considerably in solubility from the corresponding soda compound. Either the bitartrate or the sulphate, therefore, is usually preferred.

The bitartrate is ignited; the carbonaceous mass, washed with water, and the solution of carbonate of potash, thus obtained, diluted and boiled with slack lime, in the usual way, in an iron kettle; the solution of hydrate of potash, thus obtained, is boiled to dryness, and the alcoholic solution of the residue evaporated in silver dishes, to obtain what is denominated *alcoholic potash*. This product should be, and most usually is, entirely free from sulphate of potash and chloride of potassium, since it is easy to crystallize the bitartrate free from these salts.

But an almost invariable accompaniment of this alcoholic potash is a trace of silicate of potash. The solution may assume no cloudiness on the addition of solution of chlorohydrate of ammonia, or upon addition of an excess of chlorohydric acid, and afterwards an excess of ammonia; but on adding excess of chlorohydric acid, and evaporation to dryness in a platinum capsule, the aqueous solution of the residue will be found to have flakes of silica floating in it. Very few specimens that i have met with have stood this test. It is to be inferred that the soluble silicates of potash are not wholly insoluble in alcohol; but a question arises concerning the source from whence the silica is so frequently derived. It may be from the lime used, in some cases, or from silicium contained in the iron of the kettles employed I am enabled to state, in addition, that of many specimens of commercial *carbonate of potash* which I have examined, some of which purported to have been prepared from cream of tartar by the method above alluded to, none have been found entirely free from silica. I have even found traces of this impurity in crystals of commercial *bicarbonate of potash.*

This constant contamination of potash, and carbonate of potash with silica, being a very important matter in consideration of the frequent use of these two substances in chemical analysis, i have been induced to devise a means of separating the silica from the carbonate. This i have accomplished by the use of carbonate of ammonia.

An aqueous solution of the carbonate which is to be freed from silica is evaporated to dryness on the sand bath (best in a sheet iron dish), adding from time to time lumps of carbonate of ammonia. The silicate is thus converted into carbonate, and on dissolving the residue of the evaporation in water, the silica appears in the form of flakes floating in the liquid, and may be separated by filtration. This solution of carbonate of potash, free from silica, may now be used for the preparation of pure hydrate of potash, taking care to use lime which is also free from silica.

I may here introduce a few words with regard to the preservation of hydrate of potash for use in analysis. Its preservation in the solid form is evidently no difficult matter; but when we attempt to keep the solution in glass bottles for the sake of convenience in using it as a re-agent, we generally find that it very soon takes up silica from the glass. I have found, however, that flint glass bottles will preserve such a solution much longer than any other, lead glass not being easily acted upon, probably because it contains very much less silica. It might not be useless to make a trial of bottles made of thin soft iron, or sheet iron, for this purpose; but it is probable that pure *silver* is the true material for bottles, in which solution of potash is to be preserved. A very thin shell of silver might first be made, and afterwards strengthened by coating it thickly with galvanic copper

The ease with which sulphate of potash can be obtained, in a state of purity, has long ago suggested its use as a material from which to prepare pure potash. Schubert6 proposed to treat pulverized pure sulphate of potash with a concentrated solution of pure baryta, the latter somewhat in excess, and during the evaporation of the solution of hydrate of potash, thus obtained, the excess of the baryta is precipitated by the carbonic acid of the air. This, however, appears to be very expensive process. I have devised another method of treating pure sulphate of potash so as to obtain pure hydrate of potash therefrom; it consists merely in operating upon the sulphate of potash in a manner similar to that in which sulphate of baryta is operated upon to procure hydrate of baryta, that is in converting the sulphate into sulphide by the conjoined application of a reducing agent and a red heat, and to decompose the aqueous solution of the sulphide by the action of an oxide of a metal whose sulphide is insoluble, such as oxide of iron (?), oxide of copper or deutoxide of manganese. I use as a reducing agent, instead of charcoal, oil, rosin, etc., *coal gas*. This application of coal gas was proposed by dr. Wolcott gibbs. If it is found that the decomposition is not perfect, and that the solution of sulphide of potassium contains some sulphate of potash, or if a little sulphate is formed in the solution by oxidation, it is removed by the introduction of a little solution of baryta, according to the method of schubert. I am not yet prepared, however, to give the details of this method.

---

6 erd. Und mar. Jour. 26, 117.

ON THE PREPARATION OF CHEMICALLY PURE HYDRATE AND CARBONATE OF SODA.

BY HENRY WURTZ, A. M.

The remarks made in the last article with reference to the presence of silica in alcoholic potash, apply also, though not so generally, to commercial alcoholic soda. Few specimens of this product are met with which are so free from silica that it cannot be detected by saturation with chlorohydric acid, evaporation to dryness in a platinum vessel, and redissolution in water. Whatever may be the origin of the silica in this case, it is very often present.

I have selected, as the most convenient substance from which to prepare pure hydrate and carbonate of soda, a product which occurs very abundantly in commerce under the name of "carbonate of soda." It is in the form of a very fine white powder, and on examination turns out to be the ordinary monohydrated *bicarbonate* of soda.

Nao, 2 c.o^2 + h.o.

For, upon ignition, 7.756 grns. Lost, 2.7595 grns. Of carbonic acid and water, which is equal to 35.60 per cent.; bicarbonate of soda should lose 36.88 per cent. It may be mentioned, in this connection, that a preparation sent over here by button, a london pharmaceutist, under the appellation of "chemically pure carbonate of soda," upon examination turned out to be also *bicarbonate*. 2.324 grns. Lost by ignition; 0.845 grn. = 36.45 per cent.

The commercial bicarbonate above mentioned, contains, of course, all the impurities of the carbonate from which it is made, this being an inevitable consequence of the method by which it is manufactured, which, as described in knapp's chemical toohnology, is simply to expose commercial crystals of carbonate of soda to the action of carbonic acid gas, which it takes up to the extent of one equivalent, falling into a fine powder, with evolution of heat and loss of water of crystallization. These impurities, in the case of the specimen operated upon by me, were, besides considerable silica, sulphate of soda, chloride of sodium, a trace of phosphoric acid detected by monohydrate of ammonia, and a little organic matter which imparted to the mass a soapy smell.

The sulphate, phosphate and chloride are easily removed by washing with water by decantation, with a loss, however, of at least one half of the material. When the washings, after addition of excess of nitric acid, no longer react with nitrate of silver, or with chloride of barium, the mass is introduced into porcelain dishes, and dried on the sand bath; when dry it is exposed to a high sand bath heat, though not to a red heat, for two or three hours. By this treatment, not only are one equivalent of carbonic acid, and one equivalent of water expelled, but the greater part or the whole of the silicate is decomposed and converted into carbonate, so that a solution of the mass in water will now be found full of flakes of silica.

The filtered solution should now be tested for silica, and if not yet entirely free from it, must be evaporated again to dryness, with addition of lumps of carbonate of ammonia, exactly as proposed by me, in the last article, to separate silica from carbonate of potash. The residue of this last evaporation, on solution in water, filtration and evaporation in platinum, silver, or even clean sheet iron (never in glass or porcelain) dishes, will give pure carbonate of soda, from which may be prepared the pure hydrate of soda, observing the precaution of using lime which is free from silica.

REMARKS UPON SOME OF THE PREPARATIONS OF THE PHARMACOPŒIA OF THE UNITED STATES, 1851.

BY GEORGE D. COGGESHALL.

The pharmacopœia of the united states is, or should be, to the pharmaceutist of the united states, his text book and standard. In making its preparations he should not vary from the letter of its directions, unless a change of process effects a quicker, more uniform, or more elegant result; in regard to strength he should not vary at all, except upon distinct understanding with the physician prescribing, or with his customer. It is much to be regretted that perfect conformity throughout the united states, with our national pharmacopœia should not prevail, so that our citizens, traveling or removing with prescriptions, or copies of them, might not be subjected to inconvenient, and even in some cases to dangerous alterations, impairing confidence in the medicine relied upon, or involving the safety of the patient in using it. With these important considerations in view, the apothecary should, as far as circumstances permit, conform strictly to the acknowledged standard, giving up his own opinions, if need be, for the general good. But strict adherence to the formulæ of our pharmacopœia seems not to be practicable in all cases, in all localities. When there is such diversity of practice in the city of philadelphia and in new york, within five hours of each other, with intercommunication five times a day, in each of which the formation and subsequent revisions of the pharmacopœia have been of such especial interest and attention, how can it be expected that in our widely extended country, in communities diversified almost as much as those of different nations, with many local habits, set by time and many prejudices, a full and uniform compliance with the official standard should prevail.

In new york it would disappoint the physician to put ℥ss of the officinal solution of sulphate of morphia into a prescription of ℥iv cough mixture, as much, if not as unpleasantly, as it would the philadelphia physician for one of our brethren in that city to put ℥j of majendie's strength into a mixture of the same bulk. In new york the original strength of this solution has ever been preserved, notwithstanding the change made officinal in three editions of our pharmacopœia, and it is generally understood and used accordingly. With us the change has been remonstrated against, as unnecessary, because the dose can be as easily regulated as that of fowler's, or donovan's, or lugol's solution, the tinctures of aconite root, belladonna, iodine, and many other potent preparations; it may just as easily be preserved from doing mischief, and has often the advantage in mixtures of not displacing desirable adjuncts with superfluous water. It is true, that owing to the great difference in strength of the solution commonly understood here, and that of the pharmacopœia, our college has felt it incumbent to request physicians to designate the intended one, by affixing a term (in brackets or otherwise) as "maj," or "ph. U.s," to avoid the possibility of misconstruction, except in clear cases as that of the mixture above mentioned; and that we should not feel justified in dispensing an ounce of majendie's solution alone, (especially if the prescription was for "liquor morphiæ, sulphatis"—the officinal term) unless with an understanding of the strength wanted, or of the use to be made of it. This great discrepancy between what is of original and continued use and what is officinal, requires watchfulness, on our part, against occasional exceptions to the general prescription of our physicians, and in putting up prescriptions written in other places, philadelphia particularly. We must judge of the solution required, from the context.

Our pharmacopœia, in most of its formulæ, is undoubtedly entitled to our full respect and adherence, exhibiting on the part of the revising committee, laborious research and patient adjustment of details. But some of them, i think, are fairly open to criticism and susceptible of improvement. The formula given for preparing "carbonic acid water," is one by which it may safely be said, no practical man ever has made, or ever can make, the article commonly known as mineral, or soda water, the latter name given to it in its early manufacture; when a portion of carbonate of soda entered into its composition, which is now generally omitted, though the name is retained in many places. In the first united states pharmacopœia, 1820, the formula given is as follows:—

"take of water any quantity.

Impregnate it with about ten times its volume of carbonic acid gas by means of a forcing pump."

That was, probably, about the strength it was usually made at that time. It is now, generally made about one fifth or one fourth stronger. In the revision of 1830, the formula was changed as follows:—

"by means of a forcing pump, throw into a suitable receiver, nearly filled with water, a quantity of carbonic acid equal to five times the bulk of the water."

"carbonic acid is obtained from the hard carbonate of lime by means of dilute sulphuric acid."

The latter formula is repeated in the revisions of 1840 and 1850, substituting the term "marble," for "hard carbonate of lime." The strength was altered from "ten times" of the first edition to "five times," in 1830, and reiterated in 1840 and 1850. Why? "ten times" was, perhaps, sufficient in the early use of this beverage, but was hardly considered strong enough in 1830, certainly was not in 1840, and has not been since. It is difficult to conceive a reason for such change. Surely, it could not have been recommended by practical men; on the contrary it was supposed to have been made by mistake or inadvertance. It is still more difficult to find a good reason for repeating this formula in the revisions of 1840 and 1850. Upon each of the latter occasions the college of pharmacy, in new york, remonstrated against it and pointed out fully its absurdity. Carbonic acid water of that strength, it was stated, would not be acceptable as a drink to any one familiar with it, nor refreshing to the sick. The formula was also shown to be defective in several essential particulars, and where it was not defective it was wrong. But our remonstrance seems not to have been vouchsafed "even the cold respect of a passing glance."

The formula is defective in not describing the vessel in which the preparation is to be made. In other processes, not so much involving the safety of those engaged in them, the vessels are specified, as "glass," "earthen," "iron," &c. In this case it is indispensable that the vessel should be expressly and well adapted to the purpose. It should be of undoubted strength to sustain the pressure, and it should be of material not acted upon by the acid or water. These requisites should not be neglected. We need not concern ourselves much, to be sure, about "five times the bulk," but to make carbonic acid water of good quality, the "receiver" should be of sufficient strength to ensure safety, and of internal material to avoid unpleasant or injurious contamination. Copper fountains, lined with tin, are mostly used. Cast iron, lined with tin, is also used, to some extent. So far the formula is defective,—in the proportion both of water and carbonic acid it is wrong. The "suitable receiver" should not be "nearly filled with water." How near full that is, is left to the chance of different judgment in different persons; but if "nearly filled" should be understood to mean within a pint, and force enough could be applied, "the receiver" would burst before the "five times" could be got into it, though the breaking in this case would not, probably, be attended with danger to the operator, because it would be merely a dead strain without much expansive force.

I do not propose to detail the process of making soda or mineral water, "carbonic acid water," as it is properly called in the pharmacopœia. The minutiæ of its preparation may well be left to the experience and practice of the operator. But the formula given in our standard book should not be defective or wrong in prominent principles, it should accord with experience and the improvement of the times. There does not appear to be any good reason for altering the formula of 1820, which was comparatively "well enough" to that of 1830, '40 and '50, which is of no value. After designating the description of fountain required, so far, at least, as regards strength (which ought to be equal to the pressure of twenty atmospheres), and material, it should direct it to be supplied with water to the extent of about five sevenths of its capacity, in order to allow of due admixture of gas and water, and of agitation which greatly facilitates it, and the forcing carbonic acid into it to the extent of at least twelve times the bulk of the water. Thirteen or fourteen times is often employed for draught, and seventeen or eighteen times for bottling. It may be, as it has been, said that "a formula for this preparation is not of great moment." It may be so; it may, perhaps, as safely be left to the skill of the manufacturer and the taste of the consumer, as "mistura spiritus vini gallici;" but "if it be worth doing at all, it is worth doing well;" if placed in the pharmacopœia, it should be in accordance with knowledge, and the experience of practical men.

The solution of arsenite of potassa has been made by some apothecaries, with myself, for several years, by substituting 92 grs. Of bicarbonate of potassa, as the equivalent of 64 grs. Of the carbonate, by which we feel more confident of obtaining a definite compound than by the employment of the carbonate, as generally procured, which mostly contains silica and other contaminations. The resulting compound is quite satisfactory, and keeps well. We also omit the compound spirit of lavender, making up the measure of a pint with water. Our object in this is two-fold. The solution is more permanent, according to our observation, and the compound spirit of lavender only renders it (if anything) more attractive in taste and smell, to children and ignorant persons.

In making mistura ferri composita, it is peculiarly necessary to proceed exactly according to rule, both in the order of its components and in the method of adding them, to produce a correct result. In the pharmacopœia the six ingredients are set down thus:—

"take of myrrh a drachm.

Carbonate of potassa twenty-five grains.

Sulphate of iron, in powder, a scruple.

Spirit of lavender half a fluid ounce.

Sugar a drachm.

Rose water seven fluid ounces and a half."

We are directed to rub the first with the last, "and then mix with these" the fourth, the fifth, the second, and "lastly," the third.

In the written process for making a mixture, which more than most others, requires exact method, and the adding of each of its numerous components in its right order, it would seem to be desirable, for the sake of perspicuity, to set them down in the order in which they are to be used. Here we have to chase about, forwards and backwards, for the one wanted next, and to read over and over the directions, to make sure of getting them right; for few of us make this mixture so often as to be perfectly familiar with the process, without referring to the text. It is not less awkward in this case from the directions chancing to be over leaf. But the formula is otherwise defective, i think, not being quite equal to that of 1830, in which the rose water and spirit of lavender are directed to be added together. Not only should these be mixed before using, but the myrrh, carbonate of potassa and sugar should be triturated well together, and rubbed with successive portions of the mixed liquids, effecting thereby a better solution of the myrrh. The mixture, then complete, except the sulphate of iron, should be put into the vial, and the salt should, by all means, be directed to be selected in clear crystals, to avoid any per salt of iron; it should be quickly powdered in a clean mortar, and added to the contents of the vial. The result is a bluish colored mixture, soon changing to olive green. If the sulphate of iron be not properly selected, or if it be rubbed in the mortar, as inferred from the formula, the mixture is more or less brown and proportionably deteriorated. Of course, we should not "take sulphate of iron in powder."

In giving directions for making a compound, something, certainly, is to be expected from the knowledge and skill of the manipulator. But essential points should not be left to him, and a formula for a mixture, probably not very often made by apothecaries throughout our country towns, should be set down so clearly, that a person competent to put up mixtures generally, could make this one the first time he was called upon for it, without needless perplexity, and with sufficient detail of essentials to ensure its being made correctly. I have been frequently told by physicians that, even here, this mixture, requiring so much nicety of manipulation, does not appear to be made right one time in ten. This may not be so much the fault of the apothecary as of his guide. He makes the mixture but seldom, and if he make it by his pharmacopœia he does not make it as well as it can be made. For convenient use in the shop, i have the following process written out:—

"take of myrrh,

Sugar each one drachm,

Carbonate of potassa twenty-five grains,

Triturate together, and add gradually:

Rose water seven ounces and a half,

Spirit of lavender half an ounce, mixed.

Rub each portion well together, pour into the vial and add:

Sulphate of iron one scruple,

To be selected in clear crystals, powdered in a clean dry mortar, and thrown in powder into the vial; then cork, shake well, and cover the vial with buff colored paper."

I have often thought that if our formulæ, especially those that are complicated, were given in proper rotation, placing the component first to be used, first in the list, the second next, and so on, with intermediate lines of direction, which might be in smaller type or italics, it would derogate nothing from the dignity of the book, while it would facilitate the process, and might sometimes obviate misconstruction, or neglect of particulars essential to the best result.

The consideration of some few other preparations, i must defer to another number,

LETTER ON OPIUM, &C.

[The following letter, addressed to a commercial house in this city, will be found to communicate some interesting information. We print it as it is written. Perhaps our readers may derive some information from the prices given; we can make nothing of them.]

Constantinople, may 10, 1851.

To ——————— trieste,

We received your honored letter, dated messina, with great pleasure, and hasten to give you the information you desire, hoping and wishing that both an agreeable and useful connection may arise from it, for which purpose we shall not fail to give your house direct information, respecting the articles you mention. Opium is found here in different qualities, the goodness of which chiefly depends on the conscientiousness of those who prepare it. The best quality coming from some districts of asia consists of the pure juice, which flows spontaneously from the incisions made in the poppy heads, is inspissated and formed into little balls. It has eminently all the qualities which are requisite in good opium, and contains from 8 to 10 per cent, and more, of morphia. This sort is the most in request among the druggists in germany and france, to be sold by retail to the apothecaries, but scarcely forms the 8th or 10th part of all the turkish opium which comes to the market. Next to this is the ordinary quality, coming from the other provinces of asia minor; where in preparing it, they are less cautious, partly pressing the poppy heads, in order to get as much juice as possible, partly scraping the juice that has oozed out too hard, by which certain mucilaginous parts of the plant, and shavings of the rind get mixed up with it; in this way that kind of opium is produced, which is so often sold, and at trieste bears the name of tarense opium.

By this proceeding, of course, the morphia is lessened, and often in a great degree; but in the chinese market, in proportion to which, the consumption of the article in all other countries is scarcely to be reckoned, little or no regard is paid to THIS, WHICH EXPLAINS WHY THE

LATTER INFERIOR ARTICLE ALWAYS BRINGS NEARLY AS HIGH A PRICE AS THE FORMER PURE QUALITY. BESIDES THESE, SEVERAL SORTS OF ADULTERATED OPIUM ARE SOLD, SOME OF WHICH ARE PREPARED, (PRINCIPALLY FOR THE NORTH AMERICAN MARKET,) BY MIXING IN THE JUICE OF THE WHOLE PLANT, OR OTHER SUBSTANCES.—THE DIFFERENCE OF THE QUALITIES WOULD BE BEST PERCEIVED BY A COLLECTION OF SAMPLES, WHICH WE SHOULD BE GLAD TO SEND YOU, IF YOU WOULD TELL US WHERE TO DIRECT THEM. THE PRICE OF THE AFOREMENTIONED PRIME QUALITY, WHICH WE CALL "GÚEVE," FROM THE DISTRICT WHICH CHIEFLY PRODUCES IT, IS NOW 10⅔c. For the english pound, free on board. The current second quality, 10⅓c. The price of the adulterated is much lower, in proportion to the amount of the adulteration; which, however, in most cases, is not discernible by the exterior. The prices are, of course, principally regulated by the chinese market; yet the more or less considerable crop produced is not without influence. So especially now, the growers show little inclination to sell, as the new plantations are endangered by a continual want of rain.— nevertheless, probably after two months, when the new crop begins to come to market, we may be able to buy cheaper than now, if the news from china should not cause the price to rise.

As regards scammony, almost everything that has been said respecting opium is literally applicable. The difference in quality depends upon the way of preparing it, while the plant from which it is taken is always the same. The best sort is the pure dried juice, which spontaneously flows from the incisions made in the root of the plant; the next quality is produced by a strong pressure of the root. These two qualities go in commerce by the name of the 1st and 2nd scammony d'aleppo, which name, however, is wrong, as aleppo produces the 1st quality, but only in a very small quantity, whilst the greater part comes from several districts of asia minor. Then follows the so called quality of skilip, a district that produces much, but where they have the bad habit of trying to gain in the weight, by adulterating the pure substance. The adulteration is made in several ways; the least injurious of which perhaps is, THAT THEY ADD (AS IN OPIUM), THE PRESSED OR BOILED OUT JUICE OF THE WHOLE PLANT; THE NOT INCONSIDERABLE QUANTITIES OF THIS SORT, WHICH ARE YEARLY BROUGHT FROM THE INTERIOR, FIND A GOOD SALE IN EUROPE, WHICH WOULD HARDLY LAST, IF A SUFFICIENT QUANTITY OF THE BEFORE MENTIONED FINER QUALITIES WERE TO BE HAD. BESIDES THESE, A NUMBER OF OTHER SORTS ARE SOLD IN EUROPE, UNDER THE NAME OF SMYRNA SCAMMONY, WHICH CONSIST OF A HARD AND HEAVY MASS, BUT CONTAIN ONLY A VERY SMALL PART OF THE REAL SCAMMONY.

With this article it would also be necessary, as we said with the opium, to explain our statements by sending you samples, which we will do if you desire it. The finest prime sort is seldom found, and is now entirely wanting. It would sell readily at the rate of 21½c. Per pound, english. The good second quality brings according to the sort, from 18c. To 15¾c. A pound, free on board, but is also now very scarce, and will, in the course of two or three months, be more abundant in fresh quality. Of the skilip sort, there are several quantities in the market, according to the quality, at the price of 13 to 10s. 10d. An english pound, free on board.

Of the oil of roses, there is, properly speaking, only one genuine quality, with only little difference in odor, but with remarkable variation in the facility with which it congeals, which property is almost generally considered an essential proof of its being genuine, but without reason; as we have ascertained by much experience, during a long sojourn in the country where it is produced. Several reasons may contribute to this difference in congealing, but the chief one may be considered, the difference of soil, and method of preparation. We give our principal attention to the article, and have founded an establishment at kissanlik, where it is chiefly produced, through which alone we make our purchases, and must do so, in order to have the attar genuine, as we have experienced, that all the essence without exception that is sold here, second hand, is far from pure.

The common method and the one now almost exclusively adopted of adulterating it, with geranium essence, may be known TO YOU, AND THAT IT REALLY IS THE MOST IN USE, YOU MAY CONCLUDE, FROM THE PRICE OF THE GENUINE ARTICLE HAVING BEEN FOR A LONG TIME MUCH HIGHER AT THE PLACES OF PRODUCTION, THAN THE PRICE OF THAT WHICH IS SOLD AS PRIME IN EUROPE. THIS FACT HAS ONLY LATELY BEEN NOTICED IN EUROPE, THEREFORE IN THE PRICE CURRENT OF TRIESTE, FOR INSTANCE, YOU WILL FIND THE GENUINE ARTICLE NOTED, BESIDE THE PRIME ARTICLE, WITH A CONSIDERABLE DIFFERENCE OF PRICE. WHAT AT LONDON IS DESIGNATED AS PRIME QUALITY, IS ONLY A MIXTURE OF 60 TO 70 PER CENT. ESSENCE OF ROSE, WITH 30 TO 40 PER CENT. ESSENCE OF GERANIUM. SAMPLES WILL ALSO PROVE THIS TO YOU, MORE CLEARLY. THE PRICE OF THE GENUINE ATTAR IS, TO-DAY, $22\frac{3}{4}$c. For an ounce, at 10 drachms, according to which the english price current may be understood; in six or eight weeks after the preparation of the new crop, we hope to buy cheaper, but at what rate we cannot yet judge, as this depends on the produce of the crop. There is some cheaper and adulterated, and which is only bought by ignorant persons. This oil comes by caravans from the interior of asia, and in spite of all our inquiries, we could not succeed in getting any sure information, about the plant which produces it, or the method of preparation.

ON CHLOROFORM AS A SOLVENT.

BY M. P. H. LEPAGE, OF GISORS.

Hitherto, attention has been mainly directed to the manufacture of chloroform, and the study of its anesthetic properties. Many chemists, however, have casually noticed the power it possesses of dissolving essential oils, fixed fatty matters, camphor resins, (even those which dissolve with difficulty in alcohol and ether, such as copal resin, for example,) iodine, bromine, vegetable alkalies, india rubber insoluble in alcohol, and but slightly soluble in ether, and, finally, gutta percha, insoluble according to m. Vogel, in both these menstrua.

Having lately had occasion to experiment with chloroform, upon a variety of substances, i have thought it might be useful, with a view to its further application, to make known the results obtained.

1. Resinous substances, gum mastic, colophony, elemi, balsam of tolu, benzoin, are very soluble cold, in all proportions of chloroform and their solutions in this liquid form varnishes, some of which might, i think, be usefully applied, when the price of chloroform shall be diminished.

Gum copal and caoutchouc dissolve equally and almost entirely in this liquid, but more easily hot than cold.

Amber, sandarac, and shellac, are only partially soluble in chloroform, whether hot or cold. The mixture of sandarac and chloroform separates into two layers; the lower one which holds in solution a certain quantity of resin, is fluid, whilst the upper one is of a gelatinous consistence.

Olibanum dissolves with difficulty in it, either hot or cold.

Gum guaiac and scammony resin, dissolve very easily in it; whilst on the contrary, pure jalap resin is insoluble; it becomes soft by contact with the liquid, and then floats on the top, as a pitch like mass. When the resin is very pure, the lower layer of chloroform has an amber color.

Gamboge and gum dragon's blood, also yield some of their substance to chloroform. The solution of gamboge being of a magnificent golden yellow, and that of the dragon's blood of a beautiful red, these two substances might be advantageously used as varnishes.

2. Fixed fats. Oils of olive, œillettes, almond, ricinus, cod, rape, euphorbia, lathyris, croton tiglium, lard, tallow, the concrete oils of palm and cocoa, spermaceti, and probably all the fixed fats, dissolve remarkably and in all proportions in chloroform. As to wax, according to m. Vogel, six or eight parts of chloroform added to one part of this substance when pure, dissolve only .25, whence this chemist supposes, that whenever wax treated with this liquid in the above NAMED PROPORTIONS, LEAVES LESS THAN .75, IT MAY BE CONSIDERED AS HAVING BEEN MIXED WITH TALLOW OR STEARIC ACID.

I placed in a small tube, seven grammes of chloroform, and one gramme of *pure* white wax, shaking the mixture violently, at the end of six or eight hours the piece of wax had entirely disappeared, and the contents of the tube resembled an emulsion. The whole was passed through a filter of the weight of one gramme. A transparent liquid passed, which, exposed to spontaneous evaporation, left a residuum of pillular consistence weighing twenty-five centigrammes; whilst the filter which retained the portion of undissolved wax, left to the action of the air, until it no longer lost weight, was found to weigh one gramme, seventy-five centigrammes. The result of this experiment therefore, confirms the statement of the learned chemist of munich.

3. Volatile oils. All are soluble in chloroform.

4. Simple metalloid bodies. We already know that iodine and bromine are soluble in chloroform, i have further ascertained that phosphorus and sulphur are slightly so.

5. Immediate neutral principles Strynaine, piperine, naphtaline, cholesterine, are very soluble in chloroform. Pricrotoxine, slightly so. Parafine will only dissolve when warm, and on cooling, again floats on the top of the liquid. Amygdaline, phloridzine, salicine, digitaline, cynisin, urea, hematin, gluten, sugar, &c., are insoluble in it.

6. Organic acids. Benzoic and hippuric acids are very soluble in chloroform. Tannin is but slightly soluble, tartaric, citric, oxalic and gallic acids are insoluble in it.

7. Organic alkalies. Quinine, pure veratrine, emetine and narcotine are easily soluble in chloroform. Strychnine dissolves pretty well in it, and the solution, even when not saturated (one décigramme to two grammes of chloroform, for instance,) deposits, in twenty-four hours, a number of little tuberculiform crystals, which may perhaps be a modification of this alkaloid (an isomeric state), for their solution in dilute acids has appeared to me less bitter, and less easily precipitable by AMMONIA THAN THAT OF ORDINARY STRYCHNINE. BRUCINE IS ALSO QUITE SOLUBLE IN CHLOROFORM. MORPHINE AND CINCHONINE ARE INSOLUBLE.

8. Salts of organic acids. Tartar emetic, the acetates of potash and soda, lactate of iron, citrate of iron, valerianate of zinc, and acetate of lead do not dissolve in chloroform.

9. Salts with organic bases. Sulphate and hydrochlorate of strychnine, are tolerably soluble in chloroform, whilst sulphate of quinine, hydrochlorate and sulphate of morphine are insoluble.

10. Haloid salts. Iodide and bromide of potassium, the chlorides of sodium, potassium and ammonia, the iodides of mercury and lead, the yellow prussiate of potash, the cyanides of mercury and potassium do not dissolve in chloroform. Chloride of mercury is very soluble.

11. Oxysalts. The iodates, chlorates, nitrates, phosphates, sulphates, chromates, borates, arseniates and alkaline hyposulphates are completely insoluble in chloroform. The same may be said of nitrate of silver, sulphate of copper, and probably of all the metallic oxysalts.

The above facts prove: 1st that chloroform dissolves, with a very few exceptions, all bodies soluble in ether; but as it dissolves copal, caoutchouc, &c., much better than this latter substance, this property will become serviceable when the price of chloroform shall be lowered.

2nd. That contrary to what was formerly believed, it dissolves shellac much less easily than alcohol.

3rd. That it may be employed instead of ether, to separate quinine from cinchonine, narcotine from morphine, guaiac resin from jalap resin, which substances are often found mixed together in commerce.

4th. That it dissolves in large proportions strychnine, brucine, and emetine, alkaloids, which are almost insoluble in ether.

5th. Finally, that it does not dissolve tartaric, citric, oxalic and gallic acids, amygdaline, phloridzine, salicine, digitaline, hematine, gluten, &c., all which bodies are soluble in alcohol, NOR THE CHLORIDES, BROMIDES, IODIDES, OR NITRATES, SALTS, ALL SOLUBLE IN THE SAME VEHICLE.

I think it right also to add the following observation, because it tends to corroborate a fact recently stated in the *journal de chimie médicale*, by my friend and former colleague, m. Aujendre, assayer at the mint of constantinople, namely that chloroform possesses antiseptic properties. Having accidentally left in a half filled, but corked bottle, during a month (from april 10, to may 12), in my laboratory, where the variations of temperature are very frequent, some milk mixed with about a hundredth part of chloroform, i was rather surprised, on examining the milk, to find that it had preserved the fluidity and homogeneity of the liquid when freshly drawn, and that it could even be boiled without turning.—*journal de chimie médicale in l'abeille médicale.*

[note.—chloroform will preserve anatomical and pathological specimens without changing their color, or apparently their texture.]—ed. N. Y. Journal of pharmacy.

Report of a joint committee of the philadelphia county medical society and the philadelphia college of pharmacy, relative to physicians' prescriptions. (*published by order of the board of trustees of the philadelphia coll. Of pharm.*)

The joint committees of the philadelphia county medical society, and of the philadelphia college of pharmacy, appointed for the purpose of considering the means best adapted to prevent the occurrence of mistakes in the compounding of the prescriptions of physicians by apothecaries, beg leave to report that they have given to the subject all the attention that its importance demands, and present the following hints as the results of their joint deliberations. They have taken the liberty of adding, also, a few general hints on the relations that should exist between physicians and pharmaceutists.

A. *In respect to physicians.*

1. Physicians should write their prescriptions carefully and legibly, making use of good paper, and, whenever possible, of pen and ink. When obliged to write with a pencil, they should take the precaution to fold the prescription twice, so as to prevent its being defaced.

2. The nomenclature of the united states pharmacopœia is becoming annually more in favor with pharmaceutists; a statement attested by the fact that 1500 copies of the book of latin labels for shop furniture, published by the philadelphia college of pharmacy, have been disposed of within three years. Physicians are also becoming more alive to the merits of our national codex, and they are respectfully urged to familiarize themselves with its nomenclature, and to adhere to it strictly in their prescriptions.

3. The numerous treatises on materia medica, pharmacy and the practice of medicine, of english origin, that are reprinted in this country, notwithstanding they are generally interlarded with the formulæ of our own pharmacopœia, tend, nevertheless, very much to confuse the physician and apothecary, in the use and exact meaning of terms in prescriptions. To obviate the difficulties thus occasioned, the physician should, when he prescribes a medicine, which is not official, nor in common use, state on his prescription, either in a note at the bottom, or within parenthesis, following the article, the authority or work from whence it is derived, as "griffith's formulary,"—"ellis' formulary,"—"braithwaite's retrospect," etc.

4. Physicians would lessen the risk of errors in their prescriptions, and increase the chances of their detection should they be made, by observing the following hints.

1st. Write the name of the patient at the top of the prescription, unless a good reason prevents this being done; in which case, it should be expressed as for mr. G—, mrs. R—, or mrs. S.'s child, or for master t—, so as to convey to the apothecary some idea of the age of the patient.

2d. The date and name of the physician or his initials, should always be appended, and, whenever practical, the dose and mode of administering the medicine directed.

3d. When an unusually large dose of an active medicine is prescribed, as opium, morphia, elaterium, strychnia, etc., let such names be put in *italics*, and the quantity or quantities repeated in writing enclosed within a parenthesis; thus:—r morphiæ sulphatis grs. Vj. (six grains.) Div. In chart. Vj.

4th. When an active substance is to be used externally, it should be so stated on the prescription; thus, "for external application"—"to be applied to the part as directed," etc.

5th. The quantities of each article should be placed in a line with the name, and not below it and in using the roman numerals, the *i*'s should be dotted correctly.

6th. The occasional practice of writing the directions intended for the patient in *latin*, and especially in abbreviated latin, is uncalled for, and attended with some risk; it is far safer to write them in english, and without abbreviation or the use of figures, unless these are well and distinctly formed.

B. *In respect to the apothecary.*

1st. The apothecary should hesitate to dispense a prescription, the handwriting of which is so imperfect as to render the writer's meaning doubtful—especially if it involves agents of a poisonous or irritating character— unless he is able, from collateral circumstances, to satisfy himself of the intent of the prescriber. In such a case he should delay the delivery of the medicine to the patient until he can see the physician, and in doing so he should avoid committing the latter by agreeing to send the medicine when it is ready.

2d. The apothecary is justified in the same means of delay, if he, after deliberate consideration, believes that the physician has inadvertently made a mistake in the quantity or dose of the article or articles prescribed; always keeping in view the physician's reputation as well as his own. Every respectful application, in such cases, to a physician, should be met in good faith AND WITH KIND FEELING, EVEN THOUGH NO ERROR SHOULD PROVE TO EXIST.

3d. In his demeanor and language, the apothecary should cautiously avoid compromising the physician, unless it be unavoidable, in which case honesty is the best policy, and the patient or his messenger should be told that it will be necessary to have an interview with the physician previously to compounding his prescription.

4th. The apothecary is not justifiable in making inquiries relative to the patient or his disease, or remarks relative to the character or properties of the medicines prescribed, that are uncalled for, or likely to convey a wrong impression, through an ignorant messenger, to the patient, excepting it be done in a case where he has doubts in regard to the prescription, and wishes to satisfy himself, and here he should act with great discreetness.

5th. When an apothecary is asked his opinion of a physician's prescription in a manner that indicates want of faith in the prescriber, he should waive the question, unless by a direct answer he should be able to restore that confidence. When asked the nature of the ingredients, he should be guided in his answer by circumstances, avoiding to give the desired information, when he believes it would be contrary to the wish of the physician, or attended with injurious consequences. In other cases he should use his own judgment.

6th. Physicians being often unacquainted with practical pharmacy, pay little attention to the order in which the several articles entering into a prescription are arranged, with the view to facilitate the operations of dispensing. It hence becomes the first duty of the apothecary carefully to read the prescription and fix the proper order in his mind. He should, at the same time, acquire the habit of considering the quantities ordered in relation to the usual doses, and, also, the general bearing of the prescription; and a constant resort to this practice, based on due knowledge, must almost inevitably detect mistakes, if any have been made.

7th. Apothecaries should accustom their assistants to study prescriptions in this light, and to acquire such a knowledge of the doses and therapeutical uses of medicines as shall serve to guide them in avoiding errors.

8th. The apothecary, when engaged in dispensing a prescription, should, as far as possible, avoid mental preoccupation, and give his attention fully to his task. He should acquire the habit of *always* examining the label of the bottle before using its contents, and he should satisfy himself that he has read the prescribed quantity correctly, by referring to the prescription anew before weighing out each article. It is also, a useful precaution to have bottles containing mineral or vegetable poisons, distinguished by some prominent mark.

9th. As the conscientious discharge of his duty should be the aim of every apothecary, seeing that on his correct action depends, in no slight degree, the usefulness of the physician, no pains should be spared to secure the efficiency of the medicines dispensed, whether they be drugs or preparations. The latter should always be prepared of full strength, and according to the formulæ recognized by the united states pharmacopœia, unless when otherwise specially ordered.

10th. The apothecary should always label, and number correctly, all medicine dispensed by him on the prescription of a physician; he should, also, invariably, transcribe on the label, in a plain legible hand writing, the name of the patient, the date of the prescription, the directions intended for the patient, and the name or the initials of the prescriber.

11th. The original prescription should always be retained by the apothecary, whose warrantee it is, in case of error on the part of the prescriber. When a copy is requested, if as in many instances no objection can be urged, it should be a *jac simile* in language and symbols, and not a translation.

12th. In no instance is an apothecary justifiable in leaving his business in charge of boys, or incompetent assistants—or in allowing such to compound prescriptions, excepting under his immediate and careful supervision.

13th. In justice to his sense of the proper limits of his vocation, to the medical profession, and to his customers, the apothecary should abstain from prescribing for diseases, excepting in those emergencies, which occasionally occur, demanding immediate action, or, in those every day unimportant cases where to refuse council would be construed as a confession of ignorance, calculated to injure the reputation of the apothecary, and would be attended with no advantage to either physician or patient.

14th. The sale of quack or secret medicines, properly so called, constitutes a considerable item in the business of some apothecaries. Many of the people are favorably impressed towards that class of medicines, and naturally go to their apothecaries for them. It is this which has caused many apothecaries to keep certain of these nostrums, who are ready and willing to relinquish the traffic in them, but for the offence that a refusal to supply them to their customers would create. At present all that the best disposed apothecary can be expected to do, is to refrain from the manufacture himself, of quack and secret medicines; to abstain from recommending them, either verbally or by exhibiting show bills, announcing them for sale, in his shop or windows; and to discourage their use, when appealed to.

15th. Having in view the welfare of the community and the advancement of pharmaceutic science and interest, it is all important that the offices of prescribing and compounding medicines should be kept distinct, in this city and surrounding districts. All connection with, or moneyed interest in apothecary stores, on the part of physicians, should, therefore, be discountenanced. With respect to the pecuniary understanding said to exist, in some instances, between apothecaries and physicians, we hold, that no well disposed apothecary or physician would be a party to such contract, and consider the code of ethics of the college of pharmacy and the constitution of the philadelphia county medical society as sufficiently explicit on this subject.

16th. In reference to the patronage on the part of physicians of particular apothecaries, we are of opinion, as a general rule, that graduates in pharmacy should be encouraged in preference to others of the same date of business, and whilst admitting the abstract right of the physician to send his prescription where he pleases, we think that justice should dictate the propriety of his encouraging the nearest apothecary deserving of his confidence and that of the patient.

Committee of county medical society:

D. Frances condie,

Wm. Maybury,

G. Emerson.

Committee of phila. College of pharmacy:

William procter, jr.,

H. C. Blair,

John h. Ecky.

[we republish the above report from the american journal of pharmacy, as its "hints" are, in the main, practical and judicious. On one or two points, however, we differ from the author of the report. We do not think (b. Article 4th,) that the apothecary is ever justified in making inquiries relative to the disease of a patient. If his very inquiries may "convey a wrong impression to the patient, through an ignorant messenger," how can that ignorant messenger give information regarding the disease of a patient, which can guide the apothecary, himself not supposed to be versed in therapeutics, in judging of the correctness of a prescription? The apothecary, where he is in doubt, may inquire the dose and the age of the patient, and then, if he deems necessary, may have recourse to the physician himself. And in regard to the next article, when the apothecary is asked the "nature of the ingredients" in a prescription, it is wisest to refer the patient, *as a rule*, to the prescriber.]—ed. Journal of pharmacy.

NOTE ON THE DIVISION OF GUM RESINS IN POTIONS, AND IN DIACHYLON PLAISTER.

At a recent meeting of the society of pharmacy, m. Poulenc, submitted a method which he has employed for eight years in his laboratory, for suspending gum resins in medical prescriptions. It is well known how much difficulty there is in suspending either in a mixture, or lotion, one or more grammes of gum ammoniac, assafœtida, myrrh, &c. In dividing the ASSAFŒTIDA WITH YOLK OF EGG ALONE, THE MANIPULATION IS LONG; BUT IF INSTEAD OF THE EGG, WE EMPLOY 6 OR 8 DROPS OF OIL OF SWEET ALMONDS PER GRAMME, THE GUM RESIN, EVEN WHEN ENTIRE, IS EASILY REDUCED; WHEN THE OIL IS WELL MIXED, AND THE PASTE AS HOMOGENEOUS AS POSSIBLE, A LITTLE WATER IS FIRST ADDED, THEN GRADUALLY THE QUANTITY OF THE PRESCRIBED VEHICLE, AS FOR THE MUCILAGE OF A LINCTUS; THE PRODUCT OF THIS OPERATION WILL BE A SPEEDY AND VERY PERFECT EMULSION. ONE OF THE ADVANTAGES OF THIS *MODUS FACIENDI*, IS, THAT THE PRODUCT CAN BE WARMED WITHOUT DANGER OF COAGULATION, BESIDES WHICH, IT IS GENERALLY MORE EASY TO OBTAIN A FEW DROPS OF OIL OF SWEET ALMONDS, OR ANY OTHER KIND OF OIL THAN THE YOLK OF AN EGG.

M. Poulenc has recently applied the same method to the manufacture of diachylon plaister, in the following manner: take some entire pieces of gum resin, and triturate them briskly in an iron mortar, after which in a marble, or porcelain mortar, mix in the oil, and add a sufficient quantity of water to obtain an emulsion about as thick as liquid honey; strain this through a coarse cloth; there will be hardly anything left on the cloth, and the strained substance will be perfectly homogeneous. Evaporate in an earthen vessel, by the water-bath, the water which had been mixed in, and when the mass presents the appearance of a soft extract, the other ingredients of the plaister may be mixed in with the greatest ease. This plaister presents a very beautiful appearance, and exhales a very decided odour of the gum resins employed in its composition. Should it be feared that the small quantity of oil, might weaken the consistence of the plaister, m. Poulenc thinks that the quantity of turpentine might, without inconvenience, be slightly diminished.

We have tried with success the method of m. Poulenc for emulsions with gum resins; as to its further use in the preparation of diachylon plaister, we cannot speak with certainty.—there is a chemical question, which, in all cases governs the preparation of pharmaceutical agents.—*stan. Martin, l'abeille medicale.*

ESSENCE OF JARGONELLE PEAR.

BY THE EDITOR OF THE PHARMACEUTICAL JOURNAL.

The liquid sold under this name, and which has been for some time in use by confectioners, is the *acetate of the oxide of amyle.*

It is prepared with great facility by submitting to distillation a mixture of one part of amylic alcohol (better known by the name of oil of grain,) two parts of acetate of potash, and one part of oil of vitriol. The distilled liquid is to be washed with alkaline water, dehydrated by chloride of calcium, and afterwards rectified by distillation from protoxide of lead.

Its properties are thus stated by dumas:—in the state of purity it is a colorless, very limpid, volatile liquor, which boils at 257° f. It possesses an ethereal aromatic odor, somewhat resembling acetic ether; its sp. Gr. Is less than that of water. It is insoluble in water, but soluble in alcohol, ether, oil of grain, &c. Concentrated sulphuric acid does not color it in the cold; but by heating the mixture, it becomes reddish-yellow, and when the temperature is elevated, destructive reaction takes place, the mixture blackens and evolves sulphurous acid. Placed in contact with a watery solution of potash it is very slowly altered; but an alcoholic solution of this base rapidly decomposes, an alkaline acetate is formed, and the oil of grain regenerated. Its ultimate composition is

14 equivalents of carbon,	84
14 equivalents of hydrogen,	14
4 equivalents of oxygen,	32
	130

But its proximate composition is amyle, (an hypothetical radical) oxygen, and acetic acid.

1 equivalent amyle ($C_{10}H_{11}$)   71

1 equivalent oxygen,   8

1 equivalent acetic acid, ($C_4H_3O_3$)   51

[130]

Its formula is thus stated by brande, aylo, aco$_3$; by fownes, aylo, c$_4$ h$_3$ o$_3$.

Amylic alcohol, or *oil of grain*, called by the germans *fuselol*; is the hydrated oxide of amyle, aylo, ho. It is LARGELY PRODUCED IN THE DISTILLATION OF SPIRIT FROM CORN. IT IS OFFICINAL IN THE DUBLIN PHARMACOPŒIA, WHERE IT IS TERMED "*ALCOHOL AMYLICUM—FUSEL OIL*," AND IS EMPLOYED TO YIELD VALERIANIC ACID IN THE PROCESS FOR MAKING "SODÆ VALERIANAS."

From information which we have received, we have reason to believe that the use, by very young children, of articles of confectionery, flavored with essence of pear, is not without danger. A child on two occasions became partially comatose, with livid lips and feeble pulse, after eating some confectionery which it was calculated contained about one drop of the essence.—*london pharmaceutical journal, november, '51.*

On the growth of plants in various gases, especially substituting carbonic oxide, hydrogen, and light carburetted hydrogen for the nitrogen of the air.

By messrs. Gladstones. Dr. Gladstone gave the results of experiments made and still in progress, with his brother, mr. G. Gladstone. After describing the effect on some flowers, as the pansy, the crocus, &c.—a discussion ensued—mr. R Warrington suggesting that in such experiments the plants be allowed to take root well before immersing them in the gases; next, that the combined atmospheres were too much saturated with moisture, often causing rapid growth and decay; and that these flowers and roots should be compared with others grown in similar volumes of confined common air. Prof. Dumas spoke of the great, and, indeed, almost unsuspected influence of carbonic oxide gas. The judicial investigations in france had disclosed the fatal effects of this gas as being so much greater than carbonic acid gas. In the atmosphere produced by the burning of charcoal, 1-200th part of carbonic oxide was fatal, while with one-third the volume of carbonic acid the animal was asphyxiated, but afterwards revived. The chairman said that he had reason to believe that in the combustion of anthracite, much carbonic oxide gas is produced.—*pharmaceutic journal, from report of british association in the athenæum.*

EDITORIAL.

"AN ACT RELATING TO THE SALE OF DRUGS AND MEDICINES."

—We would call the attention of our readers to the following strange bill, which has been introduced into the legislature of this state:

"the people of the state of new york, represented in senate and assembly, do enact as follows:

Section 1st. It shall not be lawful for any physician, druggist, apothecary, or any person or persons dealing in drugs or medicines, or engaged in preparing any compound to be given or administered as a medicine, to offer the same for sale without first affixing or attaching thereto, in a conspicuous manner, a written or printed recipe in the english language, stating the drug or drugs, medicine or medicines, or ingredients of which it is composed, together with the proportions of each.

Section 2. Any person or persons violating the preceding section of this act, shall be considered guilty of a misdemeanor, and on conviction thereof shall be fined for each offence in a sum not less than ten dollars, nor exceeding one hundred dollars, or be imprisoned for a term not exceeding six months.

Section 3. This act shall not take effect until the first day of july, 1852.

Albany, february 6th, 1852."

On reading this bill, carelessly, we thought that it was intended to be levelled at nostroms and quack medicines. If it were so, however laudable the motives of its originators, its policy is much to be doubted. The public are not prepared for it; it would, at once, raise a clamour about selfish motives and private interests; it would never be enforced: and would tend to bring more moderate and judicious legislation into contempt. But a careful perusal of the bill shows that it applies to apothecaries and venders of medicines in the ordinary prosecution of their business.

Should it become a law, no apothecary could sell six cents worth of paregoric, or an ounce of spiced syrup of rhubarb, unless he accompanies the article sold with a detailed enumeration of the substances composing it, with the proportions of each "written or printed in the english language," without rendering himself liable to fine and imprisonment! It is not necessary to characterize such a law to druggists. It is worthy of notice, however, as an instance of that spirit of pseudo reform which is at present so rampant. As a general rule, we believe, physicians have no objection to their patients knowing the remedies they prescribe, particularly when the patients themselves are people of sense and information, but in many instances, of what use would it be to the sick man and his conclave of friends to be able to spell OUT THE INGREDIENTS OF A PRESCRIPTION? WOULD IT HELP THEM TO A KNOWLEDGE OF ITS EFFECTS? ARE THEY THE BEST JUDGES OF ITS PROPRIETY? AND IF SO, HAD NOT THE LAW BETTER PROSCRIBE EDUCATED PHYSICIANS ALTOGETHER?

And then "written or printed in the english language"! The framers of such a law could not be expected to recognize a national or any other pharmacopœia; which of the twenty trivial names, that in different times and different places have been bestowed upon the same article, should we choose? Should we follow strictly the modern chemical nomenclature, or should we take that of a few years back or should we go to the fountain head and return to the names of the old alchemists? The whole matter is unworthy serious comment.

COFFINISM.

—England for a long time supplied the united states to a great extent with quacks and quack medicines. We now begin to produce these articles not only in quantity sufficient to supply the home market, but are enabled to spare some of our surplus for the mother country. Thomsonianism has been transplanted to great britain, where it flourishes under the auspices of a man named coffin, and is thence termed coffinism. Coffin has already numerous disciples among the illiterate classes of the community. He gives instruction in his physic made easy, and furnishes his followers with certificates of their acquaintance with the mysteries of steam, hot drops and lobelia. Each of his graduates, too, pays a certain sum into a fund created to defend those of the associates, who may fall within the grasp of the law. Already several of them have been tried for manslaughter, but the "anglo saxon race," among its other peculiarities, is determined to be quacked when it chooses, and the coffinites hitherto have got off scot free.

CAMPHOR AS A STIMULANT.

—A lady who for a long time had suffered from occasional attacks of hemoptysis, and other signs of consumption, and who likewise from reduced circumstances, was subject to great moral depression, applied for advice concerning an epileptic seizure from which she had suffered for the first time on the preceding night. On inquiry it came out that she had for a long time been in the habit of taking large quantities of camphor. She had begun the practice a number of years previously, by taking the camphor mixture which had been ordered for her invalid husband. Gradually she acquired a fondness for it, and constantly increasing the dose, she, at the time of her seizure, took daily from two drachms to half an ounce. She was in the habit of taking it crude, gradually nibbling her allowance in the course of the day. She described its effects as exceedingly agreeable, renovating her strength, inspiring her with hope and confidence, and enabling her to get through with the fatigues of the day.—when not under its influence she was languid, feeble and depressed. Taking into account the condition of her lungs, her general health did not seem to have been affected by the habit.

CAVENDISH SOCIETY.

—We give place willingly to the following circular of mr. Procter, convinced that in so doing we are subserving the best interests of our readers. The names of the officers and council of the society, give ample assurance of the value of the works selected for publication.

Cavendish society, london.—president—prof. Thomas graham.

Vice presidents—dr. Faraday, prof. Brande, sir robert kane, arthur aiken, and others.

Council—jabob bell, dr. Pereira, dr. Golding bird, robert warrington, alfred s. Taylor, and others.

Treasurer—dr. Henry beaumont leeson.

Secretary—theophilus redwood.

The cavendish society was instituted for the promotion of chemistry, and its allied sciences, by the diffusion of the literature of these subjects. The society effects its object by the translation of recent works and papers of merit; by the publication of valuable original works which would not otherwise be printed, from the slender chance of their meeting with a remunerative sale, and by the occasional republication or translation of such ancient or earlier modern works, as may be considered interesting or useful to the members of the society.

Heretofore persons in this country were admitted to membership on application to mr. Redwood the general secretary of the society, at london. To facilitate communication between the society and its american members, the undersigned has been appointed *local secretary*, at philadelphia, and to whom application should be made. The payment of five dollars u. S. Currency or its equivalent, annually, entitles each member to a copy of every work published by the society for the period during which their membership continues. No member shall be entitled to the society's publications unless his annual subscription shall have been duly paid, and it is to be understood that the charges for duty and freight on the books arising from their shipment to this country are to be paid to the secretary on delivery.

The number of works published will necessarily depend on the number of annual subscribers; hence it is of great importance to the individual interest of the members that their aggregate number should be large. The society now issue two or three volumes yearly. The books are handsomely printed on a uniform plan, for members only, their publication being conducted by the council who are elected annually by ballot from among the members; every member having a vote.

Members by subscribing for all or any of the past years, may get the works issued during those years except the first volume, published by the society in 1848, entitled "chemical reports and memoirs by thomas graham, f. R. S." Which is now out of print. The other volume of that year which is the 1st volume of gmelin's handbook of chemistry, can be obtained by paying half the subscription.

The subscribers for 1849 are entitled to the 2d and 3d volumes of gmelin's chemistry—and the life of cavendish by dr. George wilson of edinburgh. The subscribers for 1850 receive the 4th and 5th volumes of gmelin's work, and those of the current year will receive the 1st volume of lehmann's physiological chemistry translated by dr. Day, and the 6th volume of gmelin.

As the sole object of the cavendish society is the encouragement of an important branch of scientific literature, all who feel interested in chemistry should assist in that object by subscribing, or using their influence with others to extend the list of members, which now amounts to more than 850. All those who may desire to become members, to examine the works already issued, or to gain further information regarding the society, are requested to apply to the undersigned.

William procter, jr.

166 south 9th street, philadelphia. October, 1851.

NEW YORK JOURNAL OF PHARMACY. MARCH, 1852.

ON THE HEAVY OIL OF WINE. BY
EDWARD N. KENT.

Having occasion to use a little of the officinal oil of wine, i applied to one of our wholesale druggists, who furnished me with an article, which i found to be useless. On testing a sample, it *mixed with water* and produced a slight milkiness. It was evidently alcohol, containing a trace only of oil. The price of this was $4 per pound.

Samples were then obtained from all of the wholesale druggists from whom it could be procured, and each of these was proved to be equally worthless, as the results of the following tests will show.

The second sample, when agitated with water, separated into two portions, one of which was aqueous and the other ethereal. The latter exposed to the air, to separate the ether by spontaneous evaporation, left a residue which was completely *soluble* in water, and proved to be alcohol. The price of this mixture of alcohol and ether was $4,50 per pound.

The third sample when agitated with water, became slightly turbid, and was dissolved. It had a pale yellow color, ethereal odor, and the sp. Gr. Was .909. A portion of it, exposed twelve hours to spontaneous evaporation in a graduated measure, lost one-eighth of its bulk, and on the application of a taper, burned with a *blue* flame. It is quite evident that this also was alcohol with a small portion of ether, and a trace of oil. The price OF THIS WAS $4,50 PER POUND, AND IT WAS LABELLED "OL. AETHERII." IT BORE ALSO THE NAME OF THE *IMPORTERS*.

The fourth sample, when agitated with water, became slightly turbid, and dissolved. It was colorless, had an ethereal odor, and the sp. Gr. Was .811. This also burned with a *blue* flame. The price of this worthless article was

$6,50 per pound. It was labelled "ol. Vini pur," and bore also the name of the *london* manufacturer.

It may be well to remark, that the officinal oil of wine, when agitated with water, separates and falls to the bottom, being heavier than water, whence its name. The sp. Gr. Of the pure oil is not less than 1.05, and it has a yellow color.

The labels on the third and fourth samples above mentioned, are alone not sufficient evidence to prove that they were *imported*, but, in addition to the label, i was informed that one of them *was recently imported*, and also that the manufacturing chemists in this country do not make or sell the oil of wine.—in view of this statement (if true) the question naturally arises: how did the above worthless articles pass the custom house under the existing law for "the prevention of the importation of spurious and adulterated drugs?"

I have examined another sample which is not offered for sale as oil of wine, but as it has properties resembling more nearly the officinal oil than either of the four samples above mentioned, it might possibly be confounded with the oil of wine. This sample had an agreeable *vinous odor*, and a *yellow* color.—when agitated with water a considerable quantity of oil separated, which was *lighter* than water. A portion of the original oil, distilled in a glass retort with a thermometer passed through a cork, inserted into the tubulare, gave about half its bulk of a colorless liquid below 180° f., which proved to be alcohol containing a small quantity of acetic ether and œnanthic ether.—the residue left in the retort had the properties of a mixture of œnanthic ether and œnanthic acid. The above article has been, extensively used (in connection with acetic ether) for the MANUFACTURE OF FACTITIOUS BRANDY, AND IS SOLD FOR ABOUT $1,50 PER OUNCE.

After having tested samples of all the different articles offered for sale under the name of "oil of wine" by the wholesale druggists in new york, without being able to find either of them worthy of the name, i prepared a little for my own use, by the following process, which is that of the london pharmacopœia:

2 lbs. Oil of vitriol were carefully mixed with 1 lb. Commercial alcohol, and distilled very slowly in a glass retort. The product consisted of two portions, the lightest of which was an ethereal solution of oil of wine measuring 6 oz. This was exposed to the air for twenty-four hours to remove the ether by spontaneous evaporation. The residue, washed with a little dilute solution of potash and dried, was pure "heavy oil of wine," and weighed half an ounce. The quantity obtained, though small, corresponds exactly with the proportion obtained by hennell at the apothecaries' hall, london, viz: 17 oz. Oil of wine from 34 lbs. Alcohol, and 68 lbs. Oil of vitriol.

By a simple calculation of the cost of manufacture, and expense of importation, it will be seen that pure oil of wine could not be imported and sold at the prices asked for the samples above mentioned. In making this calculation it will be necessary to observe that under the existing excise law, the price of alcohol in england is much higher than in the united states, and is now, i am informed, from 17 to 18 shillings sterling per gallon. The following calculation (based on the results of hennell's process) gives the cost of *pure* oil of wine, manufactured in england and imported into this country, at $35 per pound; but the spurious articles now sold for oil of wine, are offered at prices varying from $4 to $6,50 per pound.

34 lbs. alcohol (about 5 gallons) at 17 shillings sterling per gallon,	$18 70
68 lbs. oil of vitriol, at 2½ cents per pound,	1 70
Labor, fire, packing, bottle, &c.	1 50
Cost of 17 oz. oil, to the English manufacturer,	$21 90
Or per pound,	
Cost of making 1 lb. pure oil in England,	$20 61
Manufacturer's profit, say 10 per cent.,	2 06
Wholesale price in England,	$22 67
Duties paid by importer, 30 per cent.	6 80

Charges paid by importer, 10 per cent.	2 26
Cost of importation,	$31 73
Profit on importation,	3 27
Wholesale price of the imported oil,	$35 00

I regret that i have been unable to find the price of pure oil of wine quoted in the lists of any of the manufacturing chemists, but think it fair to infer that if the article is offered for sale, of english manufacture, at less than $2 per ounce, that impurity or adulteration may be suspected, and in this case, i would recommend the following process for testing its purity.

Agitate a small portion of the oil in a test tube, with an equal measure of water. If it dissolves, reject the sample as impure, but if the mixture separates into two portions, after standing at rest for a few moments, put it on a paper filter, previously well moistened with water. The water in the mixture will pass through the moistened filter, leaving ether or oil upon it. If this is colorless or very pale yellow, it should be exposed a few hours to spontaneous evaporation, to ascertain if it contains oil. But if it is yellow and heavier than water, this portion may consist of oil of wine; this, however, should be verified by observing the odor and sp. Gr. Of the oil. By carefully operating upon a *known* quantity in the above manner, the *proportion* of alcohol or ether (if present) may be easily determined.

As the efficacy of hoffman's anodyne is due to the heavy oil of wine contained in it, and as the proportion of this oil to the other constituents is small, it is particularly necessary that THE OIL SHOULD BE PURE. THE HIGH PRICE OF ALCOHOL IN ENGLAND, AND A DEFECT IN THE DIRECTIONS FORMERLY GIVEN FOR ITS PREPARATION IN THE UNITED STATES DISPENSATORY, ARE THE PROBABLE CAUSES OF THE ABSENCE OF PURE OIL OF WINE IN NEW YORK. IN RECENT EDITIONS OF THE ABOVE WORK, THE DEFECTIVE PROPORTIONS HAVE BEEN SUBSTITUTED BY THOSE OF THE LONDON COLLEGE, AND THERE IS NOW NO REASON WHY PURE OIL OF WINE SHOULD NOT BE MADE IN

THE UNITED STATES, WHERE ALCOHOL IS CHEAPER, PROBABLY, THAN IN ANY OTHER PART OF THE WORLD. I HOPE THAT OUR MANUFACTURING CHEMISTS WILL TURN THEIR ATTENTION TO THIS SUBJECT, AND DISPLACE ALL WORTHLESS CHEMICAL AND PHARMACEUTI-CAL PREPARATIONS BY SUCH AS WILL BE USEFUL TO THE PUBLIC, AND CREDITABLE TO THE MANUFACTURERS.

[the united states pharmacopœia directs two pints of alcohol (sp. Gr. .835) to be mixed with three pints of sulphuric acid (sp. Gr. 1.845); by weight rather better than 3.3 of the acid, to one part of alcohol, and gives 1.096 as the sp. Gr. Of the oil.]—ed.

PRACTICAL HINTS,
BY A WHOLESALE DRUGGIST.

The prosecution of the business of preparing and vending medicines, has been and still is too exclusively confined to the dollar and cent department.

Buyers take too much for granted. Ipecac is ipecac all the world over, and he who can sell ipecac at the lowest price is likely to sell the most and make the most money. To the credit of the craft, in part however, a manifest improvement in this respect, has taken place within the last few years, to their credit in part, i say, because the demand for good medicines has of late increased, *compelling* some druggists to furnish better qualities than they otherwise would.

It is a common remark that the late law, passed by congress, relating to the introduction or importation of adulterated and inferior drugs, has produced a more desirable state of things in OUR COMMUNITY, BY OPENING THE EYES OF CONSUMERS TO THE FACT THAT INFERIOR DRUGS ARE IMPORTED AND ARE CONSUMED. THIS IS ONLY IN PART TRUE. AN IMPROVED STATE OF PUBLIC OPINION FIRST CAUSED THE LAW TO BE PASSED; THIS, IN CONNECTION WITH THE LAW WHEN PASSED, CAUSED A FURTHER PROGRESS. THE STONE, THUS SET IN MOTION, WILL NO DOUBT ROLL ON TILL AN ENTIRE REVOLUTION TAKES PLACE BOTH WITH VENDERS AND CONSUMERS.

It is not to be supposed that the person who swallows a dose of medicine dreams that it is not of good quality, or that he would hesitate in the value of six cents when purchasing his dose, between the best of its kind and that which is comparatively inert. The root of this great evil, viz: the purchasing, selling, and administering inferior medicines is *ignorance*. The patient can have little or no knowledge of the efficacy of what is given to him to take, and to the shame of a large portion of the medical profession be it spoken, the doctor knows but little more. I speak with confidence when i say that the knowledge of the sensible properties of drugs is almost exclusively confined to the druggist and apothecary. Hence in the purchase of his supplies of medicines of the apothecary, the only guide the physician has, is the price and the word of the seller,—this ought not so to be. At this time i do not profess to offer a remedy. The object of the present communication is to offer a few practical hints to the druggist, connected with the purchase of his stock; many, if not all, desire to purchase reliable medicines, but from want of knowledge between good and bad have only the price, and the reputation of the seller to guide them.

I now propose to take up articles of general use, and suggest a few simple tests of their quality and condition, which any one can apply with such means as an ordinary drug store furnishes.

Before proceeding with this subject, however, i beg leave to urge upon every druggist and apothecary, the great importance of having, at his disposal, a set of reliable hydrometers for liquids heavier and lighter than water, and a properly constructed thermometer for determining the temperature of liquids. He will find them his right hand helps, not only for DETECTING ADULTERATIONS, BUT FOR DETERMINING THE STRENGTH OR QUALITY OF NEARLY ALL THE LIQUIDS WHICH COME UNDER HIS INSPECTION.

Certain arbitrary terms have been applied to solutions of ammonia and ethers, such as f.; f. F.; f. F. F.; and so on. These terms were originally intended to indicate the exact strength of those liquids to which they were applied; but, unfortunately, every manufacturer has a standard of his own, indicating the value of an f, or in other words these terms mean nothing, and should be banished from the books of every intelligent dealer. The hydrometer will determine the strength accurately and beyond all question, the dealer therefore should make his purchases, estimating the strength by the specific gravity either in decimals or degrees.

In detecting adulterations of essential oils, the hydrometer is invaluable. If the specific gravity of an oil does not accord with the standard, it is proof positive that the oil is not pure; the reverse, however, is not so clear. If the specific gravity does accord with the standard, it is not a positive proof that it is pure, for the reason that the adulteration may be of the same specific gravity as the oil itself.

The strength of acids such as muriatic, nitric, sulphuric, aqua fortis, and the like, is accurately determined by this means.

A set of these instruments, on which dependence may be placed, can be obtained at a price varying from $5 to $12.

Let the dealer apply these instruments (where applicable) to all his purchases, and he will soon find out what he sells and who deals honestly by him.

Magnesia (calcined). Nearly all that is used in this country is imported from england. The quality, notwithstanding the drug law, is usually quite inferior. The impurities generally are carb. Magnesia, lime, alumina and silica.

To detect carb. Magnesia, put into a vial a small portion, and add two or three times its bulk of water; after mixing them well, add a small portion of sulphuric acid—effervesence will indicate the presence of a carbonate. On the addition of an EXCESS OF ACID, THE SOLUTION SHOULD BE PERFECTLY CLEAR; WHATEVER IS DEPOSITED IS IMPURITY OF SOME KIND; IF LIME IS PRESENT AN INSOLUBLE SULPHATE IS FORMED.

The presence of moisture is indicated by the magnesia being lumpy, and when shaken, the particles do not flow among themselves easily. Good magnesia has a light, lively appearance, and is pearly white.—(to be continued.)

ON BLISTERING CERATE.

BY EUGENE DUPUY, PARMACEUTIST, NEW YORK.

The successful researches of robiquet in his labors on the cantharis vesicatoria, have demonstrated that the cristallisable neutral substance to which he gave the name of *cantharidine*, is the proximate epispastic principle of the blistering cerate on which the physician depends in most cases, where an extended and yet deep revulsive action is necessary, whether it is derived from the cantharis vesicatoria or from other members of the trachelid family. The experiments of mess. Lavini & sobrero of turin, have confirmed the supposition made by analogy, of the indentity which exists in the vesicating principle of all these coleopters, and there is a strong presumption that our commerce will soon be enriched with the beautiful cantharis, (c. Nutalli,) abounding in the midst of our rising south western states, and that it will eventually supersede the cantharis vesicatoria we obtain from abroad. If adulteration would not destroy, by its baneful influence, the advantageous form of complex extracts, we could obtain a desirable amelioration of our officinal cerate, by substituting for the powdered cantharides an equivalent proportion of the oleaginous liquid, with which they are saturated in the fresh state, and which is possessed of all the vesicating properties of the insect. That liquid is prepared in various parts of the sardinian kingdom, especially at verceil, where it is extensively used by veterinary surgeons in preference to the preparations from the powdered insect, it PRODUCING DEEPER REVULSION. IT IS ALSO USED, DILUTED IN BLAND OLEAGINOUS SUBSTANCES FOR STIMULATING THE ACTIVITY OF FEEBLE SEROUS EXUDATIONS. AS FOR THE PRESENT WE HAVE NOT GENERALLY ACCESS TO THAT NATURAL PRODUCT OF THE CANTHARIS, WE MUST SELECT THOSE INSECTS IN THE BEST POSSIBLE CONDITIONS, AND ENDEAVOR TO FIX THEIR ACTIVE PRINCIPLE IN SUCH A MANNER AS WILL DIMINISH THE

LIABILITY TO SPONTANEOUS VOLATILISATION OF WHICH IT IS SUSCEPTIBLE, EVEN AT ORDINARY TEMPERATURE.

I have been for many years in the habit of preparing a blistering plaster which, i think, has some advantages over our officinal cerate, because it fixes the volatilisable principle, and at the same time rather increases than diminishes its energy.

To the officinal plastic mixture in which the powdered cantharides have been gradually incorporated, i add about 5 per cent of a mixture containing equal parts of strong acetic acid (prepared by distillation of the acetates of copper or lead), and pulverised camphor. The acetic acid transforms the cantharidine into an acetate of the same which is not volatilized at ordinary temperatures, and the camphor diminishes the symptoms of strangury which some patients have to endure when the application of a blistering plaster is resorted to. I also usually spread the blister on adhesive plaster on account of the convenient adhesion of that material.

ON THE ADULTERATION OF CERTAIN DRUGS AND THE METHODS OF DETECTING SAID ADULTERATIONS.

BY C. TOWNSEND HARRIS, *DEMONSTRATOR OF CHEMISTRY IN THE NEW YORK MEDICAL COLLEGE.*

Since the establishment of the office of inspector of drugs in the united states custom houses, a vast amount of spurious and adulterated articles has been prevented from finding its way into our market. By reference to the report of the INSPECTOR OF DRUGS FOR THE PORT OF NEW YORK, THROUGH WHICH IS RECEIVED THE GREAT BULK OF MEDICINALS IMPORTED INTO THIS COUNTRY, SOME IDEA MAY BE FORMED OF THE ENORMOUS QUANTITY OF SPURIOUS OPIUM, JALAP ROOT, SCAMMONY, IODINE, IODIDE OF POTASSIUM, ETC. ANNUALLY INTRODUCED FROM ABROAD. WE FIND THAT IN TEN MONTHS, FROM JULY 1848 TO APRIL 1849, INCLUSIVE, 90,000 POUNDS OF ADULTERATED DRUGS WERE REJECTED AT THE ABOVE NAMED OFFICE. DURING THE YEARS 1848 AND '50, NUMEROUS SPECIMENS OF ADULTERATED ARTICLES WERE SUBMITTED TO ME FOR EXAMINATION BY DR. BAILY THE INSPECTOR OF DRUGS. FROM A LONG LIST I MAY SELECT ONE AS AN INSTANCE OF THE IMPUDENCE EXHIBITED BY FOREIGN MANUFACTURERS, IN ATTEMPTING TO THRUST UPON US THEIR VILLAINOUS COMPOUNDS, "AS STANDARD ARTICLES." I FOUND A SPECIMEN OF IODINE, PURPORTING TO BE PURE, TO CONTAIN 2 PER CENT. OF NON-VOLATILE MATTER AND *40 PER CENT. OF WATER.* THE SOLID MATERIALS MAY BE PASSED OVER AS ACCIDENTAL, BUT THE WATER IS UNDOUBTEDLY A FRAUDULENT ADDITION.

Beneficial as the establishment of this office may be in preventing the admission of any but genuine articles from abroad, in the present state of pharmaceutical regulations, it merely serves as a stimulus to the exercise of ingenuity at *home*, for producing those adulterations no longer supplied from the other side of the water. It is hardly necessary to say that rogues are to be found in every nation and in every clime, but i am justified (as i believe) in asserting that the spurious articles, at present met with in our market, are manufactured by foreigners whose métier has been destroyed by the passage of the drug bill. It is positively certain that parties who some years since conducted a factory in brussels, from which spurious sulphate of quinine, sulphate of morphine, narcotine, &c., were palmed upon the citizens of the united states as genuine, are now at work in a city not one hundred miles distant.

How is this home adulteration to be met? The appointment of a home inspector of drugs, whose duty it should be to visit, from time to time, our apothecaries' establishments, and to inspect the quality of the drugs therein, would be at variance WITH REPUBLICAN IDEAS; TOO MUCH LIKE THE EXCISE LAW OF ENGLAND SO OBNOXIOUS TO THE SEMI-REPUBLICAN INHABITANTS OF GREAT BRITTAIN. THIS QUESTION, HOWEVER, HAS BEEN SUFFICIENTLY DISCUSSED BY OTHERS MORE ABLE THAN MYSELF. THE REMEDY FOR THESE ABUSES RESTS WITH THE DRUGGISTS THEMSELVES. LEGISLATIVE ENACTMENTS ARE USELESS. THE PRESENT COLLEGE OF PHARMACY WHICH INCLUDES IN ITS LIST OF TRUSTEES, SOME OF THE LEADING PHARMACEUTISTS OF THE COUNTRY, HAS DONE MUCH TOWARDS ELEVATING THE PROFESSION. IT IS TO BE HOPED THAT THE LAWS UNDER WHICH THEY ACT WILL BE EXTENDED TO OTHER STATES, AND THAT NO APOTHECARY, UNLESS DULY LICENSED BY THE SOCIETY, SHALL HAVE ANY RIGHT TO PURSUE HIS PROFESSION WITHOUT THE DIPLOMA OF THE COLLEGE.

It is a matter of congratulation that some houses in this city, and those doing an extensive business, and of the highest reputation, have associated with themselves partners possessing a competent knowledge of chemistry. From these houses nothing can be obtained which is not up to the standard. Our apothecaries will find it to their advantage in the end, to employ persons possessing sufficient knowledge to enable them to detect adulterations in drugs, and not only that, but to be able to prepare the most difficult articles.

I shall relate in this paper some instances of *home adulterations* which have recently come under my notice. I have been furnished by retail druggists in the city with several specimens of the bitartrate of potassa. The results of the examination of five different specimens are here given:

No. 1.	Bitartrate of Potassa,	50 per cent.
	Sulphate of Lime,	50 per cent.
		100
No. 2.	Bitartrate of Potassa,	65 per cent.
	Sulphate of Lime,	35 per cent.
		100
No. 3.	Bitartrate of Potassa,	70 per cent.
	Sulphate of Lime,	30 per cent.
		100
No. 4.	Bitartrate of Potassa,	75 per cent.
	Sulphate of Lime,	25 per cent.
		100

No. 5 contains a small per centage of carbonate of potassa and a considerable amount of carbonate of lime. No weighings were made, but the amount of adulteration was apparently much less than in the other cases.

I have also had occasion to examine some specimens of iodide of potassium, procured from some of the first druggists in the city.

Specimen No. 1, contained:

	Iodide of Potassium,	64 per cent.
	Chloride of Potassium,	36 per cent.
		100
No. 2.	Iodide of Potassium,	70 per cent.
	Chloride of Potassium and Carbonate of Potassium,	30 per cent.
		100
No. 3.	Iodide of Potassium,	35 per cent.
	Chloride of Potassium and Chloride of Sodium,	65 per cent.
		100

In numerous examinations made of the bitartrate of potassa and of the iodide of potassium from foreign sources, i have never detected in the iodide of potassium more than 15 per cent of impurities, nor in the bitrate of potassa, as imported from france, more than 8 per cent. Of course the crude commercial argol always contains a small amount of tartrate of lime.

In a sample of so called "cod liver oil," submitted to me for examination by professor davis, of the new york medical college, i am unable to detect a single trace of iodine. The OIL IS RANK, *ALMOST BLACK*, AND IS EVIDENTLY A MIXTURE OF WHALE OIL AND LINSEED OIL; IN FACT IT CONTAINS NO COD LIVER OIL WHATEVER. THIS ARTICLE HAS BEEN SOLD BY A FELLOW PROFESSING TO BE A DRUGGIST AND PHYSICIAN.

It is certainly most important that druggists and their employers should possess a sufficient knowledge of chemical tests to enable them to detect sophistications. I propose to give hereafter the details of examinations of adulterated medicines and the simplest methods i can devise for the detection of such adulterations, and i trust others beside myself will turn their attention toward a subject so fraught with interest to the pharmaceutist.

ON WOORARA.
A NOTE READ TO THE ACADEMY
OF SCIENCES,

BY M. U. BERNARD, IN HIS OWN NAME, AND
THAT OF M. PELOUZE.

Woorara is a violent poison, prepared by some of the tribes inhabiting the forests bordering the upper oronoco, the rio negro, and the amazon.

Although the existence of this poison has been long known, very vague notions are still entertained regarding its component parts. Amongst the savages who sell or barter it, its preparation remains secret; and has only been made known through their priests or sorcerers. According to humboldt, woorara is simply a watery extract of a creeper, belonging to the genus strychnia. According to m. M. Boussingault and roulin, it contains a poisonous substance, analagous to a vegetable alkali, woorarine. The information given us by m. Houdet, differs from that of m. Humboldt only in this respect, that he observes, before the extract is quite dry, the indians of messaya pour on it a few drops of the venom gathered from the glands of the most venomous serpents. This last circumstance is important, as we shall see that the physiological effects of woorara must CAUSE US TO REGARD ITS MODE OF ACTION AS ENTIRELY ANALOGOUS TO THAT OF VENOMS.

Woorara is a solid extract, black, resinous looking, soluble in water. We shall have occasion hereafter to advert to its chemical properties. Our attention will now be directed to its physiological effects when exerted on living animals. Woorara resembles venom in this, that it can be eaten, that is, taken into the digestive canal of man and other animals with impunity, whilst when introduced by puncture under the skin, or in any other part of the body, its absorption is invariably attended with fatal results in all animals. This fact we have repeatedly tested. The action of this poison is instantaneous, when it is injected directly into the blood vessels. A weak, watery solution thrown into the jugular vein of a dog or a rabbit, has always produced sudden death, the animal uttering no cry, nor manifesting any convulsive agitation. The effect on the whole organization is electric, and the vital functions are arrested as by lightning. When introduced under the skin in solution or in solid fragments, its poisonous action manifests itself more slowly, and the time is varied by the dose, the size of the animal, and its species. Other things being equal, birds die soonest, then the mammalia, and then reptiles; thus, with the same specimen, birds and mammalia die in a few minutes, whilst a reptile will survive for several hours. But death is invariably accompanied by similar, and very remarkable symptoms; in the first place, when pricked, the animal apparently feels nothing. If a bird, for example, it flies as usual, and at the end of a few seconds, when the woorara is very active, it drops dead without uttering a cry, or appearing to suffer; if it be a rabbit or a dog, it runs about as usual after the puncture, without any abnormal symptom, then, after some seconds, as if fatigued, it lies down, appears to sleep, its respiration stops, and life is terminated, without a groan or sign of pain. Rarely do we see even slight contraction of the sub-cutaneous muscles of the face and body.

On examining immediately after death, the bodies of ANIMALS THUS POISONED, WE HAVE ALWAYS OBSERVED PHENOMENA WHICH INDICATE A COMPLETE ANNIHILATION OF ALL THE PROPERTIES OF THE NERVOUS SYSTEM. IT IS GENERALLY FOUND THAT WHEN DEATH HAS BEEN SUDDEN, THE NERVES RETAIN FOR SOME TIME THE POWER OF REACTION UNDER THE INFLUENCE OF MECHANICAL OR CHEMICAL EXCITEMENT; IF A NERVE OF MOTION BE EXCITED, CONVULSIONS SUPERVENE IN THE MUSCLES TO WHICH IT LEADS; IF THE SKIN BE PINCHED, IT CAUSES REFLEX MOTION. BUT NONE OF THESE ARE OBSERVED AFTER DEATH BY WOORARA. THE NERVES OF THE STILL WARM ANIMAL, IN WHOM LIFE HAS BEEN EXTINCT BUT A MINUTE, ARE INERT AS IF IT HAD BEEN DEAD AND COLD FOR SEVERAL HOURS.

Again, in animals poisoned by woorara, the blood is invariably black, and frequently so changed as to coagulate with difficulty, and not to become bright on re-exposure to air.

If we compare this effect of woorara with that of the viper, we shall observe a great analogy between them, varying only in intensity. We may further remark, that woorara, like the poison of the viper, may be introduced with impunity into the intestinal canal. We might be led to suppose from its perfect innocuousness when introduced into the stomach, that it became modified, or in a word, digested by the gastric juice, so as to destroy its deleterious properties. To verify this supposition, we caused some woorara to be digested in the gastric juice of a dog, at a temperature of between 38° and 40° of centigrade. After leaving it for forty-eight hours, we introduced it by puncture into the veins of some animals, who died with the before-named symptoms; establishing the fact, that a prolonged contact with the gastric juice in no way modified its deleterious properties. This experiment has been repeated in various ways, and on the separate parts, as well as on the living animal. We made a dog, in whose stomach we had formed a fistulous opening, swallow some fragments of woorara mixed with his food; after a little time we obtained some of his gastric juice, and on analysis found it to resemble in every respect a solution of woorara. Thus we have the singular phenomenon of an animal, carrying in its stomach, harmless to itself, a liquid WHICH WOULD CAUSE INSTANT DEATH TO ANY OTHERS WHO SHOULD BE INOCULATED WITH IT. NOT ONLY DID THE DOG WHICH SWALLOWED THE POISON EXPERIENCE NO FATAL RESULT FROM IT, BUT ITS DIGESTION WAS NOT EVEN AFFECTED BY IT; THE GASTRIC JUICE THUS MIXED RETAINING ALL ITS DIGESTIVE PROPERTIES.

These facts prove that the innocuousness of woorara when introduced into the stomach, is not attributable to the action of the gastric juice. The other intestinal liquids, saliva, bile, pancreatic juice, were attended with similar results, none of them producing by contact the least difference in the poisonous effect of woorara.

The explanation of these facts appears to be simply this: there is a want of absorption of the venomous substance through the gastro-intestinal mucous membrane. This can be shown by the following experiment:—take the fresh gastric mucous membrane of a dog or rabbit, recently killed; adapt it to an endosmometer in such a manner that the mucous surface remains outwards; then plunge the endosmometer containing sweetened water into a watery solution of woorara, and we shall find, after two or three hours, that the endosmosis will be complete. The level will have risen in the endosmometer, and yet the liquid contained in it will shew no trace of the poison, as can be proved by inoculating other animals with it.

If the experiment were to last longer, the endosmose of the poison might take place, but we should then find that the epithelium which covers its surface, had become changed, and had permitted the imbibition and endosmosis of the poisonous principle. This is so true, that if a partially decomposed membrane should be used instead of a fresh one, the endosmose of the poisonous principle takes place immediately. On the living animal, we can establish this property of the intestinal mucous membrane, and can demonstrate that amongst substances perfectly soluble in appearance there are some which when lodged on the surface of the intestinal membrane, may remain there without being absorbed, or without affecting the system. The active principle of woorara is of this kind.

It was necessary to ascertain whether other mucous membranes, besides those of the digestive organs, were possessed of this same property with regard to woorara. We have tried it successively on those of the bladder, the nasal fossæ and the eyes, and in all we have found an equal resistance to the absorption of the poisonous principle. An injection of this poison into the bladder of a dog, was retained six or eight hours, with no bad effects; but the urine voided after that time had all the poisonous properties of woorara.

One mucous membrane alone offers a remarkable exception; it is the pulmonary. This acts, in regard to the absorption of woorara, precisely like the sub-cutaneous cellular tissue, and on the introduction of some drops of the poisonous solution into the air passages, when every precaution is taken, death takes place as rapidly as when the skin has been punctured.

We readily perceive that this membrane, destined solely for the passage of the air to accomplish the phenomena of respiration, possesses a peculiar structure, and is unprovided with that protecting mucous which lubricates the other membranes communicating with the exterior. This similarity between the pulmonary mucous membrane and cellular tissue, supports the ideas which m. Majendie, long ago, promulgated on the structure of the lungs.

We shall not expatiate, at present, on the remarkable difference in the absorbent properties of the various mucous membranes of the body. We shall have occasion again to revert to the subject, and shall only state that this fact, in relation to the absorption of woorara, is not isolated, and that in the intestines, for example, many active principles, although soluble, cannot be absorbed, and are consequently forced to act locally, or as if shut up in a closed vessel.

For the present we will content ourselves with these conclusions:

1st. That woorara acts upon animals in the same manner as venom.

2nd. That its harmlessness, when injected into the intestinal CANAL, CANNOT BE EXPLAINED BY ANY CHANGE WHICH THE POISONOUS PRINCIPLE UNDERGOES, BUT RATHER BY A SPECIAL PROPERTY OF THE GASTRO-INTESTINAL MUCOUS MEMBRANE WHICH RESISTS ITS ABSORPTION.— *JOURNAL DE PHARMACIE ET CHIMIE.*

SUMBUL, OR YATAMANSI.

Sumbul, the name and therapeutical properties of which are almost unknown to french physicians, appears to have been employed in india from a very remote period. Pietro della valle, who travelled through the different countries of asia, in 1623, 1624 and 1625, mentions that sumbul is a root, and not a stem, although the arabic word, sumbul, he observes, refers to the whole plant. It appears that the word sumbul is applied in india to a plant and portions of a plant, used as a perfume, as an incense in religious ceremonies, and again, as a medicinal substance. Sir william jones thought that the true sumbul was a species of valerian, known both to the hindoos and brahmins, under the name of yatamansi. But, according to m. Granville, it appears to be an aquatic umbelliferous plant, found in the neighborhood of rivers.

It is erroneously asserted that it grows in hindostan. It is not found in any part of the indian territory, occupied by the english. The plant grows in bootan and the mountains of nepaul; and although large quantities of the dried plant have been exported, no botanist has yet been able to describe its characteristics from a living specimen. It is said that the native laws forbid the exportation of a living plant, without an order from the sovereign.

Sumbul has been described as a mass of roots and leaves of a greenish color, crumpled and pressed one against the other. This is an error, and arises from the fact of some having been first shown at st. Petersburg, which had been mixed with a STRONG DECOCTION OF THIS SUBSTANCE OF A GREENISH COLOR. SUMBUL APPEARS, ON THE CONTRARY, UNDER THE FORM OF A ROOT, THICK, HOMOGENEOUS, OF TWO, THREE, AND EVEN FOUR INCHES IN DIAMETER, CUT IN PIECES OF AN INCH TO AN INCH AND A HALF LONG, AND WHOSE SECTION PRESENTS A FIBROUS ASPECT, AND A WHITE AND YELLOWISH TINT. IT IS BROUGHT FROM THE CENTRE OF ASIA, TO MOSCOW, VIA KIATCHA. IN ALL THE GOOD SPECIMENS OF SUMBUL, THE EPIDERMIS, OR EXTERNAL COVERING, IS OF A DARK SHADE,

APPROACHING TO BROWN; IF THE COLOR BE STRONGLY MARKED, IT INDICATES THAT THE PLANT WAS OLD. THE EPIDERMIS IS VERY THIN, AND MUCH WRINKLED. THE INTERIOR SUBSTANCE IS COMPOSED OF THICK, IRREGULAR FIBRES, WHICH MAY BE SEPARATED FROM ONE ANOTHER, AFTER THE OUTER COVERING IS DETACHED, AND WHICH INDICATE A POROUS STRUCTURE, COMMON TO AQUATIC PLANTS. IF, AFTER TAKING OFF THE OUTER COVERING, WE MAKE A TRANSVERSE CUT, WE SHALL PERCEIVE AN EXTERNAL LAYER, WHITE AND MARBLED, AND AN INTERNAL LAYER, THICKER AND YELLOWISH. WITH A POWERFUL LENS WE CAN DISTINGUISH TRANSPARENT POINTS, WHICH LOOK LIKE GRAINS OF FECULA.

Two very remarkable physical characteristics demand our attention when we examine this root: first, its perfume, resembling the purest musk; then the powerful aroma which it exhales when under mastication. This odor of musk is so marked, that some had thought it owed this quality to its contact with musk, in the transportation of drugs from asia to europe; but such an idea is negatived by the fact that sumbul retains this odor, even when very old; that even when the external parts have lost it, it continues in the interior; that this odoriferous principle may be extracted from it by chemical manipulation; and again, that it has received from botanists the name of moschus-wurzel or musk-root. Its aromatic taste is also a distinguishing characteristic. The first impression on the palate is slightly sweet, this is rapidly replaced by a balsamic flavor, and then by a bitter, but not unpleasant taste.—as mastication proceeds, the mouth and throat experience a strong aromatic and pungent taste, and the breath becomes impregnated with the penetrating odor of the SUBSTANCE.—THIS FLAVOR IS STILL MORE DECIDED IN THE ALCOHOLIC TINCTURE THAN IN THE ROOT.

The chemical analysis of sumbul has occupied several german chemists, reinsch, schnitzlein, frichinger, and kalthover. According to reinsch, the root of sumbul contains, besides water, traces of an ethereal oil, two balsamic compounds, (resins) one soluble in ether, the other in alcohol, wax, aromatic spirit, and a bitter substance, soluble in water or alcohol. The solution of this bitter substance, treated with lime, and chloride of sodium, gives a sediment composed of gum, starch and saline materials. The perfume appears to be contained in the balsams, and its intensity is increased by being diluted with water. Finally, sumbul contains an acid, which reinsch proposes calling *sumbulic acid.*

Kalthover directed his attention further to its pharmaceutical uses, and obtained an alcoholic tincture of a yellowish color, musky odor, and bitter taste; an ethereal tincture, yellowish, musky, and of a sharp taste; and a substance resembling wax, precipitated after repeated decoctions in water.

It appears then, that we may obtain from sumbul for medical purposes, two tinctures, one alcoholic, the other ethereal, which seem to differ in their principles, and which may be given in drops alone, or combined with other medicines; and a bitter extract, soluble in water, which may be administered in pills. The powdered root may also be given crude, or in pills.—*(union médicale) in journal de pharmacie et de chimie.*

[sumbul has been used as an anti spasmodic and a nervine; further investigation is needed however to ascertain its true place in the materia medica. In the mean time it has been imported by one of our apothecaries, mr. Delluc, and we may soon hope to learn something more concerning its effects upon the system.] Ed. Journal of pharmacy.

OBSERVATIONS ON THE STRENGTH OF TINCTURE OF OPIUM. BY A. B. GARROD, M. D.

Professor of materia medica at university college, and physician to university college hospital.

As many discrepant statements are to be found in works on materia medica, in various dispensatories, &c. Concerning the strength of the tincture of opium of the london pharmacopœia, it may not be either uninstructive or uninteresting at least to the medical profession, to have the subject brought under notice and discussion at this society, in order that they may arrive at some definite conclusion concerning the strength of a preparation they are in the daily habit of prescribing. If we refer to the london pharmacopœia of 1836, we find the following directions for making the tincture of opium:—

Take of hard opium powdered, 3 ounces,

Proof spirit, 2 pints,

Macerate for fourteen days, and strain.

In the pharmacopœia of 1851, we are ordered to—

Take of opium powdered, 3 ounces,

Proof spirit, 2 pints,

Macerate for seven days, press out, and strain.

The only difference in the directions being that powdered *hard* opium, and digestion for *fourteen* days, are ordered in the one case, and simply powdered opium and seven days digestion in the other. If we look at the authorised edition of the pharmacopœia by mr. Philips of 1836, (and also at the present edition) we find stated, that the preparation has a deep brownish red color, possesses the peculiar odor and taste of opium, has sp. Gr. 0.952, and about 19 minims contain 1 grain of opium, which is said to be proved by the following data: 1st, by evaporating the tincture, and finding the amount of solid extract left; 2d, by ascertaining the quantity of opium remaining undissolved. The conclusion at which mr. Phillips arrived, viz: that 1 grain of opium was contained in 19 minims of the pharmacopœia tincture, has been copied into most english works on materia MEDICA, AND MOST MEDICAL MEN HAVE BEEN AND ARE STILL IN THE HABIT OF PRESCRIBING THE TINCTURE CONSIDERING IT TO BE OF THE *ABOVE* STRENGTH. WERE MR. PHILLIP'S CONCLUSIONS CORRECT?

With regard to the amount of solid extract left on evaporation of the tincture, it appears from the experiments of mr. Allchin, which are also confirmed by those which i have myself made, that 19 minims yield about 1 grain of extract; but in these cases the turkey opium of commerce must be first exsiccated; and the tinctures of commerce yield quantities varying from 1 in 19 to 1 in 28 minims of the tincture. Tincture of opium made with turkey opium in small masses not previously dried, fl. ℥ j. Gave on drying 2.7 of solid residue, or 1 grain in about 22.2 minims. Tincture of opium made with good turkey opium, previously dried and reduced to powder (pharmacopœia directions) fl. ℥ j. Gave on drying—three experiments—3.1, or 1 grain of residue in 19.3 minims.

If made with opium capable of being reduced to a state of powder, the average quantity of extract would be about 1 grain in 20 minims; this proportion would indicate that one-third of the solid ingredient (opium) is left undissolved, which was found by mr. Phillips to be the case. I believe all good specimens of turkey opium yield about this amount of residue. An experiment made within the last week at mr. Bell's establishment gave this result. If then the strength of tincture of opium be considered to be that indicated by mr. Phillips, we must assume that the undissolved portion possesses the same therapeutic effects as the dissolved portion. Is this correct?

It has been stated by some that morphia can be extracted from the residuum, and in dr. Pereira's *materia medica*, we find the following observations: "proof spirit dissolves the same constituents as water does, but it takes up a larger proportion of *narcotine, resin, oil.* I have repeatedly prepared morphia from the insoluble residue left behind in the preparation of the tincture." Again, in dr. Thomson's *dispensatory* it is stated that mr. Brande finds that the whole of the morphia is not taken up; but is found in no inconsiderable quantity in the filter. WE SUSPECT OCCASIONALLY *NARCOTINE* HAS BEEN TAKEN FOR *MORPHIA,*7 AND IN THE CASES WHERE *MORPHIA* HAS REALLY BEEN FOUND, UNLESS THE RESIDUE HAD BEEN PREVIOUSLY WASHED, AN ERROR MAY HAVE ARISEN FROM THE ALKALOID BEING CONTAINED IN THE TINCTURE OF OPIUM ADHERING TO THE DREGS, AND NOT FROM ANY CONTAINED IN THE RESIDUE ITSELF. I HAVE RECENTLY ENDEAVOURED TO ASCERTAIN THE TRUE STATE OF THE CASE, AND CHIEFLY BY MEANS OF A THERAPEUTIC INQUIRY INTO THE STRENGTH OF THE RESIDUUM. THE RESIDUE OF TINCTURE OF OPIUM PREPARED IN THE ORDINARY WAY AT UNIVERSITY COLLEGE HOSPITAL, WAS TAKEN FOR EXPERIMENT; IT WAS FIRST WASHED WITH A LITTLE COLD WATER TO REMOVE ANY ADHERING TINCTURE, AND AFTERWARDS DRIED IN A WATER-BATH. BY DIGESTION WITH ETHER, IT WAS FOUND TO YIELD ABUNDANCE OF *NARCOTINE*, AND WAS ALSO FOUND TO CONTAIN *MECONIC ACID* SUFFICIENT TO STRIKE A CLARET COLOR WITH THE PERSALTS OF IRON; BUT AT THE SAME TIME NITRIC ACID GAVE NO EVIDENCE OF THE PRESENCE OF *MORPHIA.* IT WAS FOUND ALSO BY EXPERIMENT THAT PROOF SPIRIT AT THE ORDINARY TEMPERATURE DISSOLVED BUT A VERY SMALL PORTION OF NARCOTINE; THE BULK OF THE NARCOTINE THEREFORE REMAINS IN THE RESIDUUM FROM THE TINCTURE OF OPIUM, PERHAPS UNITED WITH MECONIC ACID; FOR WHEN TREATED WITH WATER ACIDULATED WITH ACETIC ACID, BOTH *NARCOTINE* AND *MECONIC* ACID WERE DISSOLVED.

7 in the sixth edition of dr. Thomson's *dispensatory*, page 1061, the following method is given for obtaining "meconate of morphia," extracted from the *quarterly journal of science*, vol. Xx., from which it will be at once observed, that *narcotine* was mistaken for crystallized *meconate of morphia.*

"reduce good opium to powder, put it into a paper filter, add distilled water to it, and slightly agitate it; and in this way wash it till the water passes through colorless, after which, pass a little diluted alcohol through it; dry the insoluble portion (now diminished to one-half,) in a dark place; digest it, when dry, in strong alcohol for a few minutes, applying heat; separate this solution, which by boiling, and after evaporation, will yield crystallized meconate of morphia of a pale straw color."

A portion of the residue was given internally; *one grain* to a healthy adult produced no effect; *two grains* were given with no result; the dose was then successively increased to *four grains* then to *six grains*, afterwards to *thirteen*, and lastly to *thirty grains*, without causing the slightest effect on the individuals to whom it was administered; the only limitation to the quantity given being the unpleasantness of taking so large an AMOUNT OF SO BULKY A MATTER. IT APPEARS, THEREFORE, THAT THE RESIDUE IS, TO ALL INTENTS AND PURPOSES, INERT.

From these experiments, it is evident that even *should* traces of *morphia* be contained in the dregs, still the quantity must be such (when the tincture is prepared according to the london pharmacopœia) as to make no appreciable diminution of the strength of the preparation, and that the tinctura opii contains the active matter of the whole of the drug used in its formation, and therefore about 12 minims of tincture of opium possesses all the activity of 1 grain of crude opium, assuming that it loses only 12 per cent. In the drying. If dry opium is taken for comparison, 1 grain is contained in about $13\frac{1}{2}$ minims; and, therefore, *one* fluid drachm of tinctura opii contains about 5 grains of the drug, or $4\frac{1}{2}$ grains (according as it is compared with the dry or moist opium), in place of 3 grains; or 1 fluid ounce contains 40 or 36 grains in place of

24 grains usually assumed to be contained in it: a difference of strength of the highest importance when we consider the highly poisonous and powerful therapeutic action of the drug.

In the edinburgh preparation the amount of tincture containing a grain of opium is about 13½ minims, for the opium is ordered in the same proportion but not previously reduced to powder or dried. In the dublin preparation the opium is ordered to be coarsely powdered, but avoirdupois weight is used in place of apothecaries, which makes the strength of the tincture such that 12.75 minims contain *one* grain.

The error as to the strength of the tincture of opium, which is found in so many works, has been recently commented on. Thus dr. Christison objects to mr. Phillip's statements; dr. Royle also alludes to it, and so does mr. Squire, in his recent work on the pharmacopœias; and even those writers who have copied the statement must have done so without much thought on the subject, as they have calculated the strength of other preparations of opium, as that of the tinctura opii ammoniata, tinctura camphoræ composita, assuming that all the active properties of the opium used in the preparation had been taken up BY THE MENSTRUA. AND THIS IS THE CASE EVEN WITH MR. PHILLIPS HIMSELF, IN THE CASE OF THE COMPOUND TINCTURE OF CAMPHOR, WHEN HE STATES THAT *NEARLY TWO* GRAINS OF OPIUM ARE CONTAINED IN THE OUNCE, THE PHARMACOPŒIA PROPORTIONS OF OPIUM BEING 1.6 GRAINS ONLY.

I have brought the question before the society more for the purpose of eliciting the opinions of the members on the point, than with the idea of bringing forward much that is novel on the subject; if the conclusion to which we have arrived, namely, that 12 minims of tincture of opium contain all the medical properties of 1 grain of the crude drug, i think it very important that the members of the medical profession should be made fully aware of the delusion under which they have labored for so many years with regard to the strength of this important preparation.

NOTICE OF SOME VEGETABLE AND ANIMAL SUBSTANCES, NATURAL PRODUCTS OF NEW GRANADA.

BY M. J. RAF. MONZON, M. D. (*IN A LETTER TO DR. PEREIRA.*)

Sandi is a resinous gummy substance, produced in abundance by a tree known by this name, on making an incision in its bark. At first it presents itself white, or liquid like milk, and it is called in the province of barbacoas, "milk of sandi." In a few days it acquires the consistency of resinous gum. In this state it is applied to various medicinal uses in different parts of new granada, especially in the province of barbacoas, a warm and damp country near the ecuador, from whence the present sample comes. Its principal therapeutic property is *resolutive*; applied as a plaster upon lupus, fleshy excrescencies of the skin, cold and indolent tumors, &c. It produces their resolution; and this result is frequently confirmed by the INHABITANTS OF THOSE COUNTRIES. I HAVE OBTAINED IT ALMOST ALWAYS WHEN I HAVE MADE USE OF THE MILK IN SIMILAR CASES. AT PRESENT MY FATHER HAS APPLIED THIS GUM IN THE VALLEY OF CAUCA, AND WITH EXTRAORDINARY SUCCESS, FOR THE CURE OF "BOCIOS," OR OBSTRUCTIONS OF THE THYROID GLAND. HE HAS BEEN ABLE TO PURIFY IT, TAKING AWAY THE PART OF POTASS WHICH IT CONTAINS IN ITS ORIGINAL STATE, AND HAS BEEN ABLE TO GIVE IT THE CONSISTENCE AND COLOR OF GUM ARABIC; WITH THIS SUBSTANCE HE MAKES A PLASTER, WHICH DESTROYS THE "BOCIOS," WHICH SO MUCH ABOUND IN NEW GRANADA; AND ITS GENERAL BENEFITS ARE FELT AND ACKNOWLEDGED.

It is likewise used as an agent against sterility in women, applying it as a plaster upon the hypogastric region. In ulcers of a good character i have obtained frequent and quick cicatrisation by applying it in the same manner; i have also used it as a vehicle for preparing and applying blisters.

Aceite de palo (oil of wood) is produced by a tree called "manteco," in the same province. Its principal therapeutic qualities are topical and blistering. By using it as an embrocation i have destroyed the epidermis, and have thus been able to get rid of freckles and superficial stains on the face and other parts of the body. Applied in larger quantities it produces the effect of a strong blister, excoriating and inflaming the skin. This oil is used in its natural state as an ointment, on arms and instruments of steel: it destroys their temper and softens them. By decoction it loses these qualities, and might be used as an ointment without any risk. It cannot be used as a lamp-oil, because it exhales a very thick smoke and the most disagreeable smell. It has no known internal medicinal qualities; it may be classed amongst the corrosive poisons; its color is purple, its taste *sui generis*.

Leche de popa (milk of the cow-tree).—this substance, in its natural state, possesses the physical properties of animal milk. It is obtained by incision in the bark of the tree, which is very abundant in the province of barbacoas. The indians and the african race take it instead of cow milk; it is very nutritive, but has no known medicinal qualities. It is used also FOR WHITEWASHING HOUSES, COMBINING IT WITH EARTHY SUBSTANCES, BECAUSE, BEING GLUTINOUS, IT MAKES THE WHITEWASHING LAST LONGER, AND PREVENTS ITS STAINING OR RUBBING OFF.

Miel de abeja de brea (honey of the pitch bee).—this honey is extracted from the hive of a bee, very different from the one known in europe, and very much smaller. It is acid. Its medicinal qualities are for interior refrigeration. I have applied it externally for contusions and ecchymosis, caused by blows or falls, and i have always obtained a good result. The pitch is a resinous substance, of a dark yellow color, and constitutes the hive made by this bee. It has a peculiar taste and smell, is very combustible, and is used by the common people for torches. It is soluble in alcohol. I have applied it as a plaster for nervous rheumatic pains, and it has always relieved the pains and swellings.

Canedillo.—this is the name of a cane with a bitter and aromatic bark, and, in my opinion, it belongs to the family of winter's bark. It has many therapeutic qualities; amongst others it has particularly attracted my attention as an antidote against the bite of snakes and of other venomous animals. I consider it the best and safest of all the antidotes known. Put two ounces of this bark in a bottle of alcohol, allow it to macerate for three or four hours, to obtain a tincture. Use two parts of this mixture with common water; a wineglass every two hours until you allay the headache of the bitten person—an infallible consequence of the bite, cupping at the same time, and extracting the tooth, which often remains in the part, which is then to be washed and covered with lint wetted with the tincture. By this simple method i have cured hundreds, without the loss of a single life. This antidote is now generally kept by all the owners of mines, as a certain cure for bites of snakes, in preference to other antidotes formerly used. It has this advantage over them, that it may be taken in any quantity without danger. It is, besides, a tonic and anti-spasmodic. I have used it also as a febrifuge; in rheumatism (by friction); and in the windy colic, taken in the same way as for bites by snakes. FOR INDIGESTION CAUSED BY WEAKNESS, AND FOR AMENORRHŒA, FROM THE SAME CAUSE, IT IS ALSO USED.

Sandalo.—this is the bark of a tree which grows in the province of esmeraldas, in the republic of the ecuador. When burned, it produces a balsamic smell; by boiling the bark when fresh, it produces a very aromatic balsam, which, like the balsam of tolu is used in catarrh, spasmodic cough, ulcers, &c.

Note.—all these substances are indigenous in the province of barbacoas. Popa and sandi are found in great abundance. Manteca de palo (oil, or literally butter of wood), is obtained only from young trees which grow in the plains.

ON THE SODA-PYROPHOSPHATE OF IRON.

BY ALEXANDER URE, ESQ., SURGEON TO ST. MARY'S HOSPITAL.

My attention was attracted some time back by an ingenious paper of mons. Persoz on the double pyrophosphoric salts, published in the *annalen der chemie und pharmacie* for 1848. In the latter part of that paper, the author expresses an opinion that the pyrophosphoric salts are likely to prove of importance as medicinal agents. It is well known that iron is rendered very eligible for internal use, if administered in the form of a triple salt, as when combined, for example, with tartaric acid and potash; because the iron then is no longer precipitable by the alkaline hydrate. It would appear, however that the soda pyrophosphate of iron is in many respects superior as a medicine to the triple salts into which the vegetable acids enter.—thus, the pyrophosphoric salt, from being saturated with oxygen, cannot in passing through the system absorb more, whereas the latter salts under like circumstances, are constantly undergoing a process of combustion, according to millon; and by withdrawing oxygen in this manner, must necessarily impair the efficacy of the oxide of iron as an oxydizing agent. It deserves notice, moreover, that the constituent ingredients of the soda-pyrophosphate of iron are to be found in the organism.

I have prescribed this salt to various patients, and found it to act as a mild but efficient chalybeate. One little scrofulous girl, now under my care in st. Mary's hospital, for disease of the hip-joint, has taken it in solution during several months with the best effect. The remedy was accurately prepared by mr. Blyth, dispenser to the hospital, according to the subjoined directions of mons. Persoz: 32.5 grammes of green sulphate of iron in crystals are to be mixed in a porcelain capsule with 5 grammes of sulphuric acid, 30 grammes of water, and as much nitro-muriatic acid as will suffice to effect the oxidation of the protoxide of iron. The above mixture is to be evaporated to dryness in order to get rid of the free acid, and then treated with water to the amount of one litre. From 107 to 110 grammes of crystallized pyrophosphate of soda are to be dissolved likewise in a litre of water, of course in a separate vessel. The two solutions are next to be mixed together, and provided the iron solution has been rightly prepared there will be no precipitate whatever.

Each litre of liquid will contain as much iron as 16.5 of the green sulphate.

This solution is not affected by dilution with rain or distilled water, but from being faintly alkaline, is rendered slightly turbid on the addition of water impregnated with lime.

ON THE SIMABA CEDRON.

BY M. BERTHOLD SEEMANN.

A tree, which has attained great celebrity, is that called *cedron* (*simaba cedron*, planch.). The most ancient record of it which i can find is in the *history of the buccaneers*, an old work published in london in the year 1699. Its use as an antidote for the bite of snakes, and its place of growth, are there distinctly stated; but whether on the authority of the natives, or accidentally discovered by the pirates, does not appear. If THE FORMER WAS THE CASE, THEY MUST HAVE LEARNED IT WHILE ON SOME OF THEIR CRUISES ON THE MAGDALENA, FOR IN THE ISTHMUS THE VERY EXISTENCE OF THE TREE WAS UNSUSPECTED UNTIL ABOUT 1845, WHEN DON JUAN DE ANSOATIGUI, ASCERTAINED, BY COMPARISON, THAT THE *CEDRON* OF PANAMA AND DARIEN WAS IDENTICAL WITH THAT OF CARTHAGENA. THE VIRTUES OF ITS SEEDS, HOWEVER, WERE KNOWN, YEARS AGO, FROM THOSE FRUITS IMPORTED FROM THE MAGDALENA, WHERE, ACCORDING TO MR. WILLIAM PURDIE, THE PLANT GROWS IN PROFUSION ABOUT THE VILLAGE OF SAN PABLO. IN THE ISTHMUS IT IS GENERALLY FOUND ON THE OUTSKIRTS OF FORESTS IN ALMOST EVERY PART OF THE COUNTRY, BUT IN GREATER ABUNDANCE IN DARIEN AND VERAGUAS THAN IN PANAMA. THE NATIVES HOLD IT IN HIGH ESTEEM, AND ALWAYS CARRY A PIECE OF THE SEED ABOUT WITH THEM. WHEN A PERSON IS BITTEN, A LITTLE, MIXED WITH WATER, IS APPLIED TO THE WOUND, AND ABOUT TWO GRAINS SCRAPED INTO BRANDY, OR, IN THE ABSENCE OF IT, INTO WATER, IS ADMINISTERED INTERNALLY. BY FOLLOWING THIS TREATMENT THE BITES OF THE MOST VENOMOUS SNAKES, SCORPIONS, CENTIPEDES, AND OTHER NOXIOUS ANIMALS, HAVE BEEN UNATTENDED WITH DANGEROUS

CONSEQUENCES. DOSES OF IT HAVE ALSO PROVED HIGHLY BENEFICIAL IN CASES OF INTERMITTENT FEVER. THE *CEDRON* IS A TREE, FROM TWELVE TO SIXTEEN FEET HIGH; ITS SIMPLE TRUNK IS ABOUT SIX INCHES IN DIAMETER, AND CLOTHED ON THE TOP WITH LONG PINNATED LEAVES, WHICH GIVE IT THE APPEARANCE OF A PALM. ITS FLOWERS ARE GREENISH, AND THE FRUIT RESEMBLES VERY MUCH AN UNRIPE PEACH. EACH SEED, OR COTYLEDON I SHOULD RATHER SAY, IS SOLD IN THE CHEMIST'S SHOPS IN PANAMA FOR TWO OR THREE REALS (ABOUT 1*S*. OR 1*S*. 6*D*. ENGLISH), AND SOMETIMES A MUCH LARGER PRICE IS GIVEN FOR THEM.—*HOOKER'S JOURNAL OF BOTANY*.

[a large number of the cedron seeds have lately been received in new york, probably from a section of the country where they are cheaper than upon the isthmus. As a remedy for the bites of venomous reptiles, like all others of the same class, it is of little value, but from its intense bitterness, it may be expected to possess great tonic powers, and if, in addition to these, further experience shall confirm the report of its virtues as an antiperiodic, it will prove a remedy of great value.]—ed. New york journal of pharmacy.

EDITORIAL.

COLCHICUM AUTUMNALE.

—in the december number of the edinburgh monthly journal of medical science, dr. J. Mcgrigor maclagan, has published an article on colchicum autumnale, which contains little that is new, but is of interest as confirming the statements of other observers. The ordinary mode of propagation of the plant by the formation of a single new bulb is thus described. In june, "the bulb is as large as an apricot, firm, amylaceous, and extremely bitter, and having attached to it the shrivelled remains of the old bulb, and the leaves now yellow and decayed. At the end of june or commencement of july, a small bulb will be observed to have become developed upon the side of the corm at its lower part. At this time it is a little larger than a grain of wheat, and lies in a little fissure on the side of the parent bulb, a little above the origin of the radicles. It increases slowly and gradually in size till the beginning of august, when it appears as a dilatation of the flower stalk, which it then commences to put up.

In september the flower is in full perfection, the long tube of the perianth of which has raised the six partite limb to the height of from six to eight inches above the ground. The flower remains for two or three weeks, and then dies down; and nothing of the plant is seen above the surface till the beginning of february, when the leaf stalk commences to rise. If at this time the plant be taken up, the old and new bulb will still be found to be united, but the new one will be observed to have increased little in size since autumn, being still hardly larger in diameter than the leaf stalk. The bulb thus grows little during the autumn, but in winter it increases rapidly in size; in april it is like a large hazel nut, and from that time it increases still more till the end of june or the beginning of july, when it is, as dr. Christison states, as large as an apricot.

In april the leaf stalk is found perfected by a fine group of dark green leaves, generally three in number, and having within their sheath the capsules which ought to ripen their fruit in the course of the summer.

In may the old bulb will be found dry and withered, and containing very little starch; and in july if the plant be taken up, three bulbs will be found, the first now reduced to the form of a membrane, bearing no resemblance to a bulb at all; the second, arrived at full growth; and a third the progeny of the second.

In february and august, instead of one leaf stalk and flower stalk making their appearance at their respective periods, i have often remarked that two have occurred, one on either side of the parent bulb. I believe this to be one of the effects of cultivation, as i have no where seen it remarked in descriptions of the plant by botanical authors.

Dr. Christison has mentioned that the full size of a colchicum bulb is that of a small apricot. Where the plant has been cultivated however, dr. Maclagan, frequently met with them as big as large apples, and on one occasion procured one in october weighing nine and a half ounces.

He thinks that the cormus should be taken for medicinal use about the middle of july, at which time it has attained its greatest size, and is firm, amylaceous and exceedingly bitter. The bitterness is the best criterion of its medicinal activity.

A number of years ago, dr. A. T. Thomson, proposed the tincture of guaiacum as a test for the goodness of colchicum. Ten grains of the bulb were rubbed in a mortar, with sixteen minims of distilled vinegar, and immediately afterwards sixteen minims of the tincture of guaiacum were added. When the bulb was good, a beautiful cerulean color, according to dr. Thomson, was produced. Having ascertained that several specimens which he knew to be good failed in giving this characteristic color, dr. M. Proceeded to investigate the causes on which it depended. He expressed several bulbs and filtered the juice to separate the starch; a beautiful blue color was now immediately produced by the test. The blue liquid was then heated till the albumen was coagulated; the color remained with the coagulum, while the liquid was colorless. On raising the heat to 212° the blue color disappeared. The test produced no change in the starch collected on the filter. When the fluid was boiled previously to the application of the test, no blue color was produced by it either with the filtered fluid or the coagulum. From these experiments dr. M. Concludes, "1st. That albumen is the principle acted on. 2nd. That a heat above 180° destroys this action. 3rd. That the value of the test is to prove that the bulbs have been dried at a temperature not higher than 180°."

Dr. Maclagan was unable to procure colchicia, the alkaloid announced by geiger & hesse, in the crystalline form, though he followed the process they give very exactly, and consequently he doubts its crystalline nature. What he obtained was in the form of a brown resinous looking mass without smell, and of a bitter taste, the bitterness being followed by a slight sense of irritation in the throat but by nothing like the intense acrimony of veratria.

In regard to the physiological action of colchicum, dr. M. Confirms the statement of previous observers, that it markedly increases the amount of urea in the urine; and contrary to what has been maintained by some, found it likewise to increase the quantity of uric add. In an experiment related in detail, after the colchicum had been employed for six days, the amount of urea in the urine was found to be increased by nearly one half, and the uric acid was more than doubled.

Errata in the february number.

Page <u>33,</u> 13th line from the bottom—for "slack" read "slacked."

Page <u>36,</u> 17th line from the bottom—for "grns." Read "grms."

Page <u>36,</u> 11th line from the bottom—for "grns." Read "grms."

Page <u>36,</u> 11th line from the bottom—for "0.845 grn." Read "0.845 grm."

Page <u>37,</u> 2nd line from the top—for "monohydrate" read "molybdate."

NEW YORK JOURNAL OF PHARMACY. APRIL, 1852.

REMARKS UPON SOME OF THE PREPARATIONS OF THE PHARMACOPŒIA OF THE UNITED STATES, 1851.

BY GEORGE D. COGGESHALL.

In giving formulæ it is to be supposed that the purpose of a pharmacopœia is to be practical, responding to the every day wants of the associated professions of medicine and pharmacy. It would seem to be in no case of practical utility to retain a formula that is not used, and of this character i think is the one for "mucilage of gum arabic." It does not appear to be employed of the consistence directed except as a paste. Nor is this consistence understood when mucilage of gum arabic is prescribed by physicians, but by some apothecaries a solution of only one eighth, and by others, one fourth the strength is put up. If physicians are expected to prescribe, and apothecaries to compound according to the letter of the pharmacopœia, this is certainly a daily and unfortunately, owing to the want of a standard, a variable exception. The formula in our pharmacopœia is substantially the same as in those of london and edinburgh, while that of dublin is one half stronger. In the latter three it enters into other officinal preparations, but in every case it is combined with water, which appears to be a needless multiplication of the process, as the proper proportions of gum and water for the whole might as well be directed at once. Nor, is it probably used in EXTEMPORANEOUS PRESCRIPTION WITHOUT SIMILAR ADDITION OF WATER, UNLESS IT MAY BE TO FORM PILLS, FOR WHICH IT IS RARELY, IF EVER, WELL ADAPTED, OR EMPLOYED BY THE APOTHECARY WHEN IT IS PRESCRIBED, AS IT MAKES, WITH MOST SUBSTANCES, AN INTRACTABLE MASS. I HAVE BEEN TOLD BY A

HIGHLY INTELLIGENT AND WELL EDUCATED ENGLISH APOTHECARY, THAT "IT WAS FORMERLY THE PRACTICE OF ENGLISH PHYSICIANS TO PRESCRIBE ONE OUNCE OF MUCILAGE OF GUM ARABIC WITH SEVEN OUNCES OF WATER, (OR IN THAT PROPORTION,) MAKING A SOLUTION OF THE STRENGTH NOW COMMONLY USED HERE, AND THAT IT HAD BECOME GRADUALLY THE PRACTICE TO DIRECT THE WHOLE QUANTITY REQUIRED, UNDER THE TERM OF 'MUCILAGE OF GUM ARABIC,' WITH THE GENERAL UNDERSTANDING THAT THE DILUTED STRENGTH WAS INTENDED." AS THIS SEEMS TO BE NOW THE UNIVERSAL PRACTICE IN PRESCRIBING AND PUTTING UP MIXTURES, THE OFFICINAL DIRECTIONS ARE PRACTICALLY USELESS, AND LEAD TO THE ADOPTION OF VARIOUS PROPORTIONS BY DIFFERENT APOTHECARIES, TO PRODUCE THE MUCILAGE TO COMPLETE MIXTURES.

Another circumstance may be noticed. The pharmacopœia directs the use of powdered gum and of boiling water, whereas gum, in its ordinary condition or coarsely broken, and cold water make a clearer solution. Cold water is directed for the solution of the gum by the edinburgh process, and in our present formula for "syrup of gum arabic;"—if appropriate for the latter, it is quite as much so for the forming of mucilage. When the gum has been ground in a mill it appears to have been a little charred and forms a somewhat turbid solution; if powdered by hand, and rather more coarsely, its solution is clearer.

Upon the whole it seems desirable that there should be a uniform strength for the mucilage of gum arabic, prescribed by physicians in mixtures, which the officinal preparation evidently is not. Our mucilage does not enter into any other officinal preparations, and if it did, the combination of gum and water had better be made in the general process, as in our almond mixture.

"compound spirit of lavender" appears to be but seldom MADE ACCORDING TO THE OFFICINAL DIRECTIONS, OWING TO THE DIFFICULTY OF

PROCURING THE SIMPLE SPIRIT OF LAVENDER. ON THIS ACCOUNT MOST APOTHECARIES USE A PROPORTION OF THE OIL OF LAVENDER AND OF SPIRIT, VARIABLE NO DOUBT IN DIFFERENT PRIVATE RECIPES. THE OIL MAKES A DECIDEDLY INFERIOR PREPARATION, SEPARATING UPON ADMIXTURE WITH WATER, AND EVEN THE BEST ENGLISH OIL—WHICH IS PROBABLY NEVER USED—IS LESS CONGENIAL TO THE STOMACH THAN THE DISTILLED SPIRIT. BUT THE DIFFICULTY MAY BE OVERCOME, AND AN EXCELLENT PREPARATION, ESSENTIALLY THE SAME AND PERHAPS QUITE EQUAL IN QUALITY AND FLAVOR TO THAT OF THE PHARMACOPŒIA, MAY BE MADE BY THE EMPLOYMENT OF RECENTLY DRIED FLOWERS. THE FOLLOWING IS THE FORMULA I HAVE USED FOR SEVERAL YEARS, WITH AN ENTIRELY SATISFACTORY RESULT:—

Take of lavender flowers twelve ounces,

rosemary leaves,

cinnamon, bruised, each four ounces and a half,

nutmegs, bruised,

cloves, bruised, each six drachms,

coriander seed, bruised,

red sanders each three ounces,

powdered turmeric one drachm,

alcohol six pints,

water five pints and a quarter.

Mix, digest for fourteen days, express and filter.

The "syrup of gum arabic," unaccountably withdrawn from the pharmacopœia in 1840, when it had become a familiar favorite, comes to us again in the new revision, not at all improved by seclusion. It is changed in its proportions, but not for the better, as it now has too little gum and too much sugar in its composition. Of numerous formulæ by which i have made this syrup, i have always found that from our pharmacopœia of 1830, the best in proportions, consistence and flavor. It is defective however, in one point of construction, and incorrect in the use of boiling water to make the solution of gum. The syrup is probably not better in any essential particular, but it is clearer, and therefore more pleasing in APPEARANCE, WHEN IT IS CONSTRUCTED BY MAKING THE SOLUTIONS OF GUM AND SUGAR SEPARATELY, THAT OF THE GUM IN HALF THE WATER COLD, AND THAT OF THE SUGAR IN THE REMAINDER OF THE WATER BOILING, THEN IMMEDIATELY COMBINING THE TWO AND BRINGING TO THE BOILING POINT. IT MAY THEN BE EASILY FILTERED THROUGH FLANNEL.

In preparing "syrup of citric acid," it would be preferable to use, in place of the oil of lemon, a tincture made from the outside yellow part of the rind of the fresh fruit, made by covering it with pure alcohol. Two drachms of this tincture are about equivalent to four minims of the oil of lemon.

The formula for "syrup of ipecacuanha" is one of the most objectionable we have to notice, and the least calculated to answer medical wants in regard to its importance. There is a verbal error, either in the list of components or in the directions, which leads to some confusion. Amongst the former we find *"diluted alcohol,"* and in the latter, we are told to "macerate the ipecacuanha in the *alcohol, &c.*" The same error occurs in the edition of 1840. This formula is unnecessarily complex, and yields an inefficient preparation of about half the strength of the wine of ipecac, which it was intended to equal at its origin, about twelve years before its introduction into our pharmacopœia. Previously to this it had, for six or eight years, been made here of about double the strength of the wine, in accordance with the general plan of forming medicinal syrups, by combining as large a proportion of the remedial agent in them as can readily be done, to obviate at once the necessity of bulky doses, and the exhibition of undue quantities of sugar. I cannot discover the advantage of making a pint of tincture with an ounce of the root, evaporating the filtered tincture to six fluid ounces, filtering again, and then adding water to bring back the measure of a pint. If the object be to get rid of the alcohol, it is an unnecessary exposure of the soluble principles of the ipecac to heat, for half a pint of diluted alcohol, especially with four ounces of water added by way of displacement, would exhaust the root equally well; so that the evaporation need not BE CARRIED SO FAR. THERE IS NO MENTION OF A WATER BATH, WHICH SHOULD BE USED BY ALL MEANS.

We should prefer, if we could, to make all preparations which the pharmacopœia contains, in accordance with it. But when a preparation has been in such general and favorite use, for several years, as to be considered indispensable before it becomes official; and in such form is reduced to a third or a fourth of what is felt to be an eligible strength, not only without any compensating advantage, but with the positive disadvantages of greatly diluting its remedial influence, and increasing the quantity required to be taken of a nauseous medicine, there is naturally an unwillingness to yield well settled convictions of utility, and replace an important remedy, that has proved quite satisfactory, with a preparation believed to be of comparatively little value. It is not probable that, in new york, the present officinal syrup of ipecacuanha, can ever supersede the efficient and reliable one we have so long been accustomed to, nor answer the wishes and expectations of the medical profession. I append the formula proposed in a paper read before the board of trustees in 1835, seven years before one for this syrup appeared in our pharmacopœia. I have not found cause to change it in any respect. It affords about three pints of syrup, which keeps well for years at the ordinary temperatures of the shop, and of dwellings; the proportion of sugar proves to be just what is wanted for a proper consistence without crystallization, and, as a medicine, it gives entire satisfaction to the prescriber. It is as follows:—

Take of ipecacuanha, bruised, six ounces,

alcohol one pint and a half,

water one pint,

Mix, to form a tincture. Digest for ten days, filter, and add one pint of water, by way of displacement, evaporate in a water bath to two pints, add immediately:

Refined sugar three pounds and a quarter.

And bring to the boiling point.

The "compound syrup of squill" is presented in the PHARMACOPŒIA WITH TWO PROCESSES FOR ITS PREPARATION. THE FIRST IS LIABLE, THOUGH IN A LESS DEGREE, TO THE SAME OBJECTION WHICH HAS RENDERED THE ORIGINAL FORM, GIVEN BY DR. COXE, OBSOLETE, THAT IT PRODUCES A TURBID SYRUP, AND ONE THAT WILL NOT KEEP. THE SECOND PROCESS IS BETTER, BUT SCARCELY ADEQUATE, I SHOULD THINK, TO EXTRACT THE FULL STRENGTH OF THE ROOTS SO WELL AS BY THE EMPLOYMENT OF A GREATER PROPORTION OF ALCOHOL, AND LONGER DIGESTION. THE FOLLOWING PRODUCES THREE AND A HALF PINTS OF SYRUP FROM THE SAME MATERIALS, APPARENTLY STRONGER THAN IF THE BOILING, WHICH IS ONLY FOR A FEW MINUTES, WERE CONTINUED DOWN TO THREE PINTS, RETAINING A PORTION OF HONEY, FOR THE SAKE OF THE FLAVOR, AND WITH AS LARGE AN ADDITION OF SUGAR AS THE SYRUP WILL BEAR WITHOUT CRYSTALLIZATION. THE PROPORTION OF TARTAR EMETIC IS, OF COURSE, THE SAME:

Take of seneka, bruised,

squills, bruised, each four ounces.

alcohol,

water each two pints.

Mix, to form a tincture. Digest ten days, filter, and add twelve ounces of water, by way of displacement, evaporate by water bath to two pints, add:

Sugar fifteen ounces,

Honey eighteen ounces,

Boil to three pints and a half, in which dissolve while hot:

Tartar emetic fifty-six grains.

"syrup of tolu," made after the london formula, is a more elegant and better flavored preparation than can be made by any combination of the tincture. So decided is the superiority of the london process, that it is rather surprising the other pharmacopœias should not adopt it. An apothecary who does, will hardly be satisfied with the tincture-made syrup afterwards.

The "tincture of aconite root" is desired by our physicians of full saturation. The "strong tincture," to which we have been accustomed for several years, is that of fleming's process, viz: sixteen ounces of the root to a pint and a half of alcohol.

The "compound tincture of cardamom" is now first introduced into our pharmacopœia, with a change from the pleasant tincture we have been in the habit of making after the london or edinburgh formula, by increasing the proportion of cardamom, from two drachms and a half to six drachms, and reducing the caraway one fifth, which makes a tincture not near so pleasant to the taste, owing to the strong predominance of the cardamom flavor, which is rather harsh when in too great excess. As this tincture is of little medical importance by itself, and chiefly used as an agreeable adjunct to mixtures, the proportions which have been found to answer so well may still be considered preferable.

There are other cases, no doubt, in which apothecaries will find it expedient to vary the processes of carrying out formulæ, not with a view of altering the strength of preparations, but arriving at substantially the same results or better ones, from the same materials, by improved application of skill. Whoever can, by superior method, more fully develope the qualities of a substance to be acted upon, than has hitherto been done, or change the character of a preparation from perishable to permanent, from uncertain to definite, from slovenly to elegant, can accomplish something for the benefit of his art, and render it so much the more useful to the community. Most of the improvements in pharmacy have been effected by the practical apothecary, and rendered available by him, in advance of the pharmacopœia.

NOTES IN PHARMACY.

BY BENJAMIN CANAVAN.

The fact in the natural kingdom, that "nothing is destroyed," suggests an equally true axiom, as applied to the moral world, that "nothing is useless;" and, with this impression, i am induced to send the following trifles to the new york journal of pharmacy, which, if not unacceptable, it will give me pleasure to repeat "*pro re natâ.*"

Pil. Ferri comp.—this very much neglected pill, which is the prototype and should have precluded the necessity of vallet's preparation, i would beg leave to introduce, for the purpose of recommending, or rather verifying an improvement which i have sometimes adopted, in the mode of compounding it, differing from the officinal directions for so doing. We are told to "rub the myrrh with the carb. Sodæ; then add the sulph. Ferri, and again rub them; lastly, beat them with the syrup so as to form a mass." I do not hesitate to say that no amount of trituration or skill, with which i am acquainted, will enable the manipulator by this means to make the mass properly, either in a chemical or pharmaceutical point of view.—in a note the editor of the united states dispensatory informs us: "it is said the salt of iron will be better preserved, if the operator should dissolve the sulphate of iron in the syrup with a moderate heat and then add the carb. Sodæ, *stirring!* Till effervescence ceases;" this is correct in principle; but the same object is attained, and the *only* way by which the pill ought or can be properly prepared, is by triturating separately, and to solution the two salts in the necessary quantity of syrup, mixing, and again triturating until perfect decomposition is induced, and by incorporating the myrrh, form into a mass without delay. In this way you insure the existence of the intended proto carb. Ferri in the pill, which is not, or only partially the case when prepared by any other process. I would remark, en passant, that this pill presents us with the very perishable proto carb. In the most permanent form, retaining, when properly prepared, its chemical integrity unimpaired, indefinitely, and is therefore superior in this important respect to the quickly changeable mist. Ferri comp., the presence also of a larger proportion of myrrh being often a decided advantage.

Extracta liquida opii.—it has been suggested, and i believe attempted, to introduce certain preparations with the above titles, as substitutes for the demi-nostrum, known as "mcmunn's elixir of opium," which has been very extensively used, and enjoyed high favor, but of which the exact nature and mode of preparation are not generally understood, and which, either from having become too antiquated for this novelty hunting age, or its success having tempted the cupidity of avaricious persons, or from whatever cause, has been for some time diminishing in popularity, and subjected to many complaints. In all preparations of this potent drug, with which i am acquainted, ancient or modern, the great object has been, to get rid of the narcotine, which has been more or less accomplished by various processes. At present an aqueous fluid extract is said to supply the desideratum. This is merely a modification of the watery extract of all the pharmacopœias, and is no doubt as good, but no better preparation. The denarcotised tincture is superior to all of them, and the *very small* quantity of spirit contained in an ordinary dose, is scarcely an objection, and is only little more than is necessary to preserve the extract; but if deemed otherwise, a fluid extract may be prepared from denarcotised opium, *entirely free* from the peccant alkaloid, and possibly the evaporation necessary to the process, may dissipate some noxious volatile property, which would exist in a tincture, and which it is most probable the opium possesses, from the fact, among others, that *old opium* is much less prone than *new* to cause disagreeable after effects. It has been supposed that meconic acid has been the evicted principle; but this is doubtful. However, the action of heat is useful, and i think a "fluid extract of denarcotised opium," would perhaps be found to be as free as possible from objectionable effects.

Ether hydrochloric; chlorinat: or ether hydrochlorique chlorè, as the french have it, is another change, rung by m. Mialhe of paris, with the transcendental compounds of carbon and chlorine. It is a mongrel preparation, intermediate between hydrochloric: ether and chloroform, professing to have the advantage of not irritating the skin like the latter. If this be so, experience will tell, and also whether the irritation is not proportionable to the effect. With regard to such a refinement of an already infinitesimally delicate class of preparations, i should suppose it would be desirable to effect the object aimed at by them, by if possible some more palpable method, as for instance diluting chloroform either with hydrochloric ether or alcohol, to the necessary mildness, or by interposing between it and the skin, a thin *moist* layer of some substance, as bibulous paper, which would not interfere with the rigefacient effect of evaporation, and would prevent any injury arising from actual contact.

INDELIBLE INK.

BY M. GUILLER, OF PARIS.

Hitherto the various inks prepared for marking linen, have but imperfectly answered the end proposed. Some produced yellowish marks; others though blacker at first, disappeared either partially or entirely after several washings.

Again, others, in separate bottles, necessitated two distinct operations, and were thus attended with inconvenience, from the possibility of mistakes or forgetfulness, from the care required, and also from the time taken up in the operation.

In view of these difficulties, and to meet a demand constantly occurring in commerce, and in all kinds of manufactures, as well as in hospitals, and civil and military administrations, we have applied ourselves to the composition of an ink free from all these objections, and perfectly easy and certain in its application.

We shall subjoin some formulæ for the manufacture of marking inks, which represent particular improvements, as can be verified by trying them.

Formula, no. 1,

Nitrate of silver,	11 grammes,
Distilled water,	85 grammes,
Powdered gum arabic,	20 grammes,
Sub-carbonate of soda,	22 grammes,
Solution of ammoniæ,	20 grammes.

Dissolve the 22 parts of sub-carbonate of soda in the 85 parts of water; put into a marble mortar the gum, and pour on it very gradually the solution of the sub-carbonate, stirring it with the pestle to cause it to dissolve.

In the mean time, you will have dissolved the 11 parts of nitrate in the 20 parts of liquid ammonia. Mix the two solutions; put the whole in a matrass and expose it to heat. The mass which was of a dirty grey color, and half coagulated, becomes clear and brown, and when arrived at the boiling point, it becomes very dark, and sufficiently limpid to flow readily in the pen. This ink, made without heat like the two following forms no sediment, the ebullition thickening it, and besides giving the ink a very dark color, disengages the ammoniacal vapors, which attenuate the odor of the ammonia in it.

Formula no. 2,

Nitrate of silver,	5 grammes,
Water,	12 grammes,
Gum,	5 grammes,
Sub-carbonate of soda,	7 grammes,
Solution of ammoniæ,	10 grammes.

Mix as in no. 1; put the whole into a matrass and evaporate until the liquor has acquired a very dark brown tint, which will take place when it has lost about 5 per cent. Of its bulk; a more complete evaporation would form a precipitate, as the vapors would draw off too much of the ammonia.

This ink will be found excellent for marking, the character will be very black, and it will be found especially useful for applying with the stamp.

Formula no. 3,

Nitrate of silver,	17 grammes,
Water,	85 grammes,
Gum,	20 grammes,
Sub-carbonate of soda,	22 grammes,

| Solution of ammoniæ, | 42 grammes, |
| Sulphate of copper, | 33 grammes. |

First dissolve the 22 parts of sub-carbonate in the 25 parts of water, and the 15 of nitrate in the 42 of ammonia.

This done, put into the marble mortar the 20 parts of gum with the sixty parts of water which remain, stir it with the pestle, and pour on it the solution of sub-carbonate, after which, pour the whole into the solution of the nitrate; finish by adding the 33 parts of the solution of sulphate of copper.

The greater quantity of ammonia is explained by the presence of the sulphate to be dissolved.

This composition differs from the others in having a blue tinge, due to the solution of copper.

It will be readily seen that these relative qualities, given as formulæ for the production of suitable inks, may vary according as it is desirable to produce a thicker or thiner ink, or according to the material on which it is to be used, observing that if, on the one hand, the ammonia acts as a solvent, and facilitates the composition of an ink which can be used without a previous preparation; on the other hand, the evaporation of a part of the ammonia by heat, gives to the liquid a dark color which renders the writing immediately black; again, the boiled liquid greases less, and thus penetrates and spreads better on the linen without making a blot.

As to the mode of using, whether with a pen or a stamp proceed as usual, namely: pass a hot iron over the writing, to cause it more completely to penetrate the material.

ON VALERIANIC ACID AND ITS SALTS.

BY MR. J. B. BARNES.

Considerable attention having of late been directed to this class of compounds, perhaps a few practical observations relating to their manufacture, &c. Might be of interest to the readers of *the annals of pharmacy.*

Although some of the combinations of valerianic acid with bases, and the properties of those salts, have been described in the books on chemistry, yet i believe i may lay claim to the priority of the preparation of an extensive series of the combination of valerianic acid with bases.

Valerianic acid, it is well known, occurs preformed in certain plants; and it is equally well known, that it can be produced in the laboratory by artificial means. This very fact is of great interest to the investigating chemist, as it encourages him in the belief that he will, sooner or later, be able to produce artificially, not only acids, which are known to exist in the animal and vegetable kingdoms; but that he will so far imitate nature in her wonderful processes, as to produce the vegetable alkaloids, morphia, quina, &c., by the combination of their elements.

The acid employed in the preparation of this series, *for which i have had the honor of being awarded a prize medal by the jurors of the great exhibition*, was prepared, in principle, the same as that directed to be used by the dublin pharmacopœia in the preparation of valerianate of soda, namely, the oxidation of fusel oil by means of chromic acid. The formula i employed is as follows:—

Take of

Bichromate of potash,	2 parts.
Oil of vitriol,	3 parts.
Water,	4 parts.

Pure fusel oil,   1 parts.

The bichromate of potash is to be finely powdered and dissolved in the water; the solution being put into a glass retort, the oil of vitriol is gradually added, and, when quite cold, the *fusel oil* is carefully added; the contents of the vessel must be constantly agitated, and at the same time kept immersed in cold water. The deep green liquid is now distilled from a sand bath; the distillate is mixed with caustic soda, or potash, and separated from the oily fluid floating on the surface; the *valerianate of soda* is evaporated to a convenient degree of concentration, introduced into a retort, decomposed with dilute sulphuric acid, and distilled; the liberated valerianic acid is finally dried over chloride of calcium.

It is also obtained by the oxidation of oil of valerian, by means of an alkali. It is formed from fats, by treating them with fuming nitric acid; from animal nitrogenous matters, both by putrefaction and on decomposing them with strong nitric acid; and also if leucine be treated with caustic potash, or allowed to putrefy, it becomes converted into valerianic acid (no other acid being formed), ammonia and hydrogen being evolved.

It is most easily obtained in a state of absolute purity by the action of spongy platinum and atmospheric air upon potatoe fusel oil.

Valerianic acid is composed of c_{10} h_9 o_3, h o. It possesses a well known characteristic odour, an acrid burning taste, and produces a white spot on the tongue. It boils at 348° fahr., and dissolves in 26 parts water; it also forms a second hydrate.[8]

---

8 lehmann's physiological chemistry.

Combinations with the alkalies.

The potash salt was prepared by saturating the acid with liquor potassæ, and evaporating carefully until aqueous vapour ceased to be given off; it should be, while still warm, cut up and preserved in well stoppered bottles. It does not crystallize, but forms a semi-transparent colorless mass, very much resembling phosphorus in appearance. It (probably from its compactness) produces when sharply struck with any hard body a metallic sound, somewhat like that occasioned when a bell of camphor is struck in a similar manner. It is deliquescent, and very soluble.

The soda salt was prepared in the same manner as the potash salt, cut up into pieces while warm, and preserved in stoppered bottles: it is in snow-white masses composed of minute crystals; it is deliquescent, and very soluble. The ammonia salt was prepared by saturating the acid with strong liquor ammoniæ, and evaporating at a temperature not exceeding 100° fahr., until crystals appeared on the surface of the liquid. When it was set aside for further crystallization, the mother liquor was allowed to drain off, the crystals were placed upon bibulous paper, and finally dried *in vacuo*, over oil of vitriol. They are of a tabular form; when held between the fingers for a moment, they become liquid. They are deliquescent and dissolve readily in water.

Combinations with the alkaline earths.

The baryta salt was prepared by adding the acid to carbonate of baryta in excess, which had been previously mixed with water; a gentle heat was applied, and, when the disengagement of carbonic acid had ceased, the excess of carbonate was filtered off; the filtrate was evaporated very carefully, until aqueous vapour ceased to be given off, it remained a transparent gummy mass, readily soluble in water.

The strontia, lime, and magnesia salts were prepared in the same manner as the baryta salt. The two former are crystalline, and do not deliquesce by exposure to the atmosphere; they are soluble. The lime salt crystallizes in nacreous plates; it effloresces when exposed to the atmosphere; it is beautifully white.

The magnesia salt would not crystallize, therefore it was evaporated to dryness, at a temperature not exceeding 120° fahr. It forms a light white soluble powder, sweet to the taste, and strong in the characteristic odour of valerianic acid.

Combinations with metallic oxides.

The alumina, chromium, and nickel salts were prepared by the direct combination of the hydrates of those bases with the acid.

The alumina and chromium salts are in powder, and are soluble.

The nickel salt is in crystalline masses, of an apple-green color, soluble in water.

The cobalt salt was also prepared by the direct way; the flocculent blue precipitate, obtained by precipitation from nitrate of cobalt, by means of caustic potash, after being well washed, was dissolved in valerianic acid, filtered and very carefully evaporated to dryness; it occurs in masses of a rose color, and is soluble.

The manganese salt was also prepared in the direct way by mixing an excess of the hydrated oxide with water and the acid, allowing them to remain in contact for some time, filtering and evaporating at a temperature not exceeding 120° fahr., until crystals appeared on the surface of the fluids; it was set aside, and after a while, the crystals were separated from the mother liquor. The latter being again evaporated, another crop of crystals was obtained; it occurs in glistening scales of a flesh color, and dissolves very readily in water.

The valerianate of *protoxide of iron* was prepared by the double decomposition of valerianate of baryta and proto-sulphate of iron; it can only be kept in a state of solution, as least the heat and exposure to the air converts it immediately into the peroxide salt.

The valerianate of *peroxide of iron*, was prepared by bringing together neutral cold solutions of perchloride of iron and valerianate of soda, the precipitated valerianate was thrown upon a filter, well washed, to separate the chloride of sodium, and dried without heat on a porous tile; it occurs as a bright red loose powder, perfectly soluble in alcohol.

The valerianate of zinc was prepared according to the directions in the dublin pharmacopœia; it occurs in small smooth crystals, somewhat like boracic acid; it is soluble in water and alcohol.

The lead salt was prepared by decomposing freshly precipitated carbonate of lead with the acid, filtering and evaporating at a low temperature. In due time, crystals made their appearance in the fluid; but (probably from the temperature being too high) they subsequently disappeared; and, upon further evaporation, it remained in the form of a syrup.

The silver salt was produced by the double decomposition of nitrate of silver, and valerianate of soda. The valerianate of silver being very insoluble, was precipitated as a white powder; after washing with cold water, it was dried in the dark on a porous tile. By exposure to the light, it becomes black.

The salt of the suboxide of mercury was also prepared by double decomposition. It is a loose, yellowish white powder.

The salt of oxide of mercury was prepared by agitating together, the yellow hydrate of the oxide with water and valerianic acid. After some time, i obtained a colorless liquid, which, upon evaporation at a temperature not exceeding 100° fahr., yielded crystals which, however, speedily fell into a red powder. I therefore again repeated the operation, omitting the application of heat; the solution was set aside, when in the course of two or three weeks, i obtained this salt in prismatic white crystals.

The bismuth salt was obtained by the addition of valerianate of soda, to a solution of bismuth in nitric acid, which was nearly saturated with carbonate of soda. It occurs as a loose white powder.

The copper salt was obtained by double decomposition, and occurs as a beautiful green powder.

The cadmium salt was prepared in the same manner as the zinc salt. It occurs in crystalline scales, resembling in form that of zinc, but larger.

Combinations with organic bases.

The valerianate of oxide of ethyle (valerianic ether) was obtained by distilling, together, alcohol, oil of vitriol, and valerianic acid; it was well washed, dried over chloride of calcium, and re-distilled. It is an oily liquid, with a penetrating smell of fruit, and of valerian; of specific gravity, 0,894. (otto). It is miscible with alcohol and ether: it has an agreeable, cool, and aromatic taste.

I prepared the valerianate of quina, both by double decomposition, and by direct combination of the base with the acid.

That by double decomposition, was prepared by adding to a warm solution of neutral sulphate of quinine, a warm solution of valerianate of baryta; the mixture was allowed to stand for a while, and filtered to separate the insoluble sulphate of baryta; the filtrate was evaporated at a temperature of about 100°, until crystals made their appearance, when it was set aside for further crystalliza-tion. The crystals obtained by this process are in silky tufts and perfectly white.

The valerianate of quina, made by the direct combination of the acid with the base, was effected by triturating, in a mortar, freshly precipitated quina, with water and valerianic acid, until the quina had disappeared. It was then exposed in shallow dishes, to a current of air; when sufficiently evaporated, octohedral crystals were formed. Valerianate of quina in both forms dissolves readily in water.

When a solution of valerianate of quina is evaporated at a temperature of 130°, it does not crystallize, but has the appearance of an oil.

From the different appearances of this salt, it is highly probable that they each differ in composition. This phenomena is worthy of a thorough investigation.

The morphia salt was prepared in the direct way. It crystallizes in silky tufts; it dissolves readily in water.

Although but three of the salts of valerianic acid are employed in medicine, namely, those of *peroxide of iron*, oxide of zinc, and *quinine*, there appears to me no reason why those of *potash*, *soda*, *ammonia*, *teroxide of bismuth*, and *oxide of ethyle*, (*valerianic ether*), should not be employed by the physician.

In conclusion, i must express my sincere thanks to mr. Savory, for his kindness in having placed at my disposal the materials necessary for the preparation of this series.

ESSENCE OF PINE APPLE.

The above essence is, as already known, butyric ether, more or less diluted with alcohol; to obtain which pure, on the large scale and economically, the following process is recommended:—

Dissolve 6 ℔ s. Of sugar and half an ounce of tartaric acid, in 26 ℔ s. Of boiling water. Let the solution stand for several days; then add 8 ounces of putrid cheese broken up with 3 ℔ s. Of skimmed and curdled sour milk, and 3 ℔ s. Of levigated chalk. The mixture should be kept and stirred daily in a warm place, at the temperature of about 92° fahr., as long as gas is evolved, which is generally the case for five or six weeks.

The liquid thus obtained, is mixed with an equal volume of cold water, and 8 ℔ s. Of crystallized carbonate of soda, previously dissolved in water, added. It is then filtered from the precipitated carbonate of lime; the filtrate is to be evaporated down to 10 ℔ s., when 5½ lbs. Of sulphuric acid, previously diluted with an equal weight of water, are to be carefully added. The butyric acid, which separates on the surface of the liquid as a dark-colored oil, is to be removed, and the rest of the liquid distilled; the distillate is now neutralized with carbonate of soda, and the butyric acid separated as before, with sulphuric acid.

The whole of the crude acid is to be rectified with the addition of an ounce of sulphuric acid to every pound. The distillate is then saturated with fused chloride of calcium, and re-distilled. The product will be about 28 ounces of pure butyric acid. To prepare the butyric acid, or essence of pine apple, from this acid, proceed as follows:—mix, by weight, three parts of butyric acid with six parts of alcohol, and two parts of sulphuric acid in a retort, and submit the whole, with a sufficient heat, to a gentle distillation, until the fluid which passes over ceases to emit a fruity odor. By treating the distillate with chloride of calcium, and by its re-distillation, the pure ether may be obtained.

The boiling point of butyric ether is 238° fahr. Its specific gravity, 0,904, and its formula $c_{12} h_{12} o_4$, or $c_4 h_5 o + c_8 h_7 o_3$.

Bensch's process, above described, for the production of butyric acid, affords a remarkable exemplification of the extraordinary transformations that organic bodies undergo in contact with ferment, or by catalytic action. When cane sugar is treated with tartaric acid, especially under the influence of heat, it is converted into grape sugar. This grape sugar, in the presence of decomposing nitrogenous substances, such as cheese, is transformed in the first instance into lactic acid, which combines with the lime of the chalk. The acid of the lactate of lime, thus produced, is by the further influence of the ferment changed into butyric acid. Hence, butyrate of lime is the final result of the catalytic action in the process we here have recommended.

ON A REMARKABLE SPECIMEN OF DECOMPOSED CHLOROFORM.

BY JONATHAN PEREIRA, M.D., F.R.S., PHYSICIAN TO THE LONDON HOSPITAL.

In july of the present year i received from mr. Grattan, apothecary of belfast, a specimen of chloroform, accompanied with a note, from which the following is an extract:—

"some weeks prior to october 25, 1851, i received from my friend dr. M'killen a small bottle of chloroform which he had had of me two or three months previously, and which he stated was subject to very singular changes of color, despite the stopper never having been removed.

At the time he handed it to me the fluid exhibited a delicate pink tint, as though colored with cochineal, and was put aside in a glass case in my shop, of which i kept the key myself. The case was exposed to the diffused light of a large shop window but not to the direct rays of the sun.

Conceiving that the chloroform had by some unobserved means or other become accidentally colored, i took very little interest in the matter, and was not surprised to find it fade gradually, and in a short time become perfectly colorless—and i made a note to that effect upon the 25th of october, concluding that there must have been some error of observation on the part of dr. M'killen.

On the 16th of november, however, it again began to change, and the enclosed notes were made, from time to time, as i happened to have opportunity of noticing it.

I tried it under different conditions of light and temperature, without their exerting apparent influence upon it, and being unable to form the slightest conjecture as to the cause or nature of the molecular disturbance which produces these chromatic changes, have taken the liberty of forwarding it to you, should you consider it worthy of attention.

It is at present colorless, and the stopper fast in; and i would only suggest that, before removing the stopper, it might be well to observe for yourself whether changes similar to those i have noticed may not occur again.

1850.

Oct.

25. Perfectly colorless.

Nov.

16. Faint pink.

18. Fading.

25. Faint pink, as on the 16th.

26. Dirty-looking, neutral tint, without any pink.

Dec.

17. Pink again.

21. Ditto, and deeper.

27. Perfectly colorless, after having passed through various shades of pink.

1851.

Jan.

10. Again pink.

11. Faint neutral tint.

Feb.

19. Perfectly colorless. On shaking the vial, observed a deposit on its sides, like small crystals, but cannot say that they were not there before.

21. Pink and deeper than ever.

March

10. Deep pink.

12. Faint pink.

13. Colorless.

20. Colorless.

May

16. Colorless. No change having occurred between the 13th march and 16th may, concluded too hastily that the property of changing its color, upon whatever cause dependent, had been lost, for on

17. It again became faintly pinked.

19. Deeper pink.

22. Fading.

24. Fading.

31. Colorless.

June

13. Again pink.

16. Ditto.

17. Colorless.

July

2. Ditto, up to present date, when it again became pink.

3. Deeper.

5. Still very deep.

7. Fading

13. Perfectly colorless.

The foregoing changes of color were not influenced by any change of temperature between 27° and 86° fahr., nor by exposure to, nor seclusion from light. The stopper being fast, atmospheric pressure cannot have been connected therewith. Whether it may have been influenced by electrical changes, am not prepared to say."

The specimen of chloroform sent me by mr. Grattan was, in july, quite colorless, and on the sides of the bottle a few minute crystals were observed. The stopper of the bottle was, however, so firmly fixed in that i could not remove it, and i, therefore, placed the bottle on the mantel-shelf in my library exposed to diffused light, for the purpose of observing the changes which its contents would undergo.

In the course of a few weeks it began to acquire a pinkish or amethystine tint, as described by mr. Grattan. This slightly augmented in intensity for a few days, and then became somewhat paler. But for several weeks, during which it remained in the same situation, it never became colorless, though the intensity of the color was frequently changing.

The color of the liquid was precisely that of a weak solution of permanganate of potash.

Some weeks ago i placed the bottle in a dark cupboard, and at the expiration of about three weeks found that the liquid had become quite colorless. As the stopper was still immovable, i was obliged to cut off the neck of the bottle to get at the contents. I found that the chloroform had undergone decomposition, and had acquired a powerful and irritating odor, somewhat allied to, but distinct from, that of hypochlorous acid. The vapor yielded white fumes when a rod moistened with solution of ammonia was brought in contact with it, blue litmus paper was reddened but not bleached by it. A few drops of the liquid were placed on a watch glass and volatilized by a spirit lamp; they left scarcely any appreciable residue.

The crystals which lined the bottle were then examined. They were few in number, and not larger than pins' points. They were white, and when examined by the microscope, were found to be six-sided pyramids, like the crystals of sulphate of potash. Some of them were heated to dull redness in a test tube, without undergoing any appreciable change. When heated on the point of a moistened thread in the outer cone of the flame of a candle, they communicated a violet-white tinge to the flame, character-istic of a potash-salt. They readily dissolved in water, and the solution did not yield any precipitate on the addition of a solution of nitrate of baryta, showing that the salt was not a sulphate. The solution was boiled with nitric acid, and then treated with a solution of nitrate of baryta, but no precipitate was observed. Nitrate of silver produced in the aqueous solution of the crystals a white precipitate, soluble in ammonia, but insoluble in nitric acid.

Whether these crystals were in any way connected with the change of color which this sample of chloroform underwent, i am unable to determine; but i suspect not. I am anxious, however, to draw the attention of others to the subject, in the hope that larger specimens of the salt may be obtained for examination. For at present the circumstances under which chloroform frequently undergoes decomposition are very obscure. Except in this instance, i have never met with, nor heard of, any sample of chloroform which underwent these remarkable changes of color.

The chloroform was transferred into another bottle, on the sides of which a few minute crystals are now formed. But since the removal of the stopper the pink color has not re-appeared.

I have written to mr. Grattan to obtain, if possible, further information respecting this specimen of chloroform. But he tells me he has not any more of the sample, and has no means of ascertaining by whom it was made, as about the time it was purchased of him he had in his shop parcels from london, edinburgh and dublin, as well as a small quantity prepared in belfast, and he is quite unprepared to say from which of them it was taken.

I suspect that the pink color of the chloroform must have been due to the presence of manganese. If so, was this metal derived from the chloride of lime used in the manufacture of chloroform? Mr. Squire informs me that he has occasionally found the solution of chlorinated soda to become of a pinkish hue after being prepared a few days (not immediately), and that he has attributed it to some manganese carried over with the chlorine gas, as he does not remember having observed this change when the gas had been passed through water before entering the solution of carbonate of soda.

If this suspicion should prove well founded, it is obvious that the purity of the chloride of lime employed in the preparation of chloroform deserves the attention of the manufacturer.

Postscript.—subsequently to the reading of this paper before the pharmaceutical society, i have received from mr. William huskisson, jun., a specimen of pink chloroform, which, he informs me, owes its remarkable color to the presence of manganese, derived from peroxide of manganese employed in the purification of chloroform, as recommended by dr. Gregory, (see *pharmaceutical journal*, vol. Ix., p. 580.)

Mr. W. Huskisson, jun., tells me, that he has observed in his specimen neither the alterations of color nor the crystals met with in the specimen sent me by mr. Grattan.

The chairman stated, that he had never, in the various specimens of chloroform, of which his firm had always a large quantity in stock, observed the pink color described by dr. Pereira, nor had he ever seen any crystals deposited in the bottles, but he would have a more minute examination made with the view of ascertaining whether such existed. When the chloroform was first drawn over, and before it was purified, it frequently possessed more or less of a brown color, but this was quite distinct from the character described in the paper which had just been read.

Mr. D. Hanbury observed, that the use of manganese had been suggested in the process for purifying chloroform, and its presence might in this way be accounted for.

Mr. Barnes thought it desirable that the decomposed chloroform should be examined for formic acid. Although constantly subject to decomposition, no satisfactory explanation of the nature of the change had yet been afforded.

REPORT PRESENTED TO THE ACADEMY OF MEDICINE OF PARIS,

ON THE SUBSTITUTION OF AN ARTIFICIAL IO-DURETTED OIL FOR COD LIVER OIL. *BY A COMMISSION COMPOSED OF MESSRS. GIBERT, RICORD, SOUBEIREN AND GUIBOURT.*

On the 20th of august, 1850, the academy appointed a commission, composed as above, to whom was submitted a memoir, by m. Personne, entitled, "researches on the cod-liver and skate oils; and on the preparation of an ioduretted oil, by which they may be replaced as medicinal agents." A note was also submitted to us on the same subject, from m. Deschamps, and another from m. Marchall, the latter of which claimed for the author priority in the employment of ioduretted oil of almonds, as a substitute for cod-liver oil.

We proceed now to report the results of our examinations of these communications, and of the investigations to which the enquiry has led.

Cod-liver oil has long been the object of a considerable commerce arising principally from the decided superiority which it possesses over other animal oils, for the preparation of chamois leather; but it has only been within about twenty years that it has been used in medicine. It was first employed as a remedy for rheumatic pains, then for bronchial affections, and subsequently as a remedy for scrofula and consumption. It now constitutes one of the medicinal agents most extensively used, and one of those, on the action of which medical men place the greatest reliance, as a remedy capable either of curing very formidable diseases, or of retarding their fatal termination.

The most important memoir which has been published on cod-liver oil is that of dr. Jongh, in which three kinds of oil are described as met with in commerce, which are called the *black*, the *brown*, and the *white* cod-liver oil. These oils are represented to consist, principally, of oleic and margaric acids, and glycerine, and, as accessory bodies, of butyric acid, acetic acid; some principles appertaining to the bile, a non-azotised yellow or brown coloring matter, called gaduine, iodine, phosphorus, and some inorganic salts. In france, messrs. Girardin and preisser have been engaged in comparing the effects of the oil obtained from the cod with that obtained from the ray; and they advocate the superiority of the latter for medicinal use. But this superiority seems to depend, in part, on the circumstance, that the oil obtained from the livers of the ray, being carefully prepared by the pharmaciens, and being transparent, and of a light yellow color, proves less offensive to the patients than the cod-liver oil of commerce, which is generally thick, of a dark color, and has a disagreeable flavor. This, however, is scarcely admitted at the present time. Moreover, it appears from recent observations, that the above characters cannot be much depended upon for distinguishing the two kinds of oil, in consequence of their being so variable.

According to messrs. Girardin and preisser, these two oils contain iodine in the state of iodide of potassium, and in quantity much less than had been indicated by dr. Jongh. The latter author gives, as follows, the quantity of iodine in 1,000 parts of oil:—

Black cod-liver oil	0,295 parts of iodine.
Brown cod-liver oil	0,406 parts of iodine.
White cod-liver oil	0,374 parts of iodine.

Messrs. Girardin and preisser have found in a litre (thirty-five fluid ounces),

Of ray-liver oil	0,180 gramme of iodine.
Of cod-liver oil	0,150 gramme of iodine.

According to m. Gobley, a litre of ray-liver oil, prepared by direct action of the fire, contains twenty-five centigrammes of iodide of potassium. M. Goodley was unable to find phosphorus in this oil.

Such were the principal analytical results known when m. Personne presented his memoir to the academy. The uncertainty which appeared to attach to the subject, and the variations in the statements of chemists, induced him to put to himself the following questions:—

1st. Do the oils of cod and ray-liver contain iodide of potassium or iodine?

2nd. Do the different sorts of these oils contain the same proportion of iodine?

3rd. Do these oils contain phosphorus, to which their effects may be partly attributed?

For detecting the presence of the iodine, m. Personne saponified the oil with an excess of caustic potassa, incinerated the soap, and treated the product of incineration with strong alcohol. The alcohol was evaporated, the residue dissolved in water, and to this, solution of starch and sulphuric acid were added. The quantity of iodine was estimated by the intensity of the color; it is too small to be estimated by the balance.

Mr. Personne examined in this way the dark brown and thick cod-liver oil, such as is employed in the hospitals of paris; the transparent and nearly colorless oil of english commerce; and the ray-liver oil prepared by the direct action of a moderate heat, and subsequent filtration. The following are the results:—

1st. The brown cod-liver oil of the hospitals of paris contains more iodine than the fine white oil of english commerce.

2nd. It also contains more iodine than the ray-liver oil, and, moreover, the quantity present is certainly less than a decigramme of iodine in a kilogramme of oil (1 in 10,000.)

3rd. The residue of the liver, left after the preparation of the oil, contains much more iodine than the oil itself.

With regard to the question as to whether the iodine exists in cod-liver oil in the state of iodide of potassium, or directly combined with the oil, m. Personne, while he admits the difficulty of satisfactorily determining the point, inclines to favor the opinion that the iodine is directly combined with the elements of the oil.

[the different methods which have been suggested for the preparation of the ioduretted oil proposed as a substitute for cod-liver oil are described. A discussion follows of the claims of the authors, whose communications were submitted to the commissioners, for having first introduced the artificial ioduretted oil, which discussion is also omitted here as being uninteresting to our readers. The commissioners next proceed to state the result of the evidence obtained, by the medical members of the commission, of the therapeutical action of the artificial ioduretted oil.]

M. Gibert administered the ioduretted oil for periods varying from several weeks to several months, to patients suffering with eruptive complaints and scrofulous tumors; and, in some instances, found the benefit to be greater than from the use of cod-liver oil, under similar circumstances. He states, that he does not think he has tried it in a sufficient number of cases, and for a sufficient length of time, to enable him to state decidedly what its absolute value is as a specific for eruptive and scrofulous complaints; but the results he has obtained are sufficient to prove, that it is easy of administration and devoid of any injurious quality, and that it possesses a resolutive action, which renders it a valuable remedy for certain chronic eruptions and glandular swellings.

M. Ricord has employed the ioduretted oil for twelve months, in a great number of cases of scrofula, some of which were considered to be of venereal origin. He thus obtained excellent results in the treatment of strumous bubo, tubercular epididymis, and in some cases of scrofulous enlargement of the joints, etc., and other things being equal, curable cases were cured, or relief afforded, much more quickly by the use of the artificial ioduretted oil than by the natural cod-liver oil.

The average dose in which the ioduretted oil was

℥

administered was sixty grammes (ij.), which was

sometimes raised to 100 grammes ($\frac{z}{3}$ iiiss.) The patient generally took it without inconvenience. It was only in a few instances, where the dose had been raised, that vomiting, colic, and diarrhœa were produced. If the precautions which are necessary in the administration of every remedy be observed, and the degrees of susceptibility of the patients, together with all special conditions, properly studied, it may be affirmed that the ioduretted oil is a medicine of great value and that it presents considerable advantage over the cod-liver oil.—*journal de pharmacie, in pharmaceutic journal.*

EDITORIAL.

INTERNAL USE OF ATROPINE.
ABRIDGED FROM THE JANUARY NUMBER OF THE LONDON JOURNAL OF MEDICINE.

In the practice of english and american physicians, atropine (atropia) has been hitherto used chiefly as an external application, to dilate the pupil, but, as far as we know, has never been administered internally. In france, the powdered belladonna root has been strongly recommended as affording a reliable and efficient preparation; in this country, the leaves and the extracts and tincture derived from them are alone officinal. Dr. Lusanna, an italian physician, has ventured upon the internal use of atropia, and, according to our notions, in very large doses. He commences its administration in doses of one-thirtieth of a grain every three or four hours, gradually increasing the dose according to the effect produced. In some instances he went so far as to give one-third of a grain five times a day.

It may be given, according to dr. L, in solution in alcohol, or in acetic or some other mild acid. Pills and powders, from the difficulty of apportioning the dose he deems unadvisable. The alcoholic solution has a taste somewhat like that of quinine, but feebler, and not particularly disagreeable. The patient soon becomes habituated to the remedy, and the dose has to be increased. In cases of neuralgia he recommends the application of one-fourteenth to one sixth of a grain to a blistered surface, in the form of pomade. Dr. L. Carries the administration of atropia so far as to produce what we would call its toxicological effects.

1st. *Dilatation and immobility of the pupil.* Between fourteen and fifteen minutes after the exhibition of from one-twenty-fourth to one-thirtieth of a grain of atropia, the pupil becomes enormously dilated. If the remedy be persevered in the dilatation passes of, but the iris becomes immoveable, and the pupil no longer contracts on exposure to light. When the remedy is stopped, as the other phenomena produced by its exhibition subside, the pupil again becomes extremely dilated. Previous to this it commences to oscillate, contracting slightly when exposed to strong light, and dilating again in the shade. This indicates that the effects of the remedy are disappearing. The dilatation of the pupil is the last of the phenomena to subside, being sometimes met with eight days, or more after the suspension of the atropia.

2. *Disturbance of vision.* Objects at first seem hazy and ill-defined, persons are not recognized, and it is impossible to read or write. If the dose be increased, objects seem covered with a dark shade, and vision may be wholly lost. Every fresh dose has a sudden and marked effect in diminishing vision, and on its suspension the disturbance of vision disappears with equal rapidity. In one or two days the sight is perfectly restored.

3. *Disturbance of intellect.* At first the patient appears dull and stupid, then there is vertigo and confusion of ideas.

4. *Hallucinations of sight and hearing.* Objects are seen double or greatly magnified; motes and insects flit before the eyes; well known objects assume strange and monstrous forms, or horrible phantoms are seen. The hearing is more rarely affected. Buzzing, tinkling, hissing and whistling are sometimes heard.

5. *Anaesthesia.* Touch remains apparently perfect, but pain is relieved or blunted. The patient does not seem to suffer from painful tactile impressions.

6. *Dryness of the mouth and throat* were invariably felt. At first this seemed a purely nervous phenomenon, but if the medication was continued, from the diminution of the salivary secretion it became real.

7. *The appetite* is early lost, and there is no thirst; but on the cessation of the remedy it returns sharper than ever. Speech is early embarrassed and the power of swallowing early diminished, becomes finally lost.

8. *Delirium* alternating with stupor or succeeded by it, is produced by one-tenth of a grain of atropia at the commencement of the treatment, or by one-fourth of a

grain later, or by any sudden increase of the dose. The delirium is commonly gay and ridiculous; in one instance only was it mournful. When these phenomena are at all intense, they subside slowly. For several days after the cessation of the medicine, there is confusion and slowness of thought.

9. *Redness of the skin* was observed in but a single case.

10. *Torpor and paralytic tremblings.* As the patient gets under the influence of the atropia, the legs become weak and trembling, gradually lose their strength, and he is confined to bed. They may be still agitated by twitching, and convulsive movements.

11. *Paralysis of the sphincters of the rectum and bladder.* This is the highest point to which, according to dr. L., the medicative action of atropia can attain. In one case, only, the fæces and urine were passed involuntarily.

The functions of respiration, circulation, and calorification, were never affected by atropia.

After this long catalogue of serious symptoms, dr. Lusanna rather naively observes, he has never seen any truly alarming results arise from the use of atropia! Should they occur, he recommends wine as the best antidote.

CULTIVATION OF OPIUM.

—in a late number of the archives generales de medicine, will be found a short notice of a paper, read by m. Aubergier, to the french academy of science upon the cultivation of native opium. When the juice is obtained according to the methods described by m. A., the seeds continue to ripen, and the oil they yield pays the expense of cultivation. If the opium then more than repays the expense of the labor necessary to procure it, its production will be a source of profit. Now m. A., by successive improvements in his processes, has been enabled to raise the amount obtained by each laborer from a maximum of 75 to 90 grammes (1157½ grs. To 1389 grs.) To five times that quantity. The commercial value of the opium will always, therefore, more than repay the cost of manufacture. He farther finds that the proportion of morphia contained in the opium varies. 1st, with the maturity of the capsules from which it is collected, opium collected from capsules nearly ripe yielding less morphia than that obtained from those that are not so near their maturity. 2d, different varieties of the poppy yield an opium varying in the quantity of contained morphia from 15 to 17.833 per cent. Twenty specimens of foreign opium examined by m. A. Yielded quantities varying from 2.64 to 13 per cent.

The superiority of some specimens of european opium has been noticed by previous observers, and depends probably on the greater care bestowed on its preparation and on the cultivation of the plant.

CHROMIC ACID AS AN ESCHAROTIC.

Chromic acid has lately been employed in germany, both in concentrated solution and in substance, as an escharotic. The advantages it possesses are, that it is efficient, manageable, and less painful than the more ordinary applications. The concentrated solution is applied by means of a glass rod, a pencil made of asbestos, or if necessary, an ordinary hair pencil, which, if washed immediately, can be used a second time. The solid chromic acid on account of its penetrating action has to be employed with much care. All organic compounds are first oxydised and then dissolved in an excess of the acid, and this change is accelerated by an elevated temperature. Smaller animals, birds, mice, &c., were so completely dissolved by the acid within fifteen or twenty minutes, that no trace of their bones, skin, hair, claws, or teeth could be discovered. It would thus appear to be not only a gentle and gradual escharotic, but also a complete and rapid solvent. *Dublin quarterly jour. Of med. Science, from wiener medizinische wochenschrift*, 1851, no. Viii.

PUBLIC HYGEINE.

M. M. Bicourt & a. Chevalier have presented a memorial on the diseases which attack workmen engaged in the manufacture of chromsate of potash. The result of the facts presented in their memorial, proves, 1st. That workmen engaged in the preparation of bi-chromsate of potash, are subject to peculiar diseases. 2d. These diseases attack workmen who do not take snuff, and the mucous membrane of the nose is destroyed. 3d. Workmen who take snuff do not experience the same diseases. 4th. Workmen whose skin is broken in any part, suffer severely when the bi-chromsate comes in contact with the abraded surface, and should, therefore, carefully preserve the abrasions from contact with the solution of bi-chromsate. 5th. Workmen lightly clothed are exposed to some inconveniences, but these may be easily avoided. 6th. Animals are, like men, exposed to maladies caused by the bi-chromsate of potash.—*archives generales de medicine.*

CHEMICAL TECHNOLOGY;

Or chemistry applied to arts and to manufactures, by dr. T. Knapp, professor at the university of giesen; dr. Edmund ronalds, professor of chemistry at queen's college, galway, and dr. Thomas richardson, of new castle on tyne.

Illustrated with nine engravings and one hundred and twenty-nine wood cuts. Vol. Iii. London: hyppolyte bailliere, 219 regent street, and 209 broadway, new york.

Knapp's technology belongs to a class of books characteristic of the present day, and of the highest and most extended usefulness. Giving the practical details of the arts in connection with the scientific principles on which they are founded, it extends the views of the manufacturer and the economist, and places him on the right path for further improvement. To the american it presents the further advantage of ample and precise details of what is being done in great britain and on the continent of europe. All engaged in pursuits with which chemistry has any connection (and with what is it not now connected?) Will find in the various volumes of the technology, valuable information in regard to their own peculiar avocations, while the variety of its information and the copiousness of its illustrations, gives it a high interest to the general reader.

At a meeting of the college of pharmacy of the city of new york, held on thursday, 25th of march, the following gentlemen were elected officers for the ensuing year.

Geo. D. Coggeshall, *president.*

John h. Currie, *1st vice president.*

William l. Rushton, *2d vice president.*

Oliver hull, *3d vice president.*

James s. Aspinwall, *treasurer.*

B. W. Bull, *secretary.*

Trustees.

Wm. J olliffe,

John meakin,

Thomas b. Merrick,

Eugene duprey,

R. J. Davies,

Junius gridley,

Wm. Hegeman,

George wilson,

Thomas t. Green.

NEW YORK JOURNAL OF PHARMACY. MAY, 1852.

NOTES IN PHARMACY, NO. 2.
BY BENJAMIN CANAVAN.

Tinct. Ferri aetherea.—at the instance of one of our physicians, i made some of the above preparation for a lady patient of his, who, after having used the other preparations of iron "ad nauseam," had taken it with benefit in europe under the name of "bestucheff's tincture," as which, it at one time enjoyed great popularity, so that a very large sum was given to the author in purchase of it by the czarina catharine. After the composition became known it fell into disuse, almost justifying us in reversing the quotation from celsus,—

"morbos autem, non remediis, sed verbis curari."

It presents the metal in a different chemical state from what it is in the muriated tincture, viz: a very soluble deuto chloride; no acid is present and there are besides the anodyne and anti-spasmodic properties of the ethereal spirit, rendering it peculiarly appropriate in hysterical affections; and being pleasant to the taste and miscible with water, it is not at all repulsive.—supposing it may prove useful elsewhere and to others, i subjoin the formula i have used, and to which i give the preference, as being the most complete. It is original in the austrian pharmacopœia of 1820, whence it has been copied into many french formularies, under the name of "teinture étherée de chlorure de fer," and may be found with a number of other formulæ for the same preparation in the *"pharmocopée unverselle" of jourdan.*

℞   ℥

acidi hydro chlorici   iv.

Acidi hydro nitrici i.

Limatura. Ferriqs. Saturare acida.

Add the iron filings *very gradually*, and in small quantity at a time to the acids mixed together, in a porcelain mortar of ten or twelve inch diameter, and allow each portion to be dissolved before another is added, and so proceed until saturation is complete. Decant; evaporate to dryness in a sand bath; dissolve the residue in a quantity of water equal in weight to itself, and to each ounce of this solution add six ounces of sulphuric ether, agitate them well together and separate the supernatant ethereal solution, to which add four times its bulk of alcohol; finally, expose it to the action of the sun's rays until the color is altogether discharged. The dose is twenty to thirty drops.

Mucilago (gummi) acaclæ.—among the many useful hints which have appeared in the new york journal of pharmacy, in relation to several formulæ of the u. S. P., i perceive the preparation mucilage of gum arabic has been deemed worthy of a supervisory notice, and having experienced some annoyance with regard to it, arising simply from the fact that the officinal preparation has been heretofore entirely overlooked by apothecaries generally, each one instituting a formula for himself, i have been very much gratified by the result of adhering strictly to the formula of the pharmacopœia, and would take the liberty to say that as the formulæ of all the pharmacopœias of countries wherein our language is spoken are alike, it surely would not be productive of any advantage to introduce an exception to this conformity, to suit a local peculiarity, arising, to say the least, from inadvertence. Besides the thickness of the officinal mucilage is not much greater than that of syrup of gum, and is even absolutely necessary for the *chief proposes* for which it is intended or prescribed, viz: the suspension of weighty metallic oxydes, &c., and the holding balsams, oils, &c., in mixtures,—much benefit then would, so far as my experience goes, accrue from the apothecary confining himself strictly to the officinal mucilage, and as individual formulæ are based upon it, the re-compounding them from transcribed versions would be rendered more accurate.

This "whittling" away of standards, to make them correspond to the shortcomings of negligence or parsimony, has only the effect of rendering "confusion worse confounded."

Mistura amygdalarum.—being a work of some hour or so's duration to prepare the almond emulsion ab initio, it has been usual to keep the ingredients in the form of paste, from a proportionate quantity of which the mixture is made when required. The paste does not keep, becoming musty and sometimes exceedingly hard. I have therefore adopted the plan of keeping the almonds already *bleached and well dried*, in which state they do not undergo any change and thus is made all the preparation that can be, to expedite the process.

Liq. Arsenit. Potass.—on taking up, the other day, a shop bottle in which fowler's solution had been kept for some half a score or dozen of years, i perceived it to exhale a strong garlicky odor characteristic of free metallic arsenic. On examining the bottle which is of the ordinary flint glass, the inner surface presented the appearance of being coated or rather corroded, and having a metallic lustre so far up as the bottle was generally occupied by the solution, and in the upper part several specks were visible, of the same character, as if they had been produced by the sublimation of the corrosive agent. The coating was not affected by any amount of friction nor by alkalies but was slowly dissolved by acetic acid, from which iodide of potassium threw down a precipitate of iodide of lead.— deeming, therefore, the decomposition to have arisen from the lead contained in the flint glass i have since then kept the solution in green glass bottles.

LIQUOR MAGNESIÆ CITRATIS. THOS. S. WIEGAND, PHILADELPHIA.

The attention which has been given to this article by pharmaceutists, both on account of its pleasantness and its great tendency to change, has induced me to offer the following observations.

The advantage of the plan proposed is that a perfectly satisfactory article can be furnished in five or eight minutes, thus rendering unnecessary any attempt to make the preparation permanent at the expense of its remedial value. That this is the manner in which the public are supplied, save at stores where large quantities are sold, there can be but little doubt, from the experiments of professor proctor of philadelphia, detailed in the 23rd volume of the american journal of pharmacy, p.p. 214 and 216, which show conclusively that a permanent solution of citrate of magnesia must be a decidedly acid one.

Another method for making a soluble citrate has been devised by dorvault, which is published in his treatise, entitled "l'officine;" but from certain difficulties in manipulation his process cannot come into very general use.

The formula offered is—

Take, of carbonate of magnesia, in powder, five drachms, boiling water five fluid ounces, throw the magnesia upon the water in a shallow vessel, when thoroughly mixed, pour five sixths of the pulp into a strong quart bottle, fitted with cork and string for tying down; then make a solution of seven and a half drachms of citric acid in two fluid ounces of water, pour it into the magnesia mixture, cork and tie down immediately; when the solution has been effected (which will require but a minute and a half, or two minutes,) empty it into a bottle capable of holding twelve fluid ounces, containing two fluid ounces of syrup of citric acid, add the remaining pulp of carbonate of magnesia, nearly fill the bottle with water, and cork instantly, securing it with twine or wire; if the carbonate be of good quality it will be entirely dissolved in seven minutes.

Of course it is not intended that the carbonate of magnesia can be rubbed to powder, the water boiled, the bottles washed and fitted with strings and corks in the time above mentioned. My plan is to have the bottles prepared with their corks, strings, and syrup in advance, and to keep the carbonate of magnesia in a state of powder for this purpose.

[Continued From The March Number.]
Practical Hints. By A Wholesale Druggist.

Balsam peru. For many years past a factitious balsam peru has been manufactured in a neighboring city in very considerable quantities, and has entered largely into consumption; it is made by dissolving balsam tolu in alcohol. It closely resembles the true balsam, and is calculated to deceive unless subjected to a close examination. If one's attention is particularly called to it, a smell of alcohol is perceptible. It is, however, easily tested by burning in a spoon or small cup. The factitious balsam readily ignites on the application of flame and burns, as may be supposed, with a blue flame. The true balsam ignites with much more difficulty and emits a dense black smoke, and on the application of considerable heat, the air becomes filled with small feathery flakes of lamp black. This test, together with the sensible properties of appearance, taste and smell, will enable one to determine without doubt as to its genuineness.

Lac sulphuris. Sulphur precipitatum. Milk of sulphur. This preparation of sulphur is made by boiling sulphur and lime in water, and after filtering, precipitating the sulphur with muriatic acid. It differs from the ordinary sulphur in being in a state of more minute division and being softer and less brittle after having been melted.

When sulphuric acid is used to precipitate the sulphur, sulphate of lime is formed and cannot be separated from the precipitated sulphur by the ordinary process of washing, that salt being insoluble in water; for this reason muriatic acid should be used, as the salt thus formed, the muriate of lime or chloride of calcium is perfectly soluble and can be readily separated from the sulphur by washing.

The ordinary lac sulphuris of commerce, is prepared by the use of sulphuric acid, and in consequence is found to contain a very large proportion of sulphate of lime, or plaster of paris —several specimens examined were found to consist of nearly equal parts of sulphate of lime and sulphur.

The test for the above impurity is by burning in a small cup or spoon. The sulphur burns out entirely, leaving the impurity unaltered. The exact amount of impurity may be determined by weighing the substance before and after burning, and deducting the one weight from the other.

Precipitated chalk or carb. Lime. It is very important that physicians should be able to obtain this preparation of a reliable quality. A preparation purporting to be the above, but in fact nothing more nor less than sulph. Lime or plaster of paris, has, in very considerable quantities entered into consumption within a year or two past. It is difficult to determine between the two from their appearance. The test, however, is very simple and consists in treating the suspected article with muriatic acid. It should dissolve perfectly with brisk effervescence, if it be in reality pure carbonate of lime. If it consists, wholly or in part, of sulphate of lime, the whole or such part remains unaffected by the acid.

Pure muriatic acid should be used, as the commercial acid frequently contains sulphuric acid, in which case a portion of sulphate of lime is formed and remains undissolved.

Magnesia is sometimes found in this preparation, but by accident generally and not by design, as the price of the magnesia offers no inducement for the adulteration.

WEIGHTS AND MEASURES.[9]

"una fides, pondus, mensura, moneta sit una,

Et status illæsus totius orbis erit."—budeus.

"one faith, one weight, one measure and one coin,

Would soon the jarring world in friendship join."

The confusion of babel is felt most severely in the matter of weights and measures. Whether we consider the *number of names* of weights and measures, the *similarity* of names, the *discrepancy in amount* between those of the same name, or the *irregular relations* of those of the same denomination, we find a maze, the intricacies of which we cannot retain in our memory an hour after we have committed them to it. Sometimes, too, we find a farther discrepancy of a surprising nature; as if the authorised pint should not be the exact eighth of the authorised gallon, and so there should be two different quarts, one of two exact pints, and one of a fourth of a gallon, as well as a false gallon of eight exact pints, and a false pint of an eighth of an exact gallon.

---

9 universal dictionary of weights and measures. By j. H. Alexander. Baltimore. W. Menefie & co. 158 pp. 8vo.

We cannot here trace the genealogy of this multitude; chaos and old night are the ancestors of them all, except those now prevailing in france. A large number of them are of vegetable origin, from grains of wheat, carob beans, carat seeds, &c. The accino, the akey, and innumerable others seem to have had a similar origin. Most measures of length have been derived from the human form, as foot, span, fathom, nail, &c. To originate a new measure or weight has proved much easier than to preserve their uniformity when established. Here legislation has been resorted to. The arm of henry i. Was measured, and a *yard* of the same length was deposited in the exchequer as a standard. "thirty-two (afterwards twenty-four) grains of well dried wheat from the middle of a good ear" were to weigh a penny, twenty pence one ounce, and twelve ounces a pound. Science finally carried the matter one step further, and a yard is now $^{36}/_{39.13929}$ part of the length of "a pendulum that in a vacuum and at the level of mid-tide, under the latitude of london, shall vibrate seconds of mean time." The metre, a measure established by science, is $\frac{1}{10,000,000}$ part of the distance from the equator to the north pole. Measures of capacity have been still more difficult to verify, and weights, when depending upon these last, have been involved in further difficulties.—william the conquerer, enacted that 8 pounds good wheat, 61,440 grains, make a gallon. In england now, 10 pounds of water, 70,000 grains, at 60° fahr., make a gallon. In france a cubic decimetre of water, at maximum density, 39.2° fahr., weighs a kilogramme.

But the impotency of law is nowhere shown more strikingly than in its attempts to destroy spurious and useless weights and measures. Thirty of these are said to be prevalent in scotland at this day; and although magna charta required that there should be but one weight in all england, the assize of bread is still regulated by a pound,

16 of which = 17 ℔ 6 oz. Avoirdupois. Still further, it may not always occur to us that english measures, dry and liquid, need translating when their works are reprinted in the united states, as much as the french measures; for the imperial gallon, used for both dry and liquid measures, differs from both our gallons. It contains 1.2006 of our liquid gallons; our dry gallon contains 1.1631 of our liquid gallons.

But it is in the *weights of the united states* that we are more particularly interested. We will, therefore, take our leave of the rest of 5,400 and more weights and measures which mr. Alexander has ranged in alphabetical order, from

Name.	Locality.	Character.	Value.
"aam; *for wine*,	*Amsterdam*,	Liquid capacity,	41.00041 gall." To
"zuoja *piccola*,	*Udino*,	Superficial,	0.8553 acres."

Let us enquire what are the weights of the united states. we find but one unambiguous term to measure the rest by, the grain. We have then:

	Grains
1. The long ton,	15,680,000
2. The ton,	14,000,000
3. The quintal,	784,000
4. The hundred weight,	700,000
5. Quarter,	196,000
6. Pound avoirdupois,	7,000
7. Pound troy,	5,760
8. Pound apothecaries',	5,760
9. Ounce troy,	480
10. Ounce apothecaries',	480
11. Ounce avoirdupois,	437.5
12. Drachm apothecaries',	60
13. Drachm avoirdupois,	54.6875
14. Dram of the arithmetic,	27.34375
15. Pennyweight,	24
16. Scruple,	20
17. Grain,	1

A formidable array truly! From this we see that while an ounce of cork is lighter than an ounce of gold, a pound of cork is heavier than a pound of gold! Nay, further, let the apothecary go to the druggist for a drachm of opium, and he will receive and pay for a *drachm* avoirdupois, a weight unknown even to mr. Alexander, although in constant use in this city. But the moment he puts it into his mortar there is not a drachm of it! If he wishes to use a drachm in pills or tincture, he must add more than five grains to it. Could anything be more inconvenient or more prolific in mistakes? To prevent butter from becoming rancid, we are told to mix with it the bark of slippery elm, in the "proportion of a drachm (or dram) to the pound." Who can tell what it means? Six different proportions might accord with this delphic response; the most probable is 60:7000. But the grievance to which the apothecary is subject does not all consist in his buying by lighter ounces, and selling by heavier. The subdivisions by which he compounds have no reference to his convenience. Long habit alone can save him from either laborious calculation or risk of error. But still another chance of error comes

into the account. Two characters, 3 and $\mathfrak{Z}$, are joined to numerals, to indicate quantities; a mistake of these, by either prescriber or apothecary, may prove fatal. A case in point occurred a few years since, well known to many of our readers. A physician, prescribed cyanide of potassium,

by a formula in which $\mathfrak{Z}$ had been printed, by mistake, for

3 . The apothecary, instead of sending him the prescription for correction, *as he ought to have done*, put it up and sent it with the fearful monition that the dose would prove fatal—and so it did—to the prescriber himself, who took the dose his patient dared not touch. He died in five minutes, a victim to a printer's error, to his own self confidence, to want of etiquette in the apothecary, and last, not least, to an ill-contrived system of weights.

This brings us to the practical question, what is to be done? All agree that there ought to be a reform. On this point we can do no better than quote the close of mr. Alexander's preface.—"finally," says he (page vii.) "if i may be allowed, in connection with this work and its appropriate applications, to allude to certain dreams of my own, (as they may be; although i consider them capable, without undue effort, of a more prompt and thorough realisation than seems to be ordinarily anticipated,) as to the prevalence, some day, of an universal conformity of

weights and measures, i must acknowledge that such a result was one of the ends i had in view in the original collection of materials. Not that such a work was going to show more emphatically than business men feel, and reflecting men know, the importance of such an universal conformity; or that a book whose pages deal in discords, could, of itself, produce unison; but the first step to any harmonious settlement is, to see clearly, and at a glance, where the differences lie, and what they are.—if a millennial period for this world is ever to come, as many wise have deemed, and pious prayed, it must be preceded by one common language, and one common system of weights and measures, as the basis of intercourse. And the way to that is to be built, not by the violent absorption of other and diverse systems into one, but rather by a compromise into which all may blend. When the earth, in her historical orbit, shall have reached that point, (as it stood ere mankind were scattered from the plain of shinar) and not till then, may we begin to hope that her revolutions will be stilled, and that before long the weights and measures of fleeting time will be merged and lost in the infinite scales and illimitable quantities of eternity."
We are not sure that we precisely understand the last sentence, and we are sure we dissent entirely from the one that precedes it. No compromise can be of service in bringing about a uniformity in weights and measures. We must either make a better system than the best extant, and ask all men to adopt it, or if the best that human ingenuity and science can devise is already in use, so much the better; let us adopt it with all our heart. Is the french system this best one? We believe it is, nor have we ever heard it called in question.—why then speak of a new one as desirable? We fear the suggestion is the offspring of a national vanity, which ought to be beneath us. We would not oppose such a motive even to the introduction of the centigrade thermometer, which is much more inconvenient than fahrenheit's, and has *no one* advantage over it in any respect; still less should it bar the progress of a system against which no fault can be alleged, but that it is *foreign*.

We agree with our author that the introduction of a new system is much easier than is generally supposed. It will not be like the change of a monetary system, where the old coins remain, mingled with the new, to perpetuate the old names.—the change could be, by law, effected next new year's day, and all inconvenience from it would be over in a month, save some awkwardness from habit, and two more serious difficulties. One is from the human propensity to *bisection*. Thus the old hundredweight of 112 pounds is bisected down to 7 pounds, and the grocer will sell half this quantity, $3\frac{1}{2}$ pounds, at a cheaper rate than he will sell 3 pounds or 4. Unfortunately in bisecting 100 we run down too soon to the fractions $12\frac{1}{2}$ and $6\frac{1}{4}$. The french have been obliged to give way to this propensity, and divide the kilogramme in a binary manner, with an unavoidable irregularity, reckoning $31\frac{1}{4}$ grains as 32. Would that $32 \times 32 = 1000$! Our only remedy is to change the radix of numeration from 10 to 16, a thing impossible but to a universal dictator. The other difficulty is in our measure for land. This must remain in all surveyed tracts in such a shape that 40 acres, and also 5 acres, shall be some multiple of unity.

But shall the apothecary wait the action of government?—this is neither necessary nor desirable. Some relief he ought to have speedily. If he dare not make so great an advance as to adopt the french system, (his truest and most honorable policy,) let all subdivisions of the avoirdupois pound be discarded, except the grain. Introduce the chemists' weights of 1000, 500, 300, 100, 50, &c. Grains, and let all prescriptions be written in grains alone. This, perhaps, is the only feasible course.

We must return once more to our author before taking leave of our readers. The motive for making the collection was one that strikes us as new. It was for ethnological and historical purposes. As the carat points to india as the origin of the diamond trade, so we find in the names, mode of subdivision, and amount of weights and measures evidences of the migrations of races, and of the ancient and obsolete channels in which trade once flowed. The care with which mr. Alexander seems to have corrected these tables, and adjusted the discordant elements of which they are composed, and corrected the discrepancies between them, makes them more worthy of reliance than anything that has preceded them, and leaves little to be desired that is within the reach of human attainment. After the alphabetical arrangement, are given the weight and measure systems of the "principal countries of the world," beginning with abyssinia and ending with würtemberg. And we have only to add that the mechanical execution of the volume is worthy of the care and labor the author has spent upon it, unsurpassed, in fact, by any book made for use we have ever seen.

QUINIDINE.

BY MR. ROBERT HOWARD.

This alkaloid, which gained a prize in the great exhibition, has scarcely yet attracted much attention. Some of the cheaper barks now largely imported from new grenada contains so much of it that it is, perhaps, as well that it should be more studied. The *cinchona cordifolia*, from this part of the continent, is particularly rich in it. It is, however, contained in larger or smaller quantities in the bolivian and peruvian barks—the *cinchona calisaya, boliviana, rufinervis,* and especially *ovata*.

Referring your readers to a very able paper in your journal,10 i beg to add a few facts from my own observations.

---

10 *pharmaceutical journal,* vol. Ix., p. 322, january, 1850.

The sulphate of quinidine, or β quinine as it is called by some, (van heijninger and others,) is so like the sulphate of quinine, that the eye or the taste can with difficulty distinguish them. It forms the same light fibrous crystallization, and occupies as large a bulk. It corresponds in appearance with the description given by winckler, of "chinidine." (see *pharm. Journ.* For april, 1845, vol. Iv., p. 468.) He notices that it has "a remarkably white color and a peculiarly faint lustre." Its most striking characteristic is its extreme solubility. Pure sulphate of quinine requires nearly thirty times its weight of boiling water for solution, whilst the sulphate of quinidine dissolves in four parts. On the other hand the pure alkaloid crystallizes readily out of proof spirit and out of ether, whilst quinine does not crystallize out of either. A very good test for the presence of cinchonine in sulphate of quinine is also capable of being applied to detect the presence of β quinine. On this point i would refer for very interesting details to a paper by m. Guibourt, in the *journal de pharmacie* for january in this year.

In your journal of april, 1013, i gave a test for sulphate of quinine, to which i would again advert, because subsequent experience has proved it to be a tolerable easy, and at the same time exact means of ascertaining its purity. Put 100 grains in a florence flask with five ounces of distilled water, heat this to brisk ebullition; the sulphate of quinine ought not to be entirely dissolved; add two ounces more water, and again heat it to ebullition; ought to make a perfectly clear solution. If this be allowed to cool for six hours, and the crystals carefully dried in the open air on blotting paper, they will be found to weigh about ninety grains, the mother-liquor may be evaporated and tested with ether, when any cinchonine or β quinine will be easily detected. On examining sulphate of quinine of commerce from several leading manufacturers, i have found all of them give, within a grain or two, the same result, and, in each, indications of a β quinine, though to an unimportant extent.

The above quantity of water (seven ounces) readily dissolves 800 grains of sulphate of β quinine; and if 100 grains of this salt are dissolved in seven ounces of water, the crystals as above weigh only fifty-four grains, thus leaving forty-six grains in solution instead of about ten grains.

The medical effects of β quinine deserve investigation, the chemical constitution and the taste appear to indicate a great similarity if not identity.

ON THE ADULTERATION OF SULPHATE OF QUININE, AND THE MEANS OF DETECTION.

Mr. Zimmer, manufacturer of sulphate of quinine in frankfort-on-the-maine, has published the following circular and paper to his correspondents abroad:

Frankfort-on-the-maine, feb. 6th, 1852.

You are doubtless, aware that various and partly spurious kinds of sulphate of quinine have for some time past found their way into the market. The substance now frequently mixed with quinine is quinidine. But little positive is as yet known of the medicinal properties of this alkaloid, and whatever may be the result of future experiments, its arbitrary substitution is, under any circumstances, unwarrantable, and renders all fair and honest competition almost impossible.

The importance of the subject has induced me to address a few words to you, that i may submit a simple experiment by means of which the most usual adulterations of quinine may readily be detected.

I have the honor to be, with much respect, &c.
C. Zimmer.

The high price of genuine bolivian *cinchona calisaya*, through the monopoly of its export, has given occasion to imports, from other districts, of *cinchonas*, the quality of which widely differs from that of the calisaya, inasmuch as they contain principally quinidine. The lower prices of these barks, regardless of their different constituents, have brought them quickly into use in many factories of quinine, whereby a large quantity of quinine, containing quinidine, has got into the market, causing an undue depreciation in the price of quinine.

The existence of this third cinchona-alkaloid is now established beyond a doubt by ultimate analysis, by the peculiarity of its salts, and by important distinctive tests;

and there can be no further question, that quinidine must, equally with cinchonine, be distinguished from quinine. The external characters of sulphate of quinidine differ from those of sulphate of quinine; it has a greater specific gravity and less flocculent crystallization. In dry warm air it parts with its water of crystallization, without deliquescing or losing its crystallized aspect; lastly, it is far more soluble than sulphate of quinine in cold water and in alcohol.

One of the distinctive properties of the three alkaloids in question, *viz.*, their behavior with ether—places in our hands a ready means of detecting the mixture of cinchonine and quinidine, with quinine. Schweitzer (*lond. Med. Gazette*, vol. Xxi., p. 175) has already employed ether for the detection of cinchonine with complete success, and his process has, with justice, been subsequently quoted in most manuals, as it answers its purpose completely; cinchonine is known to be entirely insoluble in ether, whatever may be the quantity of ether employed. The solubility of quinidine in ether, as compared with that of quinine, is but slight; ten grains of pure sulphate of quinine dissolve in sixty drops of ether, and twenty drops of spirit of ammonia, while only one grain of sulphate of quinidine is soluble in the same quantity of the fluid; and in proportion quinine containing quinidine will always be less soluble than pure sulphate of quinine.

Guided by this fact i can recommend the following simple and very convenient process for the detection of quinidine and quinine:—

Ten grains of the salt to be examined is to put into a strong test tube, furnished with a tight-fitting cork, to this are to be added ten drops of diluted sulphuric acid, (one acid and five water) with fifteen drops of water, and a gentle heat applied to accelerate the solution. This having been affected, and the solution entirely cooled, sixty drops of official sulphuric ether with twenty drops of spirits of ammonia, must be added, and the whole well shaken while the top is closed by the thumb. The tube is then to be closely stopped and shaken gently from time to time, so that the bubbles of air may more readily enter the layer of ether.

If the salt examined be free from cinchonine and quinidine, or contain the latter in no greater proportion than ten per cent., it will be completely dissolved; while on the surface, where contact of the two layers of clear fluid takes place, the mechanical impurities only will be separated (in which respect the various sorts of commercial quinine differ.) After sometime longer the layer of ether becomes hard and gelatinous, after which no further observation is possible.

From the above statement respecting the solubility of quinidine in ether, it appears that the ten grains of the salt to be examined, may contain one grain of quinidine, and still a complete solution with ether and ammonia may follow; but in this case the quinidine will shortly begin to crystallize in the layer of ether. The last trace of quinidine may be yet more definitely detected by employing, instead of the ordinary ether, some other, previously saturated with quinidine, by which means all of the quinidine contained in the quinine must remain undissolved. It is particularly requisite in performing this last experiment to observe, after the shaking, whether all has dissolved, for owing to the great tendency of quinidine to crystallization, it may become again separated in a crystalline form, and be a source of error.

If more than a tenth of quinidine or cinchonine be present, there will be found an insoluble precipitate at the limits of the two layers of fluids. If this be quinidine, it will be dissolved on the addition of proportionately more ether, while cinchonine will be unaffected.

It is expressly to be remarked, that the necessity for testing sulphate of quinine, in search of other fraudulent adulterations is not superseded by the above described process.

We have particularly to determine upon the absence of inorganic substances, which may be effected by subjecting to red heat on a platinum dish, or simply by solution in alcohol. Gypsum, chalk, magnesia, &c., will be left undissolved. Boracic acid will be dissolved by alcohol, but its green flame will indicate its presence in the alcoholic solution when ignited.

The absence of organic substances, such as salicine, sugar, stearic acid, &c., may be inferred from the formation of a colorless solution with pure concentrated cold sulphuric acid; it is as well to leave the sulphuric acid to act for some hours.

The presence of sal-ammoniac may be detected by the addition of caustic potash to the suspected salt, when, if present, it will be known by the diffusion of the ammoniacal odour.—*pharmaceutical journal, march, 1852.*

REMARKS ON THE ENVELOPEMENT OF PILLS.

BY DORVAULT.

The envelopement of pills is a minute question, an accessory in this form of administering medicines, but as it is a frequent cause of trouble to practitioners, and as their successful operation is often due to their peculiar mode of exhibition, we shall perhaps be pardoned for devoting a short space to the subject.

In order that pills may not adhere to one another, they are rolled in an inert powder, such as marsh-mallow, liquorice, and above all, lycopodium. Carbonate of magnesia is now particularly used for pills of turpentine and copaiba. To disguise the peculiar odour of the pill mass, german practitioners use iris powder, or cinnamon.

To render pills more pleasing to the eye, as well as to disguise their taste, instead of rolling them in the before named powders, they are frequently covered with gold or silver leaf. The mode of doing this is too well known to need repetition. We will only remark that those pills which contain iodine, bromine, sulphur, iodides, bromides, sulphides, salts of mercury, gold, platina, &c., cannot be silvered.

These methods conceal but imperfectly the unpleasant taste and smell of certain pillular compounds. M. Garot, to obviate this inconvenience, has proposed to cover pills with a layer of gelatine, by means of a process which he has made public, and into the details of which we think it needless to enter. The gelatinous layer conceals the bad taste and smell perfectly, but it is attended with one inconvenience; in time it shrinks, cracks, and the pill mass exudes. Besides, much skill is required in its manipulation. After gelatinization comes sugaring. This is frequently preferable to the former modes, and can be equally well applied to pills of a repulsive taste and smell, (copaiba, turpentine, musk, assafœtida, &c.,) or to those which are changed by air or light, (proto salts of iron,) or deliquescent, (iod-hydrargyrate of iodide of potassium,) or caustic, (croton oil.) It can extemporaneously be performed in the following manner:—put the pills into a vase with a round bottom, or into a box lined with silver, moisten them with a little syrup of sugar, clear mucilage, or white of eggs, agitate them so as to moisten them uniformly; add a mixture of equal parts of gum, sugar and starch; again rotate them, so as equally to enclose all the pills. If a first layer be not sufficient, add a second and third in the same manner. Dry them in the air or in a stove. In damp weather, these pills should be enclosed in corked bottles. Gelatine of carragheen or caseine dried and powdered may be substituted for the above powdered mixture. This method is more expeditious than gelatinisation, and it has besides the advantage of the material being always perfectly soluble. Collodion has been proposed for enveloping pills, but seems never to have been used.

The last method we shall call *toluisation*. It appears to possess many decided advantages over the others. M. Blancard, its originator, employs it particularly for pills of proto iodide of iron. It is to induce its more general use that we make these remarks. The following is the mode of proceeding, which can be modified to suit the daily wants of practice:

Dissolve one part of balsam of tolu, in three parts of ether, (the balsam which has been used in the preparation of syrup of tolu will answer perfectly;) pour some of this tincture into a capsule containing the pills, to favor the evaporation of the ether. When the pills begin to stick together, throw them on a mould of tin passed through mercury, or simply on a plate, taking care to separate those which stick together. Set them in the air to dry. The drying may be completed in a stove of moderate heat, especially if several layers have been found necessary. This mode of enveloping may take the place, or nearly so, of all the others. An important point in it, is, that it resists the effects both of damp and dryness on the pill mass. Its balsamic odour is generally agreeable; but should it not be so, the tolu might be replaced by some inert resin soluble in ether, as mastic tears for example. The layer of resinous matter is so thin, that we apprehend no obstacle in its influence on the medicine.

We will, however, make one general remark, namely: that as each method possesses some peculiar advantages, we thought it right to give them all.—*bulletin gen. Ther. Med. Et chir. January, 1852.*

ON THE APPLICATION OF ORGANIC CHEMISTRY TO PERFUMERY.

BY DR. A. W. HOFFMAN. PROFESSOR TO THE ROYAL COLLEGE OF CHEMISTRY, LONDON.

Cahours' excellent researches concerning the essential oil of gaultheria procumbens (a north american plant of the natural order of the ericinæ of jussieu,) which admits of so many applications in perfumery, have opened a new field in this branch of industry. The introduction of this oil among compound ethers must necessarily direct the attention of perfumers towards this important branch of compounds, the number of which is daily increasing by the labors of those who apply themselves to organic chemistry. The striking similarity of the smell of these ethers to that of fruit has not escaped the observation of chemists; however, it was reserved to practical men to discover by which choice and combinations it might be possible to imitate the scent of peculiar fruits to such a nicety, as to make it probable that the scent of the fruit is owing to a natural combination identical to that produced by art; so much so, as to enable the chemist to produce from fruits the said combinations, provided he could have at his disposal a sufficient quantity to operate upon. The manufacture of artificial aromatic oils for the purpose of perfumery is, of course, a recent branch of industry; nevertheless, it has already fallen into the hands of several distillers, who produce sufficient quantity to supply the trade; a fact, which has not escaped the observation of the jury at the london exhibition. In visiting the stalls of english and french perfumers at the crystal palace, we found a great variety of these chemical perfumes, the applications of which were at the same time practically illustrated by confectionery flavored by them. However, as most of the samples of the oils sent to the exhibition were but small, i was prevented, in many cases, from making an accurate analysis of them. The largest samples were those of a compound labelled "pear oil," which, by analysis, i discovered to be an alcoholic solution of pure acetate of amyloxide. Not having sufficient quantity to purify it for combustion, i dissolved it with potash, by which free fusel oil was separated, and determined the acetic acid in the form of a silver salt.

0,3080 gram. Of silver salt = 0,1997 gram. Of silver.

The per centage of silver in acetate of silver is, according to

Theory.	Experiment.
64,68	64,55.

The acetate of amyloxide which, according to the usual way of preparing it, represents one part sulphuric acid, one part fusel oil, and two parts of acetate of potash, had a striking smell of fruit, but it acquired the pleasant flavor of the jargonelle pear only after having been diluted with six times its volume of spirits of wine.

Upon further inquiry i learned that considerable quantities of this oil are manufactured by some distillers, from fifteen to twenty pounds weekly, and sold to confectioners, who employ it chiefly it flavoring pear-drops, which are nothing else but barley-sugar, flavored with this oil.

I found, besides the pear-oil, also an *apple-oil*, which, according to my analysis, is nothing but valerianate of amyloxide. Every one must recollect the insupportable smell of rotten apples which fills the laboratory whilst making valerianic acid. By operating upon this new distillate produced with diluted potash, valerianic acid is removed, and an ether remains behind which, diluted in five or six times its volume of spirits of wine, is possessed of the most pleasant flavor of apples.

The essential oil most abundant in the exhibition was the pine-apple oil, which, as you well know, is nothing else but the butyrate of ethyloxide. Even in this combination, as in the former, the pleasant flavor or scent is only attained by diluting the ether with alcohol. The butyric ether which is employed in germany to flavor bod rum, is employed in england to flavor an acidulated drink called pine-apple ale.

For this purpose they generally do not employ pure butyric acid, but a product obtained by saponification of butter, and subsequent distillation of the soap with concentrated sulphuric acid and alcohol; which product contains, besides the butyric ether, other ethers, but nevertheless can be used for flavoring spirits. The sample i analyzed was purer, and appeared to have been made with pure butyric ether.

Decomposed with potash and changed into silver salt, it gave

0,4404 gram. Of silver salt = 0,2437 gram. Of silver.

The per centage of silver in the butyrate of silver is according to

Theory.   Experiment.

55,38   55,33.

Both english and french exhibitors have also sent samples of cognac-oil and grape-oil, which are employed to flavor the common sorts of brandy. As these samples were very small, i was prevented from making an accurate analysis. However, i am certain that the grape-oil is a combination of amyl, diluted with much alcohol; since, when acted upon with concentrated sulphuric acid, and the oil freed from alcohol by washing it with water, it gave amylsulphuric acid, which was identified by the analysis of the salt of barytes.

1,2690 gram. Of amylsulphate of barytes gave 0,5825 gram. Of sulphate of barytes. This corresponds to 45,82 per cent. Of sulphate of barytes.

Amylsulphate of barytes, crystallized with two equivalents of water, contains, according to the analysis of cahours and kekule, 45,95 per cent. Of sulphate of barytes. It is curious to find here a body, which, on account of its noxious smell, is removed with great care from spirituous liquors, to be applied under a different form for the purpose of imparting to them a pleasant flavor.

I must needs here also mention the artificial oil of bitter almonds. When mitscherlich, in the year 1834, discovered the nitrobenzol, he would not have dreamed that this product would be manufactured for the purpose of perfumery, and, after twenty years, appear in fine labelled samples at the london exhibition. It is true that, even at the time of the discovery of nitrobenzol, he pointed out the striking similarity of its smell to that of the oil of bitter almonds. However, at that time, the only known sources for obtaining this body were the compressed gases and the distillation of benzoic acid, consequently the enormity of its price banished any idea of employing benzol as a substitute for oil of bitter almonds. However, in the year 1845, i succeeded by means of the anilin-reaction in ascertaining the existence of benzol in common coal-tar-oil. In his essay, which contains many interesting details about the practical use of benzol, he speaks likewise of the possibility of soon obtaining sweet scented nitrobenzol in great quantity. The exhibition has proved that this observation has not been left unnoticed by the perfumers. Among french perfumeries we have found, under the name of artificial oil of bitter almonds, and under the still more poetical name of "essence de mirbane," several samples of essential oils, which are no more nor less than nitrobenzol. I was not able to obtain accurate details about the extent of this branch of manufacture, which seems to be of some importance. In london, this article is manufactured with success. The apparatus employed is that of mansfield, which is very simple; it consists of a large glass worm, the upper extremity of which divides in two branches or tubes, which are provided with funnels. Through one of these funnels passes a stream of concentrated nitric acid; the other is destined as a receiver of benzol, which, for this purpose, requires not to be quite pure; at the angle from where the two tubes branch out, the two bodies meet together, and instantly the chemical combination takes place, which cools sufficiently by passing through the glass worm. The product is afterwards washed with water, and some diluted solution of carbonate of soda; it is then ready for use. Notwithstanding the great physical similarity between nitrobenzol and oil of bitter almonds, there is yet a slight difference in smell which can be detected by an experienced nose. However, nitrobenzol is very useful in scenting soap, and might be employed with great advantage by confectioners and cooks, particularly on account of its safety, being entirely free from prussic acid.

THERE WERE, BESIDES THE ABOVE, SEVERAL OTHER ARTIFICIAL OILS; THEY ALL, HOWEVER, WERE MORE OR LESS COMPLICATED, AND IN SUCH SMALL QUANTITIES, THAT IT WAS IMPOSSIBLE TO ASCERTAIN THEIR EXACT NATURE, AND IT WAS DOUBTFUL WHETHER THEY HAD THE SAME ORIGIN AS THE FORMER.

The application of organic chemistry to perfumery is quite new; it is probable that the study of all the ethers or ethereal combinations already known, and of those which the ingenuity of the chemist is daily discovering, will enlarge the sphere of their practical applications. The caprylethers lately discovered by bouris are remarkable for their aromatic smells (the acetate of caryloxide is possessed of the most intense and pleasant smell,) and they promise a large harvest to the manufacturers of perfumes.—*annalen der chemie.—in an. Of pharmacy.*

ON TESTS FOR THE IMPURITIES OF ACETIC ACID.

Pure acetic acid is colorless, possesses strong acid properties and taste, and no empyreumatic flavor. It should have, according to the new london pharmacopœia, a specific gravity of 1.048, and one hundred grains should saturate eighty-seven grains of crystallized carbonate of soda; consequently the pharmacopœial acid consists of thirty-one per cent. Of the anhydrous acid, and sixty-nine per cent. Of water. It should leave no residuum by evaporation. Sulphuretted hydrogen, nitrate of barytes, ferrocyanuret of potash, and nitrate of silver, should produce no precipitate in it. When it contains empyreumatic matter, which besides being evident to the smell, concentrated sulphuric acid causes its color to darken. Sugar, in a more or less changed condition, is frequently one of the impurities of the german diluted commercial acid, and may be recognized by the taste of the residuum left upon its evaporation.

When sulphuretted hydrogen produces in acetic acid a milky turbidity, it shows that sulphurous acid is present, the presence of which is due to the decomposition of coloring and other organic matters, contained as impurities in the acetates, from which the acetic was prepared, when treated with sulphuric acid. The turbidity is caused by the separation of sulphur from the sulphuretted hydrogen, and from the sulphurous acid by reason of the hydrogen of the former combining with the oxygen of the latter, and forming water (wittstein.) If the sulphuretted hydrogen produces a black precipitate, either lead or copper may be present. The lead may be recognized by sulphuric acid giving a precipitate of sulphate of lead; and the copper, by the blue reaction which ensues, with an excess of ammonia. Sulphuric acid can be readily known when present by nitrate of barytes producing a white precipitate, insoluble in mineral acids. Nitrate of silver detects muriatic acid by throwing down a white precipitate, which changes, under the influence of light, to a violet color, and is insoluble in nitric acid, but soluble in ammonia.

Ferrocyanuret of potassium will indicate the presence of salt of iron when by its addition, a blue precipitate results.

The above tests are not applicable to the same extent to detect the impurities of the brown vinegar of commerce, because manufacturers are allowed by law to add to it a small per centage of sulphuric acid, and there are always sulphates and chlorides and other salts present in it, derived from the water used in its manufacture; therefore, in testing for its impurities, an allowance must be made for those which arise from the necessary process of the manufacture, and those considered only as adulterations which are over and above such fair allowance. To detect such impurities as cayenne pepper, &c., it is merely necessary to neutralize the vinegar with carbonate of soda, when their presence will be palpably evident to the taste.

Acetic acid may be purified by distillation from those substances which are not volatile. By adding acetate of lead previously to its distillation, sulphuric and muriatic acids can be separated from it; and sulphurous acid can be removed by peroxide of manganese, which converts it into sulphuric acid. It can be freed from empyreumatic impurities by agitation with charcoal, subsequent filtration and distillation.

The strength of acetic acid and vinegar cannot be determined by the specific gravity. The power of saturating an alkaline carbonate is the best criterion of the quantity of anhydrous acid present in any given sample. This method will only give correct results when the acid is pure, or when the quantities of free mineral acids have been estimated previously by precipitation, so as to make the necessary deductions for their saturating power when the acid is neutralized with an alkaline carbonate. It would be well if pharmaceutists were more frequently to try the strength of their acetic acid, which is constantly sold with very plausible labels, about one part of the acid to seven parts of water, making the distilled vinegar of the pharmacopœia, which statement we have oftentimes proved to be a very pretty fiction.—*an. Of pharmacy, march, 1852.*

A TEST FOR ALCOHOL IN ESSENTIAL OILS.

J. J. Bernoulli recommends for this purpose acetate of potash. When to an etherial oil, contaminated with alcohol, dry acetate of potash is added, this salt dissolves in the alcohol, and forms a solution from which the volatile oil separates. If the oil be free from alcohol, this salt remains dry therein.

Wittstein, who speaks highly of this test, has suggested the following method of applying it as the best:—in a dry test tube, about half an inch in diameter, and five or six inches long, put not more than eight grains of powdered dry acetate of potash; then fill the tube two-thirds full with the essential oil to be examined. The contents of the tube must be well stirred with a glass rod, taking care not to allow the salt to rise above the oil; afterwards set aside for a short time. If the salt be found at the bottom of the tube dry, it is evident that the oil contains no spirit. Oftentimes, instead of the dry salt, beneath the oil is found a clear syrupy fluid, which is a solution of the salt in the spirit, with which the oil was mixed. When the oil contains only a little spirit, a small portion of the solid salt will be found under the syrupy solution. Many essential oils frequently contain a trace of water, which does not materially interfere with this test, because, although the acetate of potash becomes moist thereby, it still retains its pulverent form.

A still more certain result may be obtained by distillation in a water bath. All the essential oils which have a higher boiling point than spirit, remain in the retort, whilst the spirit passes into the receiver with only a trace of the oil, where the alcohol may be recognized by the smell and taste. Should, however, a doubt exist, add to the distillate a little acetate of potash and strong sulphuric acid, and heat the mixture in a test tube to the boiling point, when the characteristic odor of acetic ether will be manifest, if any alcohol be present.

CHEMICAL EXAMINATION OF RESIN OF JALAP. BY B. SANDROCK.

It is a well known fact that when resin of jalap is treated with ether, we obtain two kinds of resin, one soluble, and the other insoluble in ether. Dr. Kayser chose first for his analysis that part of the resin which is insoluble in ether. This resin, purified by means of charcoal, was friable, almost colorless, without smell or taste, insoluble in ether and water, but easily dissolved by spirit of wine; the alcoholic solution reddens litmus slightly. The resin, again precipitated by water, was perfectly soluble in solution of caustic ammonia and acetic acid. This resin was dissolved with difficultly in cold solutions of caustic potash and soda, but was perfectly soluble when hot, and could again be readily precipitated from the alkaline solutions by acids. The solution of this resin, in ammonia was of a bright brown color, and became neutral by volatizing the superfluous ammonia. It is consequently a resinous acid, which is distinguished from other resinous acids, by the facts that it does not precipitate the bases from metalic salts, such as nitrate of silver, sulphate of copper; it afforded only a precipitate when acted upon by basic-acetate of lead. A question arose, whether the resin of jalap, dissolved in alkaline fluids, undergoes any changes in its constitution. To answer this question, kayser undertook several analyses, the results of which were as follows: the uncombined resin of jalap gave c 42, h 35, o 20.—the resin, precipitated by oxide of lead, gave c 42, h 36, o 21. It is evident that resin of jalap, combined with the bases of salts, acquires the elements of one equivalent of water. Dr. Kayser, has named the unchanged resin of jalap, rhodeoretin, and that modified by bases of salts, hydro-rhodeoretin.

By dissolving rhodeoretin in absolute alcohol and submitting the solution to the action of chlorine, and subsequently adding water to it, kayser obtained an oily fluid, dark yellow, possessing a pleasant smell, easy to be volatilized by heat, soluble in water, which he called rhodeoretin oil.

The part of the resin soluble in ether, possesses eminently the disagreeable smell of jalap, a prickly taste; its solution reddens litmus, and in drying leaves a greasy spot on paper; it is soluble in alkaline fluids. If the alcoholic solution is allowed to stand, mixed with water, for a lengthened period, prismatic crystalline needles are precipitated. According to these properties, kayser includes the soluble jalap resin among the fatty acids. Sandrock in general agrees with kayser; but, according to his analysis, the jalap can be resolved in three different resins, one soluble in ether, the second obtained by precipitating the alcoholic solution by oxides of lead; the third remains unprecipitated in this solution.

That part of the resin which is insoluble in ether, but is precipitated from the alcoholic solution by oxide of lead, sandrock calls alpha resin; that which is not precipitated, beta resin; that part which is soluble in ether he calls gamma resin.

The alpha resin agrees in its properties with buchner's and herberger's jalapine. Sandrock calls ipomic acid, the produce of this resin when treated by boiling carbonated alkaline solution; and the one obtained in the same way from beta resin, jalapic acid. The gamma resin forms in ether a yellow solution, and a purple one in concentrated sulphuric acid.—*archiven der pharmacie.*

ON THE PREPARATION OF CHLOROFORM FROM THE ESSENCES OF LEMON, COPAIBA, PEPPERMINT AND BERGAMOTTE.

BY M. CHAUTARD, PROFESSOR OF CHEMISTRY AT THE LYCEUM OF VENDOME.

M. Chautard, after having completed his experiments for the production of chloroform by means of oil of turpentine instead of alcohol, led by analogy, proceeded to try by a similar method to prepare it by means of the essences of lemon, bergamotte, copaiba and peppermint, and succeeded. However, the quantity of essences upon which he acted was too small to carry on a minute analysis. In the meanwhile, his researches led him to discover formic acid in the calcareous residuum of the operation. It was already known, m. Chautard observes, that oil of turpentine, when old and exposed a long time to the action of the air, was transformed into formic acid, which observations is due to m. Wappen. On the other hand, m. Schneider, by collecting the volatile products of the oxidation of turpentine, by means of nitric acid, detected therein the presence of acetic, metacetic, and butyric acids. Finally, a few years ago, mr. William bastick11 showed that hypo-chlorite of lime, by reacting upon neutral unazotised bodies, such as sugar, starch, &c., gave rise to the formation of a certain quantity of formate of lime; hence, turning to advantage the details given by this chemist, m. Chautard continues—i thus have carried on my operation:—

---

11 "journal de pharmacie," 3ᵉ serie, 1. 14.

After having ascertained, by means of the solution of indigo, that the residuum contained in the alembic did not contain any hypochlorite of lime, the presence of which would have prevented the extraction of formic acid, i threw the whole upon a cloth, and added sulphuric acid to the filtered liquor to precipitate the lime retained in a state of chloride or formate.—this liquor, after having been filtered anew, was distilled, and the product was a mixture of formic and hydrochloric acids, which i saturated by means of carbonate of soda. By subsequent evaporation to dryness, i succeeded, by adding afterwards a little water, in separating the formate of soda from the chloride. By means of the formate of soda, i proved the principal properties of formic acid, and besides, produced from it the formate of silver, which is decomposed by a boiling heat, leaving a precipitate of metalic silver.

In finishing this communication, i must observe that fixed oils, treated in the same way by hypochlorite of lime, do not produce chloroform; however, the reaction which occurs is so strong, and indicative of interesting results, that it induces me to continue my experiments.—*journal de pharmacie.*

ON DRY EXTRACTS.
BY DR. MOHR.

Every one is aware of the utility of possessing dry extracts, particularly of narcotic plants, so as to be able to administer them as powders. This able pharmaceutist gives the following formula for their preparation; and as it seems to answer all purposes, and is adopted in berlin, and other continental towns, it deserves to be made public.

Take of any extract, and of powder of licorice equal parts, mix them well in a mortar; when well mixed, put the paste in an earthenware evaporating dish, and then put this vessel over an iron pan, which has been filled with chloride of calcium, previously dried in the vessel by a strong fire without melting; the iron vessel must have a cover to enclose both vessels, so that the chloride of calcium can absorb the vapor from the extract without communication with the air, and must be put on as soon as the extract has been placed on the chloride of calcium. Let it stand for some days. Remove the extract, and add an equal weight of licorice powder to it in a mortar, mix well, and preserve it in bottles.

EDITORIAL.

PHARMACEUTICAL CONVENTION.

The apothecaries of the united states are in an anomalous and exceptional position. Exercising functions which concern the life and health of those who require their services, the public expects them to possess the experience, the varied requirement, the high moral qualities which the proper exercise of their profession demands; yet this same public, itself incapable of discriminating between knowledge and ignorance, furnishes them no aid in the pursuits of their studies, and yields them no protection against quackery and imposture. Everything is left to the spirit of trade, and to the laws of supply and demand. The advances that have been made in pharmacy have come from within itself, unaided by any assistance from the state governments, and looked upon often with coldness or distrust by the public. In this way, in some of the large cities, with the influence of the sister profession of medicine, something has been done; but, even there, how much remains to be accomplished before pharmacy can assume the rank it holds in france and germany!

As heretofore, so now, the best and the only prospect of progress in the profession lies in itself. It best knows its necessities and requirments, and it can best devise the remedies that will meet them. It is in the union of its members, in mutual association and intercourse, in the formation of a public opinion of its own, which, operating first upon the members of the profession, will necessarily have its weight upon the public opinion of the community, that lie our best hopes. Pharmacy is at once a liberal art, and a trade. In individuals, particularly in a community like ours, the spirit of trade is apt to be in the ascendant. Science is estimated at its money value, for what it brings in, rather than for what it is. But when the best men of a profession meet together, science resumes its proper position; they are encouraged in their noblest aims, and that encouragement is spread widely among their fellows. Individuals struggling, isolated throughout the country, feel that there is a tribunal to which they can appeal, and by which they will be judged, and its influence will be felt too by another class, as a restraint, if not an encouragement. Success, obtained by worthy means, loses much of its value, when it costs the esteem of those with whom we are most intimately connected.

It is from such considerations that we look upon the approaching convention at philadelphia, as a step in a very important movement. A great deal depends upon its success, and every one who has the interest of pharmaceutical science at heart, should do all he can to promote it.

To prove all that is hoped for by its friends, the convention should be a national one, not only in name, but in reality. Every institution and society entitled under the requisitions of the call, should appoint delegates, and above all, they should appoint delegates who will attend. But there are many apothecaries scattered through the country, in places not entitled to appoint delegates, who may be enabled to be present at the meeting of the convention, and we are glad to see that our philadelphia brethren are prepared to welcome them in a liberal and cordial spirit. They will both receive and communicate benefit. Their presence will add weight and authority to the convention; while, independent of its official proceedings, they cannot but derive advantages from acquaintance and intercourse with the numerous able members of the profession who will, as delegates, attend the meeting.

Great care should be exercised in the selection of delegates; they should not only, above all, be men who will attend, but men who have at heart the position and advancement of pharmaceutists.

We hope that their election will take place as early as possible, that they may have time fully to consider the objects of the convention, and the wants and wishes of the institutions they represent. It would be well, too, if early notice of their election should be communicated to mr. Proctor, or some other of the members residing at philadelphia, and their names should be published. The convention will have much to discuss and determine upon, while its duration will necessarily be limited. Were the names of its members early announced, an interchange of opinion might take place between, not to forstall the active of the convention, but to promote and expedite it. For this purpose, if deemed desirable our own columns are freely tendered.

NEW YORK JOURNAL OF PHARMACY. JUNE, 1852.

ON THE PREPARATION OF PURE BARIUM COMPOUNDS. BY HENRY WURTZ.

The preparation of the compounds of barium in a state of absolute purity is a subject which has not generally received much attention from pharmaceutical chemists, in consequence of the hitherto limited application of these compounds, except in chemical analysis. The time, however, is undoubtedly close at hand, when new developments in the arts, will create a demand for pure barium compounds, as well as for very many other products now considered as pertaining exclusively to the laboratory. Indeed, efforts have already been made to introduce the *chlorate of barytes* to the notice of pyrotechnists as a means of producing a green fire unequalled in beauty, and the pure carbonate has been for some time in use in england, in the manufacture of superior varieties of plate and flint glass. The precipitated or purified native sulphate is also preferred as a water color pigment to white lead, being far more durable than the latter. I may here be permitted to mention a practical application of the carbonate which has occurred to myself. I have found that sulphate of lime is totally precipitated from its solution by mixing therewith an equivalent quantity of the precipitated or finely pulverized natural carbonate of barytes, of course with the formation of sulphate of barytes and carbonate of lime. It is by no means improbable that this property may be made available in removing sulphate of lime from spring or sea water which is to be used in steam boilers, thus preventing the formation of the troublesome incrustation which so often occurs, especially when it is considered that the sulphate of barytes which would be formed, might easily be reconverted into carbonate and used over again. Again, sulphate of lime might be removed in the same way from the brine in salt works, thus contributing to the purity of the salt produced.

Recent improvements in chemical analysis have greatly increased the usefulness of barium compounds in the laboratory, especially of the carbonate, to which the late investigations of professor h. Rose, and of ebelmen have given a place in the very first rank among the reagents valuable to the chemist. Any suggestion, therefore, concerning the preparation of barium compounds in a pure state, cannot be considered as useless.

The sulphate of baryta is the only compound which occurs in sufficient abundance to be an economical source of the other barium compounds, and the enormous though illegitimate use of this substance in the adulteration of white lead, is so far fortunate as to render it an easy matter to obtain it in any required quantity, already in a state of fine powder which is so desirable in chemical operations.

The sulphate of baryta is always reduced to the state of sulphide of barium, by exposing it to a red heat in intimate admixture with some carbonaceous substance, such as powdered charcoal, rosin, oil or flour. It is exceedingly difficult, however, if not impossible, to effect in this manner a complete decomposition of the sulphate. Indeed, it is probable that in most cases the quantity of sulphide obtained, is not more than half that which is equivalent to the sulphate employed. A modification which promises to be far more economical was proposed by dr. Wolcott gibbs. His proposal was to submit the sulphate to the action of a current of common coal gas at a red heat. It is evident that in this way a perfect decomposition may readily be accomplished, especially if the powdered sulphate is stirred during the operation, so as to expose fresh surfaces to the action of the gas.

The mass obtained after the reduction of the sulphate is submitted to the action of boiling water, and a solution obtained, which, according to professor h. Rose,12 contains principally hydrate of baryta and sulphohydrate of sulphide of barium bas. Hs. Formed by the reaction of equal equivalents of water and proto-sulphide of barium. It almost invariably contains also a quantity of lime, probably in the form of sulpho-hydrate of sulphide of calcium, or of hydrate of lime, proceeding from the almost constant concurrence of sulphate of lime with native sulphate of baryta. From the presence of this lime originates the principal difficulty in preparing pure barium compounds from this substance. Thus when the carbonate is prepared from the solution by precipitation, with carbonate of soda, or a current of carbonic acid gas, it is found contaminated with carbonate of lime, which is fatal to its use as a reagent in analysis. Also in examining many specimens of commercial *chloride of barium*, which is prepared from this solution by the addition of chloro-hydric acid, boiling to separate sulpho-hydric acid gas which is evolved, filtration to separate the sulphur which is precipitated and crystallization, i have always found it to contain a small quantity of chloride of calcium, which i have found it impossible to separate entirely by repeated recrystallizations. It has been proposed13 to separate the chloride of calcium from chloride of barium by the use of very strong alcohol, in which the latter when anhydrous, is insoluble. This method is rather expensive and troublesome as it involves the evaporation to dryness of the chloride of barium solution, the reduction of the previously ignited residue to a very fine powder and digestion in strong alcohol. Attempts were made after some previous experimentation, in which it was found that an aqueous solution of *oxalate of baryta* precipitated chloride of calcium, but not chloride of barium, to separate the lime from a chloride of barium solution by addition of oxalate of baryta, or simply of a little oxalic acid, but it was soon found that oxalate of lime was somewhat soluble in a solution of chloride of barium, so that a solution of oxalate of baryta, gave no precipitate in a mixture of solutions of chloride of barium and chloride of calcium. It was found also that the precipitate formed by a little oxalic acid in a lime solution, could be re-dissolved by addition of chloride of barium. It may also be mentioned, though irrelevant to the subject, that it was found that oxalate of lime was soluble in solutions of chloride of calcium, of ammonia, and of chloro-hydrate of ammonia.

---

12 poggendorff's annalen, 55,416.

---

13 gmelin's handbuch, 2,158

The well known property of carbonate of baryta which the recent investigations of professor h. Rose have rendered so important in the analysis of phosphates, of completely precipitating lime from its solution by a sufficiently long contact therewith, furnishes us, however, with a perfectly easy and cheap method of purifying the chloride of barium solution. In fact a solution of chloride of barium to which chloride of calcium has been added, having been treated with a little carbonate of baryta, and allowed to stand in contact with it for two days, with occasional agitation, was found on filtration to be free from lime. The only objection to this method, is the considerable length of time required; but i must here describe an elegant modification which was communicated to me by dr. Wolcott gibbs, and tested by him in his laboratory; that is to add first to the solution of chloride of barium containing lime, a little solution of hydrate of baryta and then to pass through it a current of carbonic acid gas. The precipitate immediately formed contains of course all the lime.

The only impurity which is prevalent in commercial chloride of barium besides lime, is strangely enough, a trace of *lead* which is almost always present and sometimes in such quantity that the solution is immediately blackened by sulphuric acid.[14] this is, however, very easily removed, either before or after the separation of the lime by the process of dr. Gibbs, by passing a little sulpho-hydric acid gas into the solution, gently heating for a short time and filtering.

Commercial chloride of barium thus purified is probably the most convenient source of the other compounds of barium when required pure. Thus pure carbonate of baryta may be prepared from it by precipitation with carbonate of ammonia, or with carbonate of soda, which is free from silica, sulphuric acid and phosphoric acid.[15]

---

[14] it may be that leaden pans are used for the evaporation or crystallization of the commercial chloride of barium, which would sufficiently account for the presence of lead in the product.

---

[15] new york journal of pharmacy, 136.

RESULTS OF THE EXAMINATION OF SEVERAL PARCELS OF ALEPPO SCAMMONY.

BY B. W. BULL.

Since the publication of an article upon virgin scammony in a previous number of this journal, i have had an opportunity of examining four different varieties of scammony received from constantinople, under the names, aleppo scammony, first; aleppo scammony, second; tschangari scammony and skilip scammony.

No. 1. *Aleppo scammony, first.* This occurs in large amorphous pieces weighing one or more pounds; is not covered with any calcareous powder. The fractured surface presents a dark greenish resinous appearance. The specific gravity will be found below. The caseous odor is not so decided in this specimen as in some of the other varieties, confirming, as will be seen from its composition, as adduced farther on, the remark made in the article above alluded to, in regard to the insecurity of relying upon the odor as a means of judging of the quality of scammony.

No. 2. *Aleppo scammony, second.* Of this a sample of about one pound was received. This is in amorphous pieces; it differs from the previous specimen in its fracture which is non-resinous and horny, it is of a much lighter color, and has a grayish tinge. The scammony odor is more decided. This variety receives the prefix *aleppo* improperly, as it does not come from that locality, and is said to be made by pressing the root, though the quantity of insoluble organic matter which it contains, seems to indicate some other impurity, intentionally added.

No. 3. *Tschangari scammony*, derives its name from the place of production. It appears to be a variety not found in market here. It resembles in fracture the last mentioned, and is like that, in amorphous pieces. Its odor is more decided than that of any of the others.

No. 4. *Skilip scammony*. This specimen appears to have undergone some deterioration, and evinces a disposition to mould. Some of the pieces are marked exteriorly, as if placed in a bag when soft, and dried in this way. It is destitute of the caseous odor, and has a mouldy smell. Fracture, non-resinous, and grayish, like the last mentioned varieties.

These three latter varieties are always to be obtained in constantinople, we are informed, while the first quality aleppo, is only produced in small quantity, and is soon out of market.

The difference in composition of the different varieties will be found annexed, the numbers referring to those given above. All of them indicate the presence of starch by the test with iodine.

	No. 1.	No. 2.	No. 3.	No. 4.
Specific gravity,	1.150	1.325	1.339	1.311
	Per cent.	Per cent.	Per cent.	Per cent.
Resinous matter, water, and loss.	86.88	55.42	64.10	34.00
Vegetable substance, insoluble in ether,	8.10	38.00	23.17	59.43
Inorganic matter,	5.02	6.58	12.73	6.57
	100.000	100.000	100.000	100.000

New york, may, 1852.

WHAT IS MONESIA?

BY E. DUPUY, PHARMACEUTIST, NEW YORK CITY.

Dorvault in the *officine* gives it "as the product of a foreign bark never found in commerce, but described by mr. Bernard derosne, (who, according to the same authority is the only possessor of it,) as being found in voluminous thick pieces, filled with extractive. The color is dark brown, excepting the epidermis which is grayish. It contains tannin and a red coloring matter, analoguous to cinchonic red, also an acrid one and salts." Virey attributed it to a *chrysophi lum.*; martens says it is the *mohica* of the brazilians; according to mr. Constant berrier, it bears in that country sundry other names: *furanhem, guaranhem, buranché*, etc. Duchesne in his *répertoire des plantes utiles et vénéncuses du globe*, and descourtils in his *flore médicale des antilles* mentions the *cainito chrysophillum* the bark of which is tonic, astringent and febrifuge. In examining some extract of monesia i was struck with the striking resemblance in its properties with the extract of logwood, (*hematoxylon campechianum*) both possessing the same astringent sweetish taste, precipitating salts of iron, etc. Descourtils, who practiced medicine for a long time in the west india islands, says "it is recommendable in dysentery and diarrhea after the inflammatory period." And to that effect prescribes the decoction of one ounce of the wood or a drachm of the extract added to an infusion of orange tree leaves, or cascarilla bark, per diem. Besides, dr. Wood in the u. S. Dispensatory, mentions its frequent use in some parts of the united states, "in that relaxed condition of the bowels, which is apt to succeed to cholera infantum," and also in the same complaints as mentioned by descourtils. Though both the decoction of the wood and the solution of the extract are officinal in our national pharmacopeia, so far as my means of observation go, they are seldom, if ever, prescribed in new york, and yet i have repeatedly prepared solutions of the monesia, prescribed by our city practitioners. The extract of log-wood being so similar in its medicinal action, i am strongly inclined to think that it is the same substance, though perhaps obtained from other sources; and as the price of it is so much higher than that of the other, it would be desirable to obtain the results of comparative experiments made to test their relative value, and whether the extract of *hematoxylon campechianum* should not be prescribed as answering for all therapeutical purposes, the mysterious monesia of derosne?

THE PHARMACOLOGY OF MATICO: WITH FORMULA FOR ITS PREPARATION.

BY DORVAULT.

As matico is daily attracting more and more the attention of practitioners, its pharmacology demands consideration. It is well known that this new peruvian plant has been lauded as an efficacious remedy in leucorrhea and gonorrhea, as a vulnerary, and above all as an excellent hemostatic, both external and internal.

We shall, in the present paper, content ourselves with making known the principal pharmaceutical forms which this substance is capable of assuming, reserving all other considerations for a later period. A long and careful experience will be needed to establish the relative value of each of the subjoined forms.

POWDER OF MATICO.

Matico can be easily reduced to an impalpable powder. This powder is of a yellowish green, and its odor, when fresh is more fragrant than that of the plant itself. To preserve it well, it should be kept in well stopped bottles.

Matico powder can be advantageously used externally in sprinkling over bleeding parts, in plugging the nasal fossœ and in epithems for contusions. Internally it may be used moistened with a little sweetened water under the form of electuary or in pills.

INFUSION OF MATICO.

Bruised matico,	10 to 20 grammes.
Boiling water,	1,000 grammes.

Let it infuse until cold and strain it. This infusion is amber-colored, and possesses the aromatic odor of the plant. It is not unpleasant to take, but may be rendered more agreeable by the addition of sugar, or an appropriate syrup.

For external use, lotions, embrocations, lavements and injections, 30, 40 or even 50 grammes of matico may be used to the same quantity of water, and it may be submitted to a slight decoction. If, in this mode of operation, it parts with some volatile oil, it gains a small portion of resin.

DISTILLED WATER, OR HYDROLATE OF MATICO.

Bruised matico,	100 parts.
Water,	1,000 parts.

Draw off by distillation, 500 parts of hydrolate.

The product is colorless throughout the distillation, except the first few drops, which are milky.

Hydrolate of matico has an odor of turpentine stronger than the plant itself. It is covered with globules, or a light layer of a volatile oil, almost colorless, and of the consistence of castor oil.

If the volatile oil be, as authors have advanced, one of the active principles of matico, then the hydrolate must be to a certain extent efficacious. The hemostatic waters of binelli, broechieri, tisseraud, &c., over their property to the volatile oil of turpentine.

The hydrolate may be employed both externally and internally.

EXTRACT OF MATICO.

The one which appears to us the preferable is the hydro-alcoholic. Introduce some rather coarse matico powder into the apparatus for lixiviation, pour on it the alcohol at

56° so as to imbibe all the powder, leave it 24 hours, open the lower cock, pour the same alcohol over the same matico, until the latter is exhausted, and then evaporate the liquid in the vapour bath, till it is brought to the consistence of an extract. The product is black, with a marked odor of matico, and a bitter taste. It is only partially soluble, either in alcohol or water.

The extract of matico may be used internally in the form of pills, lozenges, syrup and electuary, and externally, dissolved or softened in the form of plasters, embrocations, plugs, lavements and injections.

Matico furnishes about ¼ of its weight of the hydro-alcoholic extract.

SYRUP OF MATICO.

Bruised matico,   100 parts.

Water,   1,000 parts.

Distil till you obtain 100 parts. Draw off the residue from the retort, press the matico, add to the product 700 parts of sugar; mix it so as to have by the addition of the hydrolate a syrup of ordinary consistence; filter it by demarest's method.

Thus prepared, matico syrup is brownish, limpid and of an aromatic taste, which is not disagreeable; it contains all the principles, active, volatile or fixed, of the substance.

It may be administered pure, or diluted with water. It is one of the easiest and most efficacious modes of administering matico in cases of internal hemorrhage or of flour albus.

It represents 1-10 of its weight of matico. The spoonful being 30 grammes, would represent 2 grammes, the tea spoonful being 5 grammes, would represent ½ gramme.

MATICO PILLS.

Powdered matico,	20 grammes.
Powdered marsh mallow	2 grammes.
Syrup of gum,	Q. S.

Make secundum artem 100 pills rolled in lycopodium. They are of a dark green. The weight of each pill from 40 to 50 centigrammes, each containing 20 centigrammes of matico, give from 2 to 25 daily.

EXTRACT OF MATICO PILLS.

Hydro-alcoholic extract of matico, 10 grammes.

Divide secundum artem into 100 pills, which will each contain 10 centigrammes. They are blackish. Being smaller they possess the advantage of being more easily swallowed.

OINTMENT OF EXTRACT OF MATICO.

Extract of matico,	5 grammes.
Weak alcohol,	5 grammes.
Lard,	20 grammes.

Make an ointment, secundum artem.

TINCTURE OF MATICO.

| Bruised matico, | 100 parts. |
| Alcohol at 85°, | 400 parts. |

Macerate for 10 days, express and filter. The tincture may also be obtained by lixiviation from the powder

It is used both internally and externally as a vulnerary; it must in the first instance be diluted with water.

Matico not being poisonous, practitioners can trace its application through the widest range.

We will again repeat that we only give these formulæ that they may be experimented on; we shall hereafter give further comments on the choice to be made amongst them.—*bulletin thèr: 30th january, 1852.*

CHEMICAL RESEARCH ON CROTON OIL.

BY M. DUBLANC. DIRECTOR OF THE LABORATORY OF THE CENTRAL PHARMACY OF THE PARISIAN HOSPITALS.

Some interesting researches have been instituted to ascertain,

A. Whether the croton oil contains within itself an acid volatile at a low temperature?

B. Is this acid the principle of its action, and can it be preserved if it be separated from the oil, and diminished if it be allowed to evaporate?

In order to answer both questions, the following operations have been instituted by this chemist.

The seeds of croton, deprived of their husks, ground at the mill, and subject to pressure, yield a certain quantity of oil.—if the residuum be mixed with double its quantity of alcohol and pressed again, it yields a liquid which is a mixture of oil and alcohol. This liquid, when distilled, will yield more oil. Both oils are filtered, after having been allowed to settle.

The produce of this first operation is the natural croton oil, such as it exists in the seeds, which is of a brown amber color, viscid, having a peculiar smell, and possessed of great acidity, by which if applied to the skin, it produces an irritation varying in intensity according to its quantity, and the duration of time during which it has been applied. One drop, for instance, causes a blister in twelve hours.

If a piece of litmus paper be dipped in this oil, it turns red, and re acts acid; and the red color, though not deep, resists the action of the air and of a hot furnace.

The oil obtained by distillation from a solution in alcohol is rather more dark, viscid, and acid, than that obtained by simple expression.

The blue paper dipped in the oil obtained by distillation, reddens, and retains the color under the same circumstances as the former.

The second operation, however, offers already a fact which is of great value in deciding the question about the acidity of the croton oil. If you dip the litmus paper in the fluid which is gained by distillation, no traces of a change of color is visible; when, on the other hand, if you dip it in the oil which remains in the distilling apparatus, it changes the color as quickly as if dipped in the oil previous to distillation. The same is the case if the residuum is again acted upon with water or alcohol, the distilled fluid has no traces of acidity.

However, since the contrary opinion is entertained by good authorities, we must add other facts in corroboration of our own.

Croton oil was extracted by the action of ether upon the seeds. The ethereal solution containing croton oil in suspension was acid: it was placed in a glass vessel with two openings. One of them admitted a straight tube, and reached to the bottom of the vessel, admitting the introduction of external air: the other communicated with woulfe's apparatus, composed,

1. Of the globular tube after liebig, containing blue solution of litmus.

2. Another globular tube filled with alcohol.

3. An angular tube in connection with a large vessel full of water, giving an inferior running to the liquid, and causing the air to pass across the thick layer of ethereal oil, to lead the volatile principles in contact with the liquor destined to retain them. The apparatus being arranged, it was put in action by causing the water to run which was contained in the large vessel. The vacuum having begun, air was introduced to the bottom of the ethereal liquid, keeping up this action till the ether was totally evaporated. Consequently, the air has agitated the liquid long enough to remove in a state of vapour all the ether which was contained in the mixture. Nevertheless, the tincture of turnesol, which opposed the passage of the vapours of ether and water, did not change into red, which would have

happened if the volatile principles should have contained any acid. Neither did the alcohol which was acted upon by the same current exhibit any sign of acid. The air saturated with ether arrived in the vessel to replace the water had no acid property; its action upon the eye-lids and nostrils was pungent and irritating, but not that of an acid. Another experiment was made with the same apparatus, having always in view to cause a great quantity of air to pass through croton oil. But this time, instead of causing the current to pass through a mass of ethereal solution, it was caused to pass through pure croton oil. The large vessel was this time not quite filled with water, allowing space to introduce on its upper part two sponges, one filled with oil, the other with ether. Things being thus arranged, the liquid was set running, and the air rushed through the oil, coming in at the bottom of the liquid and spreading through the surface, causing a lengthened ebullition. The mass of air employed in this operation was not below two centimetres. The tincture of litmus contained in the globular tubes was not altered; the oil contained in the sponge was neither acid, pungent, or corrosive. The ether acted upon by too much air had disappeared, the sponge was dry. These two proofs appear to be conclusive, and to show that the croton oil does not contain an active volatile acid, otherwise it would have been made manifest by being carried away by the ether in the first case, or by its proper volatility in the second.

Is it, however, possible to separate the active volatile principle from the mere neutral oil? It has been said by several authors that the croton oil was composed of two different oils, but this was a mere statement which required to be proved by facts. To solve this problem, the oil employed in the experiments was obtained by means of ether. The seeds of croton yield by expression 35 per cent.; treated by ether, they yield from 52 to 55 per cent. If treated by ether, the ether obtained by distillation is free from acid, all the acid remaining in the oil. When a certain fixed quantity of this oil is put in contact with ten times its weight of strong alcohol, the alcohol dissolves 6 per cent. Of its own weight, and the oil 50 per cent.

The portion of the insoluble oil has lost its color, its smell, a part of its pungency, and all its acidity.

The portion of oil which has been dissolved in alcohol, when separated from this menstruum by evaporation, is more viscid, more colored, more pungent, and acid. The oil which is not dissolved, can be acted upon again by alcohol; by this second operation, it yields some parts to the alcohol, and the remainder loses all its specific qualities. The action of alcohol upon oil in successive operation, can be followed up to its last limits.

Twenty volumes of oil mixed with 100 volumes of alcohol, will be followed by the reduction of five volumes of oil. In the next operation, when the alcohol is renewed, the volume of the columns of oil lowers only three volumes instead of five. By a fourth operation, the oil loses not a single volume. When reduced to this state, the croton oil is slightly amber-colored, without smell, taste, or acidity; it can be taken in the mouth without causing any sensation. It is soluble in all proportions in ether. Its specific gravity is, 92 compared with that of water.

Thus we find by experiments an evident proof of the co-existence of a sweet oil with the pungent croton oil.

All the specific properties of the croton oil are carried over in that dissolved by alcohol.

Is it possible by further processes to separate these active principles from the oily matter that contains them?

To solve this question we resorted to the following experiment:—

We took two kilogrammes of croton oil, and for several days we left it in contact with half a kilogramme of alcohol. A distinct separation took place. The upper part, composed of oil and alcohol, did not represent the exact quantity employed; which is explained by the power which the oil has to dissolve 10 per cent. Of alcohol. The upper part being decanted, it was necessary to remove the alcohol, to avoid the inconvenience which might have arisen by employing heat for this purpose. Water was added to this liquid, which having become turbid, ether was added. Thus the oil came with the ether to the surface. The ether was removed by free evaporation. During this lengthened process, the effluvia was so pungent as to affect the eyes and nostrils of the operator, and cause blisters to rise on his face. The oil thus obtained is dark-brown, opaque, thick, possessed of a strong smell and acidity. Applied to the skin, it causes almost instantaneous pain, followed by a blister. It is soluble in all proportions in alcohol and ether. Mixed with nine parts of its volume of olive oil, it forms a liquid possessing specific qualities stronger than those of common croton oil.

These facts prove the mobility of the active principles of croton oil, and the possibility of succeeding in obtaining them free from all fatty matter by chemical ingenuity, a task which will be the object of further experiments.

The results from the above experiments are the following:—

1. That the croton oil does not contain a volatile acid.

2. That the sensible acid in croton oil is fixed or retained in the oil, and cannot be separated from it by a heat at 212° fahr., or even by distillation.

3. That the acrid volatile principle, which exists in this oil, possesses not the qualities of an acid, and has hitherto withstood the chemical operations which were instituted to extract it.

4. That the active principles of croton oil are capable of being separated from one part of the oil, and concentrated in the other.

5. That croton oil is not homogeneous in its composition, but is formed of two parts, one inert, of which alcohol is unable to dissolve more than one-tenth, and a more soluble part, which carries with it all the active principles.

6. That the greatest degree of concentration of the active principles, is by acting upon a large quantity of oil with a small quantity of alcohol.

7. That either may be usefully employed in manufacturing croton oil.—*repertoire de pharmacie.—from the annals pharmacy*, 1852.

ON ALOINE, THE CRYSTALLINE CATHARTIC PRINCIPLE OF BARBADOES ALOES.

BY JOHN STENHOUSE, L.L.D., F.R.S.L., & E.

About two months ago i received from my friend, mr. Thomas smith, apothecary, edinburgh, a quantity of a brownish yellow crystalline substance which he had obtained from barbadoes aloes. Mr. Smith's process consisted in pounding the previously dried aloes with a quantity of sand, so as to prevent its agglutinating, macerating the mass repeatedly with cold water, and then concentrating the liquors *in vacuo* to the consistence of a syrup. On remaining at rest in a cool place for two or three days, the concentrated extract became filled with a mass of small granular crystals of a brownish yellow color. This is the crude substance to which mr. Smith has given the name of aloine, and which appears to constitute the cathartic principle of aloes. The brownish yellow crystals obtained in this way are contaminated with a greenish brown substance, which changes to brownish black on exposure to the air, and still more rapidly when it is boiled. In order to purify the crystals of aloine, therefore, they must first be dried by pressure between folds of blotting-paper, and then repeatedly crystallized out of hot water till they have only a pale sulphur yellow color. The aqueous solutions of aloine must on no account be boiled, but simply heated to about 150° f., as at 212° f. Aloine is rapidly oxidized and decomposed. By dissolving the purified crystals of aloine in hot spirits of wine, they are deposited, on the cooling of the solution, in small prismatic needles arranged in stars. When these crystals have a pale yellow color, which does not change when they are dried in the air they may be regarded as pure aloine.

Aloine is quite neutral to test-paper. Its taste is at first sweetish, but soon becomes intensely bitter. Aloine is not very soluble either in cold water or in cold spirits of wine; but if the water or the spirits of wine are even slightly warmed, the solubility of the aloine is exceedingly increased: the color of these solutions is pale yellow. Aloine is also very readily dissolved by the carbonated and caustic fixed alkalies in the cold, forming a deep orange yellow solution, which rapidly grows darker, owing to the oxidation which ensues. The effects of ammonia and its carbonate are precisely similar. When aloine is boiled either with alkalies or strong acids, it is rapidly changed into dark brown resins. A solution of bleaching powder likewise gives aloine a deep orange color, which soon changes to dark brown. Aloine produces no precipitate in solutions either of corrosive sublimate, nitrate of silver, or neutral acetate of lead. It also yields no precipitate with a dilute solution of subacetate of lead; but in a concentrated solution it throws down a deep yellow precipitate, which is pretty soluble in cold water, and is therefore difficult to wash. This precipitate is by no means very stable; and when it is exposed even for a short time to the air, it becomes brown.

When powdered aloine is thrown, in small quantities at a time, into cold fuming nitric acid, it dissolves without evolving any nitrous fumes, and forms a brownish-red solution. On adding a large quantity of sulphuric acid, a yellow precipitate falls, which, when it is washed with water to remove all adhering acid and then dried, explodes when it is heated. It plainly, therefore, contains combined nitric acid. I could not, however, succeed in obtaining this compound in a crystalline state, as when it was dissolved in spirits, it appeared to be decomposed. When aloine is digested for some time with strong nitric acid, much nitrous gas is evolved, and it is converted into chrysammic acid, but without the formation of any nitro-picric acid, as is always the case when crude aloes is subjected to a similar treatment. A quantity of aloine was boiled with a mixture of chlorate of potash and muriatic acid. The acid solution was evaporated to dryness, and digested with strong spirits of wine. The greater portion of the spirits was removed by distillation; and the remainder, when left to spontaneous evaporation; yielded a syrup which could not be made to crystallize. Not a trace of chloranil was produced.

When aloine is destructively distilled, it yields a volatile oil of a somewhat aromatic odor, and also a good deal of resinous matter. When aloine is heated on platinum foil it melts, and then catches fire, burning with a bright yellow flame, and emitting much smoke. It leaves a somewhat difficultly combustible charcoal, which, when strongly heated, entirely disappears, not a trace of ashes being left.

A quantity of aloine dried *in vacuo* was analyzed with chromate of lead in the usual way.

I. 0.2615 grm. Aloine gave 0.5695 carbonic acid and 0.14 water.

Ii. 0.2415 grm. Aloine gave 0.5250 carbonic acid and 0.126 water.

	Hydrated aloine.		Found numbers.	
	Calculated numbers.		I.	Ii.
34 c	2550.0	59.47	59.39	59.24
19 h	237.5	5.54	5.97	5.79
15 o	1500.0	35.09	34.64	34.97
	4287.5	100.00	100.00	100.00

The formula derivable from these analyses is $c_{34} h_{19} o_{15}$, which, as we shall presently see, is $= c_{34} h_{18} o_{14} + ho$, or aloine with one equivalent of water.

The aloine which had been dried *in vacuo* was next heated in the water-bath for five or six hours, and was also subjected to analysis.

I. 0.251 grm. Aloine dried at 212° f. Gave 0.550 carbonic acid and 0.128 water.

Ii. 0.2535 grm. Aloine dried at 212° f. Gave 0.564 carbonic acid and 0.129 water.

Iii. 0.234 grm. Aloine dried at 212° f. Gave 0.521 carbonic acid and 0.114 water.

	Calculated numbers.		I.	Ii.	Iii.
34 c	2550	61.07	60.51	60.67	60.72

18 h	225	5.39	5.66	5.65	5.42
14 o	1400	33.54	33.83	33.68	33.86
	4175	100.00	100.00	100.00	100.00

The aloine employed in these analyses was prepared at three different times. These results give $c_{34} h_{18} o_{14}$ as the formula of anhydrous aloine, that dried *in vacuo* being a hydrate with one equivalent of water.

When the aloine was allowed to remain in the water-bath for more than six hours, it continued slowly to lose weight, apparently owing to its undergoing partial decomposition by the formation of a brownish resin. The loss of weight gradually continued for a week or more, but became very rapid when the aloine was heated to 302° f., when it melted, forming a dark brownish mass, which when cooled became as hard and brittle as colophonium. It still, however, contained a good deal of unaltered aloine, as i ascertained by crystallizing it out with hot spirits and analyzing it. Much of the aloine, however, had been changed, most probably by oxidation, into a dark brown uncrystallizable resin.

Brom-aloine.—when an excess of bromine is poured into a cold aqueous solution of aloine, a bright yellow precipitate is immediately produced, the amount of which increases on standing, while at the same time the supernatant liquid becomes very acid from containing free hydrobromic acid. The precipitate, after it has been washed with cold water to remove adhering acid, is dissolved in hot spirits of wine; and on the cooling of the solution it is deposited in bright yellow needles radiating from centres, which attach themselves to the bottom and sides of the containing vessel.

The crystals of brom-aloine are considerably broader than those of aloine, and have a richer yellow color and a higher lustre. Brom-aloine is quite neutral to test-paper, is not so soluble in either cold water or cold spirits of wine as aloine, but dissolves very readily in hot spirits of wine.

I 0.421 grm Substance dried in vacuo gave 0.547 carbonic acid and 0.103 water.

0.856 grm. Gave 0.848 bromide of silver = 42.16 br.

Ii. 0.300 grm. Substance gave 0.391 carbonic acid and 0.078 water.

0.661 grm. Substance gave 0.649 bromide of silver = 0.2762 br. = 41.78 per cent.

	Calculated numbers.		I.	Ii.
34 c	2550.00	35.73	35.43	35.53
15 h	187.50	2.62	2.71	2.86
14 o	1400.00	19.63	19.70	19.83
3 br	2998.89	42.02	42.16	41.78
	7136.39	100.00	100.00	100.00

The brom-aloine employed in these analyses was prepared at two different times. It is plain therefore from these results, that this bromine compound is aloine, $c_{34} h_{18} o_{14}$ in which 3 equivs. Of hydrogen are replaced by 3 equivs. Of bromine.—the formula of brom-aloine therefore is $c_{34} h_{15} o_{14} br_3$.

When a stream of chlorine gas was sent for a considerable time through a cold aqueous solution of aloine, a deep yellow precipitate was produced. It contained a great deal of combined chlorine; but as it could not be made to crystallize, it was not subjected to analysis. In the present instance, and in those of several other feeble organic principles, such as orcine, chlorine appears to act some what too strongly, so that the constitution of the substance is destroyed, and merely un-crystallizable resins are produced. Bromine, on the other hand, is much more gentle in its operations, and usually simply replaces a moderate amount of the hydrogen in the substance, so that, as in the case of orcine and aloine, crystalline compounds are produced.

It has long been known to medical practitioners, that the aqueous extract of aloes is by far the most active preparation of that drug. The reason of this is now very plain, as the concentrated extract of aloes obtained by exhausting aloes with cold water consists chiefly of aloine, by much the larger portion of the resin being left undissolved. Mr. Smith informs me, that from a series of pretty extensive trials, from 2 to 4 grs. Of aloine have been found more effective than from 10 to 15 grs. Of ordinary aloes. Aloine is, i should think, therefore, likely ere long, to supersede, at least to a considerable extent, the administration of crude aloes.

I endeavored to obtain aloine by operating on considerable quantities of barbadoes, cape and socotrine aloes. These were macerated in cold water, and the aqueous solutions obtained were concentrated to the state of thin extracts on the water-bath. I was quite unsuccessful in every instance. The impurities contained in the extracts in these different kinds of aloes appear, when in contact with the oxygen of the air, to act upon the aloine so as effectually to prevent it from crystallizing. Aloine can only, therefore, be obtained in a crystalline state by concentrating the cold aqueous solution of aloes *in vacuo*; though, after the aloine has once been crystallized, and it is freed from the presence of those impurities which appear to act so injuriously upon it, the aloine may be quite readily crystallized out of its aqueous solutions in the open air.

Though aloine has as yet only been obtained from barbadoes aloes, i have scarcely any doubt that it also exists both in cape and socotrine aloes. The amount of aloine in cape aloes, is, however, in all probability, much smaller than in either of the other two species; for cape aloes is well known to be a much feebler cathartic, and to contain a mass of impurities. In corroboration of this opinion, i would refer to the fact already mentioned in a previous part of this paper, viz. That when aloine is digested with nitric acid, it is converted into dr. Schunck's chrysammic acid. Now it has been satisfactorily ascertained that all the three species of aloes yield chrysammic acid, of which in fact they are the only known sources. Cape aloes, as might have been expected, yields by far the smallest amount of chrysammic acid together with much oxalic and some nitro-picric acids. There appears, therefore, great reason to believe that all the three kinds of aloes contain aloine.

Since the above was written, i have learned from mr. Smith that he has not succeeded in obtaining crystallized aloine from either cape or socotrine aloes. Mr. Smith does not doubt that both of these species of aloes also contain aloine, though, most probably contaminated with so much resin, or some other substances, as prevents it from crystallizing. What tends to confirm mr. Smith in this opinion is the observation he has made, that when the crude crystals of aloine are allowed to remain in contact with the mother liquor of the barbadoes aloes, they disappear and become uncrystallizable. I have also observed a similar occurrence in the mother-liquors of tolerably pure aloine. These become always darker and darker; so that if we continue to dissolve new quantities of aloine in them, at length scarcely any of it crystallizes out, and the whole becomes changed into a dark-colored magma.

In the year 1846, m. E. Robiquet published an account of an examination he had made of socotrine aloes. By treating the concentrated aqueous solution of this species of aloes with basic acetate of lead, he obtained a brownish yellow precipitate, which was collected on a filter and washed with hot water. On decomposing this lead compound with sulphuretted hydrogen and evaporating the solution to dryness, he obtained an almost colorless varnish, consisting of a scaly mass, which was not in the least degree crystalline. M. E. Robiquet subjected his substance, which he called aloetine, to analysis, and obtained the following result:—

8 c =	27.7 per cent.
14 h =	10.8 per cent.
10 o =	61.5 per cent.

$$\boxed{100.0}$$

It is plain, therefore, that m. E. Robiquet's aloetine, if it really is a definite organic principle, which i very much question, is certainly a very different substance from the aloine which has formed the subject of the present notice.—*london and edinburgh philosophical magazine.*

ON HENRY'S MAGNESIA.

BY DR. MOHR.

In england, under this name is sold a calcined magnesia, at a very high price, which is not to be obtained in any other way. Many english travelers, as well as most of their countrymen, believe that they possess a very large knowledge of medicines, because such things as blue pills, calomel, sweet spirits of nitre, and laudanum they administer without medical advice, and bring this magnesia with them to our shops when they wish a recipe to be dispensed, which contains calcined magnesia as one of the ingredients. By such opportunities, i became acquainted with the purity and beauty of this preparation, and its peculiar silky gloss and whiteness. With a view to discover its method of preparation, i made the following research:—

By heating to redness the ordinary carbonate of magnesia, it is not to be obtained. The ordinary magnesia of commerce, which produces by a red heat a fine calcined magnesia, i exposed in a crucible, to a strong white heat. It solidified, and was of a yellow color, and had become so hard that it was only with the greatest labor that it could be powdered and sifted. Prepared in this way, it cannot be used. I now prepared some carbonate of magnesia, observing that henry's was very dense, without reference to that result, which was very fine, by precipitation in the heat. The process by which the flocculent magnesia of commerce is obtained, is not explained in any chemical works. Pure sulphate of magnesia, free from iron, was dissolved in distilled water, and a solution of carbonate of soda added to it as long as anything was precipitated by a boiling heat. The ebullition was continued until the mixture ceased to evolve carbonic acid, and set aside for decantation. When decanted, fresh distilled water was added to the precipitate, and the whole again boiled, and afterwards placed on a filter and washed with hot distilled water, until the liquid passing from the filter gave no trace of sulphuric acid. The precipitate, when pressed and dried, was very white and dense. It was exposed to an intense white heat in a closely-covered hessian crucible for one hour. When the crucible was opened, i found a beautifully white magnesia, finely granulated. Where it had come in contact with the crucible, it had acquired a yellow color, from the peroxide of iron contained in the crucible. The yellow portion alone adhered firmly to the crucible and the rest was perfectly white, and readily removed. In acids, this magnesia was with difficulty dissolved, although ultimately completely soluble therein. By a repetition of this process, an identical result was obtained. The magnesia thus produced in small lumps exhibited by transmitted light a slight rosy tint, and by reflected light, a very white color. In these respects, it agrees perfectly with henry's. To determine its comparative density, a cubic inch measure was filled with its powder, and weighed. As the results of three trials, it contained respectively 10,74, 11,19, and 11,18 grammes of the powder. Two experiments with henry's magnesia gave 7, and 7,2 grammes. Three of the carbonate of magnesia, prepared by heat, gave 12,68, 12,9, and 12,5 grm. One of the ordinary calcined magnesia gave 1,985 grm.; and one of the ordinary carbonate of magnesia, 1,4 grm.

The calcined magnesia, as above prepared, contains some hard particles, which are very difficult to pulverize. In attempting to powder them, i remarked that this magnesia, which was washed before being burnt until no traces of sulphuric acid could be detected, now afforded an evidence of a small portion still being present. This same observation i have previously made in the preparation of oxide of zinc. To remove this contamination, i recommend that carbonate of magnesia should first be lightly burnt, and then well washed with hot water, and again burnt with a very strong heat.

The above determinations of the density of the magnesias must not be confounded with their specific gravity. To ascertain the latter is a task of great difficulty, for rose, in attempting it, obtained such discrepant results, that he has withheld them. The specific gravity of henry's magnesia, as near as it could be ascertained, is from 2,50 to 2,67. The magnesia prepared according to my process, gave 3,148 as its specific weight.—*buchner's repertorium, in annals of pharmacy.*

MEDICINE AND PHARMACY IN BRAZIL.

In the entire brazilian empire, there are two national faculties of medicine, termed *escola imperial de medecina*, one established at rio de janeiro, the other at bahia—the present and former capitals of brazil. Both are constituted exactly alike in laws, forms, number of professors, modelled, with very trifling difference, after the constitution of the *ecole de médecine* of paris. Each college consists of fourteen professors, and six substitute professors, with a director and a vice-director, answering to our own dean and vice-dean of the faculty. The latter are named by government, from a triple list sent up by the professors every third year, and discharge the ordinary duties of their chairs, being only exempt from attending the examinations. They possess a limited controling power over their college, and constitute the official channel of communication with government and public bodies, on all matters relating to public health, prisons, &c. The duties of professor-substitute are explained in the name. When illness, or public employment—the latter not unusual in brazil—interferes with the duties of the professor, his chair is supplied by the substitute: both are appointed, as in france, by *concours*. Most of the older members have graduated in portugal, scotland, france, or italy. Both classes receive a fixed income from the state, and derive no emolument whatever from pupils and examination fees, &c. Which are applied to public purposes connected with the college. The income of the professor was fixed at twelve hundred *mil-reis* per annum—(about three hundred pounds) when first established; and that of the professor-substitute at eight hundred *mil-reis*. Both enjoy the right of retirement on their full salary, after twenty years' service, or when incapacitated by age or infirmities. A travelling professor is elected by *concours* by the faculty, every four years, for the purpose of investigating, in the different countries of europe, the latest improvements and discoveries in medicine and the collateral sciences, an account of which he regularly transmits, in formal reports, to his college. His expenses are defrayed by the state.

The medical faculty consists of the following chairs:—1, physics; 2, botany; 3, chemistry; 4, anatomy; 5, physiology; 6, external pathology; 7, internal pathology; 8, materia medica; 9, hygiene; 10, operations; 12, midwifery; 13, clinical medicine; 14, clinical surgery.

In addition to the professors, there is a secretary (medical), treasurer, librarian, and chemical assistant—all elected by the faculty.

The order of study is as follows:—first year, medical physics and medical botany; second year, chemistry and general and descriptive anatomy; third year, anatomy and physiology; fourth year, external pathology, internal pathology, pharmacy and materia medica; fifth year, operative medicine and midwifery; sixth year, hygiene, history of medicine, and legal medicine.

All examinations are public, and the subjects are drawn by lot.

The titles conferred by the faculty, are only three, viz., doctor in medicine, apothecary, and midwife. The latter is specially educated and examined.

In each chief city there are commonly three or four large hospitals—the misericordia, or civil hospital, possessed of ample funds from endowments, legacies, and certain taxes; the military and naval hopitals; and in rio, bahia, and pernambuco, leper hospitals. There are also infirmaries attached to convents. Private subscriptions to institutions are utterly unknown.

The academical session lasts for eight months—from 1st march to 30th october—lectures being delivered daily (with some exceptions) by the professors or their substitutes. The professors of clinical medicine and surgery have the right of selecting their cases from the misericordia hospital.

The student, previous to matriculation, must take his degree in arts; and the curiculum is the same for all, viz., six years to obtain the degree of doctor in medicine. The examinations are conducted as in paris. For the degree of doctor in surgery—which, however, is not essential—a subsequent and special examination must be undergone, as in france.

All students are classified, on entering college, into *medical* and *pharmaceutical*; and both are obliged to obtain the degree in arts before they can be matriculated, and to have completed their sixteenth year. The pharmaceutical student obtains his diploma of pharmacy after three years study; while that of medicine can only be obtained after six years. The student of pharmacy is obliged to repeat the courses of medical physics, botany, chemistry, pharmacy and materia medica; while one course only of each is required from the medical pupil. The pharmaceutical student is obliged to attend for three years in a pharmacy, after the conclusion of his academical studies. He then undergoes an examination by the faculty, and publicly defends a thesis to obtain his diploma. His duty afterwards, as apothecary, is strictly limited to the sale of drugs, and the compounding of prescriptions. He is never consulted professionally; and, did he attempt to apply a remedy for the cure of any disease, he would be immediately fined fifty *mil-reis* by the municipality, for the first, and an increasing fine for every subsequent offence; and, did he still persist, his licence would be withdrawn. On the other hand, the medical practioner is strictly prohibited from the compounding or sale of medicines, in any shape or form.—*dundas's sketches of brazil.*

CHEMICAL EXAMINATION OF
BROOM. (CYTISUS SCOPARIUS D. C.)

BY DR. STENHOUSE.

The broom plants examined by dr. Stenhouse, had an uncommonly bitter taste. The watery decoction, evaporated down to a tenth part, leaves a gelatinous residue, which consists chiefly of scoparin. This is a yellow colored substance, which, when purified, can be got in stellate crystals, and is easily soluble in boiling water and spirit of wine. Dr. Stenhouse, from five ultimate analyses, assigns it to the constitution $c_{21} h_{11} o_{10}$.

Scoparin is, according to an extensive series of experiments by dr. Stenhouse, the diuretic principle of broom, which has been recognised by mead, cullen, pearson, pereira, and others, as one of the most efficacious remedies in dropsy. The dose for an adult is 5 or 6 grains. Its diuretic action begins in 12 hours, and the urine under its use is more than doubled in quantity.

From the mother liquor of the crude scoparin, dr. S. Obtained, by distillation, a colorless oily liquid, which, when purified, was found to be a new volatile organic base spartein. This has a peculiarly bitter taste, and possesses powerful narcotic properties. A single drop dissolved by means of acetic acid, affected a rabbit so much, that it lay stupified for 5 or 6 hours. Another rabbit, which took four grains, first went into a state of violent excitement, then fell into sopor and died in three hours. The author observes that shepherds have long been acquainted with the excitant and narcotic action of broom.

The proportion of scoparin and spartein, varies very much in plants grown in different localities, which probably explains the very different accounts given by practitioners of its activity as a drug. The author suggests that it would be better to employ pure scoparin free from admixture of spartein.—*edin. Monthly jour. Of medical science.*

EDITORIAL.

POISONING BY TINCTURE OF ACONITE.

—the frequent use of the strong tincture of aconite root, as an external application, has, as might have been expected, given rise to repeated accidents, from the accidental or careless internal administration of that powerful substance in an overdose. An instance has occurred within a day or two, where an attendant administered a tea-spoonful of the tincture, which had been directed to be used as a liniment for a rheumatic affection. An emetic of sulphate of zinc was administered by the physician, and within five minutes after the poison had been swallowed, free vomiting was produced. This continued for several hours, though the external application of mustard poultices to the pit of the stomach, and the administration of strong coffee, with small doses of laudanum, were employed to check it. The man was naturally very stupid, and could give no clear account of his sensations. He made no complaint of his throat, until his attention was directed to it, when he said it was sore and that he had difficulty in swallowing. He had a strange, as he termed it, bursting sensation in his limbs, with constant sickness and retching, and great debility. He looked alarmed and anxious, and was restless. The pupils were at first dilated, then nearly natural, and afterwards again dilated. The extremities were cold and moist, the pulse early intermitting and weak, became extinct at the wrist, and the action of the heart was feeble and irregular. Stimulants were administered internally, but could not be retained, brandy and water with carbonate of ammonia was afterwards given in injections, per anum. And the temperature of the extremities maintained by mustard poultices, and the application of heat. After an interval of seven or eight hours the pulse again became perceptible, and the man gradually recovered.

The characteristic symptoms produced by poisoning with aconite, are a peculiar numb tingling sensation produced in the tongue and lips, a sensation in the throat, as if the palate were enlarged and elongated, and resting upon the root of the tongue, irritability of the stomach, a numb creeping or tingling sensation felt in the limbs, or over the whole surface, and depressed action of the heart, and consequent prostration and coldness of the extremities. Death when it occurs, seems to depend on the depressing effect produced upon the heart. From this it would seem that the proper treatment would be, 1st, to promote the evacuation of the poison by mild means. 2nd, to maintain the circulation, by keeping the patient as quiet as possible in a horizontal posture, by the application of sinapisms and external warmth to the extremities, and by the administration of stimulants by the mouth or when they cannot be retained, by the rectum, and 3d, to control, if possible, the vomiting.

Pereira states that aconite, when dropped in the eye, or when taken internally in poisonous doses, produces contraction of the pupils, and that with the exception of opium, it is the only article which does so. In the above case, and in one other, which was likewise seen by the writer, the pupils were dilated, and the same condition was observed in several cases which have been communicated to him.

The above case is note-worthy from the great severity of the symptoms endangering the patients life, which followed the administration of a single tea-spoonful of the poison. It must have been absorbed too, with great promptness, since the vomiting, which took place in five minutes afforded no relief. This probably depended on the stomach being empty at the time. Much of the difference observed in the effects produced by the same dose, too, doubtless depends on the variation of the strength of the tincture, caused either by the employment of different formulæ in its preparation, or by the occasional use of decayed and inferior roots in making it.

SPURIOUS SULPHATE OF QUININE.

—we understand that the article referred to in the subjoined note, has likewise been offered for sale in this city. It bears the label of pelletier, delondres & levaillant. We hope our western friends will be on their guard against this atrocious swindle.

TO THE EDITOR OF THE NEW YORK JOURNAL OF PHARMACY:—

Dear sir,—i would direct the attention of druggists and apothecaries to an article sold in new york, purporting to be quinine, put up so as to resemble the french.

It has somewhat the appearance of that article, but upon examination will be found to be totally devoid of bitterness, &c. I should suppose it to be mannite.

I am led to believe that 500 ounces have already been shipped to the west, and some has been sold in this vicinity.

I hope that your numerous subscribers may profit by this hint, and that the parties selling the same as quinine, may be frustrated in their nefarious traffic.

Your obedient servant, r. J. D.

Brooklyn, may 28, 1852.

MAGANESE.

—some attention has lately been given, lii fiances, to a variety of preparations of maganese. Maganese is commonly found associated with iron in minute quantities. It appears to be an invariable constituent of the blood, and in certain diseases, in which the iron, normally contained in that fluid, is deficient, the maganese would seem to be deficient in similar proportion. It is said that the preparations of maganese, given in connection with those of iron, in such diseases, produce effects which cannot be obtained from iron alone. Various formulæ have been offered for its administration. Commonly similar salts of the two articles, as the sulphate, lactate, carbonate, &c., are given together, the manganese being to the iron in the proportion of from $\frac{1}{2}$ to $\frac{1}{3}$. The subject would seem to deserve further inquiry.

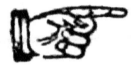

OUR EXCHANGES.

—owing to a variety of circumstances, the journal has not been forwarded with proper regularity to the editors of the journals in our own country, with whom we would desire to exchange. Exchanges and books intended for us should be directed "to the editor of the new york journal of pharmacy," care of george d. Coggeshall, 809 broadway, or of t. B. Merrick, no. 10 gold street. *Foreign exchanges* may be sent through the house of h. Bailliere, london, or j. B. Baillere, paris.

NEW YORK JOURNAL OF PHARMACY. JULY, 1852.

NOTES IN PHARMACY, NO. 3.

EXTR. LIQ. CUBEBÆ.

—the formula for this preparation, made officinal in the lately revised u. S. Pharmacopœia, appearing to me to afford rather an ethereal oil, than what may be properly called a fluid extract, i am induced to make known the process which i have been accustomed to adopt, during some years, to obtain what i conceive to be a true extract, containing, in an agreeably administrable form, all and the whole of the properties belonging to the berry, and which has given much satisfaction in practice, particularly to patients, some of whom who have had extensive experience in the use of anti-gonnorrhæl compounds, i have heard state that it is the only thing of the kind they had ever taken which was not disagreeable to the stomach. I take of

Pulv. Cubeb. Crud.   i

Ether. Sulph.

Sp. Vin rect.

Aquæ puræ āā q. S.

The coarsely powdered cubebs, being lightly packed in a displacement funnel, i pour upon it as much of a mixture of equal parts of ether and spirit of wine, as it will imbibe, and, having covered closely the top of the apparatus with moistened bladder, and corked the lower aperture, allow it to stand for twenty-four hours. I then uncork it, and after it has ceased dropping, displace the remainder with sp. Vin. Rect. Until the original quantity (generally a pint,) be obtained; this i set aside in an open and shallow vessel to *evaporate spontaneously*, until all the ether, and most of the spirit has passed off, reducing the quantity to about one half. I then obtain, by displacement with diluted alcohol, another pint of the liquid, exposing it in the same manner, until three-fourths of the quantity is evaporated spontaneously as before; again another pint is obtained by displacement with water, (this will be a proof spirit tincture,) which is added to the former, and allowed to lose by the same means, about one-fourth, or sufficient to leave a resulting quantity of one and a half pints, which will contain about eight ounces of alcohol. The displacement with water is continued to exhaustion, when enough fluid will be obtained to raise the quantity, when added to that already prepared, to two and a half pints, which is transferred to a proper bottle, and there is dissolved in it sixteen ounces of white sugar, yielding, in toto, three pints of fluid extract, equal to one pound of the berries, one F

3   Э

I of which represents   J of the dry powder. The dregs, when dried, are destitute of sensible properties, appearing to be merely ligneous remains, and the loss in weight, when time is had, may be easily calculated and compared with the recorded analyses. The extract has the appearance of a somewhat thick, brownish colored liquid, possessing the peculiar taste and smell of the cubebs in a remarkable degree, remaining homogeneous for some time after agitation, and showing after settling a large proportion of the oleaginous constituents of the berry. Having aimed more at efficiency than beauty in this preparation, i claim for it the former rather than the latter, and if it should not invite the eye, it will be found very agreeable to the palate. Fluid extract of valerian may be prepared by the same process, and, indeed, all those of a volatile nature, whose active principles are soluble in any of the above menstrua.

UNG. AQUÆ ROSÆ.

—the great trouble with this preparation is, that the water will separate from it after a time, giving it a lachrymose and unhandsome appearance. This defect is completely remedied by using *only one half the quantity* of aq.

Rosæ, by which a better consistence and much nicer preparation is obtained, and one more, in accordance with the soubriquet "cold cream," which is given to it by the fair sex, for whose use, as a cosmetic, it is far superior to the *highly scented*, and irritating fancy article of the same name. It is also an admirable unirritating, cooling, dressing for surgical use; but i would remark, *en passant*, that it is a very unfit medium for the composition of ointments, for which purpose it is sometimes prescribed to the annoyance of the apothecary. In such cases the physician should be apprised that the addition of a drop of oil of rose to simple cerate would answer his purpose much better, as the odor only is the quality desired. I think the above note might not be undeserving the attention of the next revisers of the pharmacopœias.

UNG. PERUVIAN.

It is sometimes difficult to make this ointment smooth, as, though readily miscible at first, continued trituration causes the balsam to separate, and like the colored person who "the more he was called, the more he would not come," the more it is rubbed, the more it separates. This hostility to union is readily overcome by the addition of ten drops or so of alcohol for each drachm of the balsam. It is perhaps unnecessary to state that this difficulty will not be had when the balsam is adulterated with alcohol—a good practical test of the purity of the article.

PHARMACEUTICAL ETHICS.

—morality being at present in the ascendant, as it should always be, it may not be inappropriate, though more important than practical, to "make a note" of some fashionable practices prevalent amongst the more ostentatious pharmaceutists of the day, savoring much more strongly of "quackery," to use a vulgar phrase, than art unions, &c. Are pronounced by legal wisdom to do of the "lottery." I allude, for example, to the system of *getting up*, under some mystified appellation, certain preparations, as "brown's elixir," "white's essence," or "black's compound,"—something or other, which are merely the ordinary preparations of the shop, or could easily be prepared if they were worth the trouble, but under *assumed names*, are heralded forth at the *ne plus ultra* of pharmaceutical perfectibility. I do not envy a reputation so acquired, nor do i wish to speak of it in that spirit, but to point out its inconsistency with correct principles, and designate it as unworthy of honorable ambition. Such preparations generally "hail" from some obscure place or person, but are occasionally dabbled with by others who should give themselves to better things. It is self evident, from the nature of his calling, that the exclusive duty of the apothecary *per se*, is to make, as faithfully or skilfully as he may, the various preparations of the pharmacopœia, as therein set down, when he is called upon to do so, and to compound accurately the prescriptions of the physician. If, by long experience or increased skill, he may have been led to any real discovery or improvement, the minutiæ of which he does not choose to divulge, (the reverse of which would be the more generous,) its nature should be stated, when relating to a preparation, in terms distinct enough at least, to convey an idea of its real composition and medical properties: thus tinctures should not be misnamed essences or extracts; fluid extracts, or concentrated infusions, elixirs; syrups, panaceas, &c. Thus avoiding the inconsistency of condemning, if not morally, at least *constitutionally*, the more open mountebank who plunders your pockets, while the beam is in your own eye. It is also perhaps worthy of remark that the necessity does not appear any longer to exist of retaining those prescriptively excellent preparations made by some, no doubt, very respectable apothecary in london, claiming, with a dozen others, to be the sole possessor of the original receipt. They are imported at a very high price, and as the composition of most, perhaps all, is, or can be known, might be made by any apothecary here as well as in london. Some of them might be deserving of adoption into the pharmacopœia, as have been dover's powder, daffy's elixir, &c. Already. It is said by connoisseurs in wines, that madeira is very much improved by crossing the line; but i am not aware that pharmaceutical preparations are at all benefitted by crossing the ocean. Their *genuineness*, too, has become a by-word. By the way, i was gravely informed by a certain importer, the other day, of whom i enquired concerning one of these *genuine* articles, that it was obtained directly from the inventor. I was at a loss to imagine the "modus transitûs," nor had i the hardihood to enquire, the good man having been gathered to his fathers scores of years ago.

VARIOUS ARE THE UNWORTHY PRACTICES, ONE OR TWO OF WHICH ARE THUS CURTLY ALLUDED TO, DESERVING OF A MORE STUDIED NOTICE AND SEVERE CENSURE, THAN I AM ABLE OR WILLING TO GIVE THEM. SUCH MATTERS, THOUGH NOT EXACTLY "PUTTING MONEY IN THE PURSE," SHOULD BE ATTENDED TO. THE PURGING OF OUR PROFESSION—FOR IT IS ONE—OF THEM, WOULD BE A HIGHLY MERITORIOUS SERVICE.

CHLORIC ETHER.

BY J. F. HOLTON, PROFESSOR OF BOTANY IN THE NEW YORK COLLEGE OF PHARMACY.

In the early part of this century, some chemists in holland found a peculiar oily fluid of very fragrant smell, resulted from the action of chlorine on olefiant gas. It is generally known as the dutch liquid; it has been called also chloric ether and bichloric ether. Its composition is $c_4 h_2 o_2$.

In 1831, mr. Samuel guthrie of sackets harbor, in this state, distilled alcohol from the so called chloride of lime, and obtained a product so closely resembling the dutch liquid that he though it identical. From some relations to formic acid, it was afterwards called chloroform, and chloroformid. Its composition is $c_4 ho_3$. In 1847, anaésthetic properties brought chloroform prominently before the public. We find an article by prof. B. Silliman, jr., in the american journal of science, new series, vol., 5, p. 240, in which it is stated that "the terms chloric ether, bichloric ether, perchloride of formyle, dutch oil and oil of dutch chemists, are all synonyms of chloroform."

In a recent visit of the writer at new haven he saw a prescription of "chloric ether." Being reminded of the singular error in the journal printed there, he inquired into the nature of the article dispensed. It proved to be a solution of chloroform in alcohol, and on his return to this city he found the same practice here to a small extent. The proportions in the article bearing this name vary greatly; often it seems that the mere contents of the wash-bottle are in this way disposed of, containing of course a large proportion of water. Mr. Currie, one of our most careful and consciencious chemists, usually prepares it so as to contain 10 per cent. In bulk of chloroform. A more convenient formula would be, chloroform 1 part, alcohol 10 parts. Some such article under the name of tinctura chloroformi ought to have place in our pharmacopœia.

But to our confusion the term chloric ether is applied to yet another, and entirely a different body, formed by the distillation of alcohol and hydrochloric acid, the composition of which is $c_4 h_5 o$. This is also called hydrochloric ether and muriatic ether.

But to neither of these four substances does the name chloric ether properly belong. Were there such a thing, it would be obtained from the action of chloric acid on alcohol, a reaction which is prevented by the decomposition of the chloric acid by the alcohol, to which it gives part of its oxygen, forming acetic acid.

This subject is not of so much importance intrinsically as it is by way of illustrating the extreme importance of rigid adhesion to systematic nomenclature as the only means of saving us from dangerous errors and inextricable confusion.

ON THE PREPARATION OF PURE MAGNESIA.

BY HENRY WURTZ, M. A.

The preparation of few substances presents such difficulties as that of *pure magnesia*.

It seems, however, at first glance, that the cheapness and general purity of the sulphate which occurs in commerce, would render this an easy task. Unfortunately, however, no simple process has yet been proposed for obtaining pure magnesia from the sulphate. The usual course is to precipitate from the boiling solution with carbonate of soda, and to expel the carbonic acid from the magnesia alba thus obtained, by ignition. On trying this process, however, it was found that the carbonate of magnesia thus precipitated could not be freed from soda by washing. After an enormous quantity of hot distilled water had passed through it on the filter, the slight residue left by evaporation of the washings, still gave the soda tinge to flame.

It is true that the trace of the soda compound thus retained might probably be washed out of the magnesia after its ignition, but the difficulty and tedium of the operation of washing the very voluminous precipitate, together with the expense attendant upon the necessity of using *pure* carbonate of soda, to avoid the presence of silica, phosphoric acid, and other impurities, which, if present, would inevitably contaminate the magnesia, induced me to reject this method. In fact this method, which was formerly almost used universally by analysts for the *determination* of magnesia is now rejected by them, except in some unavoidable cases.16

16 *h. Ross's handbuch*, last edition, 2, 33.

The substitution of carbonate of ammonia for carbonate of soda is inadmissible with any regard to economy, on account of the existence of the soluble double sulphates of ammonia and magnesia. A trial was made to decompose sulphate of magnesia by mixing its anhydrous powder with a large quantity of carbonate of ammonia, and igniting, but the only trace of decomposition which appeared was a slight alkaline re-action of the aqueous solution of the mass.

I must here mention an impurity which i have met with in commercial sulphate of magnesia, and this is a double sulphate of magnesia and potash, which occurs in small crystals, apparently rhombohedrons, among the rectangular prisms of the epsom salt. It may probably be separable by recrystallization, though this, with sulphate of magnesia, is rather a difficult affair.

The method which i adopted for preparing pure magnesia was the ignition of the nitrate prepared from the commercial *magnesia alba*. The impurities in the commercial carbonate which i made use of were sulphate and chloride, a surprisingly large quantity of silica, a trace of phosphoric acid easily detectable by molybdate of ammonia, oxide of iron, alumina, lime, alkalies and some organic matter. A small excess of this impure article was added to commercial nitric acid and the whole boiled; the silica, oxide of iron, alumina and phosphoric acid were thus separated by the excess of magnesia and the filtered solution contained no trace of either of them; the solution was slightly colored by organic matter.

Either of two methods may now be adopted for separating the *lime*.

One is to add a late excess of ammonia, then a little oxalic acid, and filter. To this method, besides the expense of so large a quantity of *pure* ammonia the necessity of the subsequent decomposition and expulsion by heat of the very large quantity of nitrate of ammonia formed is a serious objection.

Unsuccessful attempts were made to separate the lime by adding oxalic acid immediately to the neutral solution of nitrate of magnesia. It was found upon experiment that oxalate of lime is somewhat soluble in a solution of nitrate of magnesia.

The other method, which is preferable, consists in adding to the solution a little sulphate of magnesia, and then a quantity of alcohol, but not enough of the latter to produce any immediate precipitation. If a precipitate is formed immediately, water is added, for, singularly enough, it was found that the liquid filtered from this first precipitate still contained lime. In the course of time the sulphate of lime separates in the form of small crystals.

The filtered liquid is now evaporated in porcelain dishes, and the residue transferred to porcelain crucibles, or still better, to platinum dishes, and the nitric acid expelled by a gentle heat. By a slight modification i have succeeded in shortening this operation very much, that is by adding, from time to time, powdered carbonate of ammonia to the mass, and stirring with a glass rod, or a platinum spatula. When no more red gases are evolved the heat is raised to redness for a few minutes. The mass thus obtained requires washing with pure water to separate alkaline salts and some sulphate of magnesia which it still contains.

Magnesia thus prepared was found, by a most rigid qualitative analysis, to be perfectly pure. I am aware, however, that the process is a troublesome one, and it is very much to be desired that some one would present us with a simple and direct process of obtaining pure magnesia from the sulphate.

ON TINCTURE OF
IPECACUANHA.

BY G. F. LEROY, OF BRUSSELS.

Officinal preparations during reposition or preservation, when placed in situations proper to preserve them from all changes, yet undergo such important modifications, that the pharmaceutist is frequently obliged to reject them as worthless. We are accustomed to consider alcoholic tinctures, by reason of the vehicle used in their preparation, as amongst the most stable of officinal preparations; and therefore very few pharmacologists have observed the changes they undergo. Amongst those whose attention has been drawn to the subject, i may particularly cite: 1st, baumé, who has remarked that tincture of saffron deposits a substance analagous to amber.—(*elements of pharmacy*, 2d *ed.* 1789.)

2nd. Guibourt, who presented to the academy of medicine at paris, some observations on the changes in its composition which tincture of iodine undergoes according to the time when it was prepared, (year 1846.)

3rd. Bastick, with the desire of ascertaining the nature of the changes to which alcoholic preparations are subject, placed various tinctures, during several months, in situations similar to those of a pharmacy, that is to say, exposed to a temperature varying from 60° to 80° fahrenheit, in bottles half filled, and to which air was, from time to time, admitted.

On examining them, some time afterwards, he found that most of them had undergone active fermentation in a greater or less degree, and that the alcohol had gradually become converted into acetic acid. The tinctures had generally lost their color and taste, and contained *a precipitate which was partially re-soluble* in a proportion of alcohol corresponding to that which had been decomposed.—(*pharmaceutical journal and transactions*, 1848.)

The tinctures prepared with weak alcohol are the most subject to this species of change.

4th. Tincture of kino changes so with time, that it passes from the liquid to the gelatinized state. This change even affords an excellent test when it is suspected that catechu may have been substituted for kino in this preparation.— (*dorvault, officine*, 1850, 3d. Ed.)

In general, pharmacologists consider that tinctures only deteriorate by the evaporation of the alcohol used in their preparation, and that this evaporation has the effect of concentrating them too much, and of giving rise to the precipitation of a part of the principles which were held in solution.

I do not entirely concur in this opinion; on the contrary, i believe that, in many cases, the precipitates which are formed in the tinctures, do not arise from the evaporation of a part of the vehicle, but from a modification which takes place in a part of the principles held in solution, and which, becoming less soluble, or even insoluble, are precipitated.

Amongst these precipitates i shall place that which is almost uniformly found in tincture of ipecacuanha.

Druggists generally are aware that this tincture, shortly after its preparation, throws down a deposite of a yellowish white color, very light, and increasing daily; that when separated by filtration a new deposit immediately commences, and recourse must again be had to filtering.

It is only after three or four filterings, at intervals of five or six weeks, that the formation of this deposit can be arrested. In the course of july of this year, i prepared from the *belgian pharmacopœia*, some tincture of ipecacuanha, to be used in the preparation of some syrup of the same.

Desiring to follow the different phases which it presents, and to study, as far as possible, the nature of the precipitate formed in it, (for as yet i believe that no research has been directed to this subject.) I took advantage of the opportunity which this preparation afforded me.

About six weeks after its preparation, this tincture contained a deposit which was yellowish white, tolerably abundant, very light, and rising on being shaken.

I again suffered the precipitate to form, and after some days, i decanted the clear liquor, and threw the deposit on a filter. I afterwards mixed the decanted liquors and that which was filtered, in a bottle.

The precipitate remaining on the filter, i repeatedly washed. I put it to dry spontaneously, but perceiving, after twenty-four hours, that it was becoming the prey of a number of little cryptogami, formed in the same manner as in animal gelatine which dries slowly in the air, i hastened the desication by carrying the filter into a medium of from 30° to 35° centigrade.

This deposit, during the process of drying, loses its hydrogen, changes color, becoming reddish brown, and is slightly translucid, when very dry it is friable.

The quantity obtained in this first filtering, weighed 5 grains of the netherland weights, or 0,3250 milligrammes; from an ounce or 32 grammes of roots, employed towards the end of october, i again saved the deposit which was formed: it weighed 1 grain, netherland, or 0,065 milligrammes.

At present, at the end of november, a third deposition is taking place, and will be collected to be added to the others.

During the whole time the tincture had no effect either upon blue or red litmus paper.

Physical properties. The precipitate is solid, friable, of a reddish color, slightly translucent, without taste.

Chemical properties. Ether, alcohol, water, cold or boiling, have no action upon it; dilute hydrochloric, sulphuric and nitric acids, have no action when cold. Concentrated nitric acid, when cold, produces no effect upon it, but if heated to ebullition it attacks it actively, becoming of a brownish red color. Put in a glass tube closed by one only of its extremities, the other being furnished with two pieces of litmus paper, the one becomes blue, the other red. If the tube is placed in the flame of a spirit lamp, in a few instants the matter swells and the reddened paper becomes again blue.

Placed on a slip of platina, and exposed to the flame of a spirit lamp, it swells, giving out a strong odor of burnt animal matter; it burns without flame and leaves a white ash. This ash treated by reagents, has the characteristics of lime.

As may be seen by this short exposition, the deposit is by no means a product resulting from the evaporation of a part of the alcohol, which holds in solution the principles that are deposited, but a particular organic matter united to lime, which is formed at the expense of the azotized principle contained in the roots of the ipecac. What is the azotised principle which concurs in the formation of this substance? Certainly it is not one of those which are commonly met with in vegetables, otherwise the phenomenon which is observed in the tincture of ipecac would be observed in the tinctures made with the other roots. Is it the emetine which is decomposed? If that be the case, the tincture of ipecac would be considered rightly an uncertain preparation.

From the character assigned by m. Willigh to his ipecacuan acid, as well as to the tribasic salt of lead, (journal de chimie et de pharmacie, octobre, 1851,) it will be readily understood, how i at first thought, without, however, having made any serious researches, that it might be this acid united with the lime, to which the precipitate was owing. But the analysis made by that chemist, which denotes the absence of nitrogen in its composition, does not permit us to entertain this idea.

As will readily be perceived, my researches are far from complete, as i had not a sufficient quantity of the precipitate at my disposition. But while waiting to complete them, i did not wish to delay acquainting the learned world with a fact which appears to me extraordinary and until now unique, and at the same time to call to it the attention of those better situated than myself to pursue such researches.—*presse medicale belge.*

ON THE MODE OF ASCERTAINING THE PURITY OF ESSENTIAL OIL OF BITTER ALMONDS.

Mr. Redwood laid before the meeting some samples of *oil of bitter almonds*, prepared by different makers, together with the results of experiments he had made with the view of ascertaining whether or not they had been subjected to adulteration.

He stated, that his attention had been directed to the subject by more than one of the dealers in this article, in consequence of its having been represented that some of the samples had been adulterated with alcohol, an inference which had been drawn from the fact that the suspected samples had a much lower specific gravity than others met with in commerce.

He had been furnished with five samples from different makers, the specific gravities of which were as follows:—

1. 1052.4

2. 1055.2

3. 1067.

4. 1081.

5. 1082.2

The merchants having no better mode of testing the quality of this oil than by its flavor, its specific gravity, and other physical characters, it was important to ascertain what reliance could be placed on this class of observations. It was well known that spirit was sometimes mixed with it, the effect of which would be to reduce its specific gravity, and this addition, to the extent to which it would be likely to be made, would not impair the flavor of the oil, or alter its sensible characters in any other way than is above stated. The light oils were, therefore, very naturally suspected to have been reduced with alcohol.

The experiments he had made in reference to this subject had fully satisfied him that the specific gravity of essential oil of bitter almonds, within certain limits, could not be relied on as affording evidence of purity or adulteration. The specimens on the table, to which he had already referred, although differing in specific gravity to the extent of nearly thirty grains in the thousand grain-measures, he believed to be all free from adulteration.

Before describing the tests which he had found to afford the most satisfactory indications, he described the proximate constituents of the crude oil, which vary considerably in proportion in different samples, and hence the differences in density and in some of the properties of the oil.

According to liebig and gregory, crude oil of bitter almonds consists of *hyduret of benzoyle, hydrocyanic acid, benzoic acid,* and *benzoine,* and these probably are not its only constituents. Of these the two first may be said to be essential constituents, and the others accidental, being the result of changes which the hyduret of benzoyle, or true oil of bitter almonds, undergoes.

The *hyduret of benzoyle* has the ordinary characters of an essential oil. When pure it is a colorless, transparent liquid, the specific gravity of which is 1043. It possesses the peculiar almond flavor, and is not poisonous. This, which is the true oil of bitter almonds, ought to constitute about eighty-five or ninety per cent. Of the crude oil. When oil of vitriol is added to pure hyduret of benzoyle the mixture acquires a dark reddish brown color, but no other visible change takes place.

If the hyduret of benzoyle be exposed to the air it speedily becomes oxidized, and by the substitution of an atom of oxygen for one of hydrogen it is converted into benzoic acid. The *benzoic acid* present in oil of bitter almonds is the result of this transformation, and sometimes it occurs to such an extent that it is deposited from the oil in crystals Benzoic acid is not colored by the action of oil of vitriol.

Benzoine is also a product of a remarkable change which hyduret of benzoyle, when mixed with hydrocyanic acid, is liable to undergo. Like benzoic acid, it is a solid crystalline body, but unlike benzoic acid, when mixed with oil of vitriol, it forms a violet colored compound.

The characters and properties of *hydrocyanic acid* arc too well known to require notice. It is this constituent, which is sometimes present to the extent of eight or ten per cent., that gives to oil of bitter almonds its poisonous properties.

In examining oil of bitter almonds, with the view of determining whether it be pure or not, it is necessary to consider the influence on the action of the reagents employed, of variations in the number and proportions of the several constituents present. This is especially the case with reference to the use of oil of vitriol as a test.

On adding *oil of vitriol* to the samples of oil under notice, it was found that it formed with all of them a clear but very dark colored mature, from which no separation took place. The color of the mixture thus produced, however, differed to a greater or less extent in each case. The lightest of the oils produced a reddish-brown color, similar to that afforded by pure hyduret of benzoyle, while the heaviest oil formed a bright red mixture, having a shade of violet, and those of intermediate density gave intermediate shades of color.

These results, viewed in connection with the differences of density in the different specimens, were at first thought to indicate that the light specimens had some admixture foreign to the oil, but on examining the action of the test on pure hyduret of benzoyle and the other legitimate constituents of the crude oil, it was evident that such an inference could not be justly drawn, and, indeed, suspicion now seemed rather to attach to the heavy oil. Subsequent experiments, however, showed that the light oil distils at a lower temperature than the heavy, and that if the heaviest specimens were distilled with water, the first portions that passed over produced precisely the same reaction as the light specimens above referred to, while the last portions that passed over, and especially the oil obtained from the water by distilling it, after saturating it with common salt, produced with oil of vitriol a splendid crimson color, the purity and intensity of which could hardly be surpassed.

It thus became pretty evident that the differences in the reaction of oil of vitriol with the different specimens of oil under notice, arose from variations in the circumstances under which the oils were distilled, and it seemed probable that the heavy oil had been obtained by distilling the almond cake with water, to which a large quantity of salt had been added, so as to raise the point of ebullition, while the light oil either was the product of a process in which less salt had been added to the water, or consisted of the first portions distilled.

In order to obtain more satisfactory evidence of the absence of spirit, or other foreign substance, from these samples of oil, *nitric acid* was used as a test. If oil of bitter almonds be mixed with about twice its volume of nitric acid, of specific gravity 1.420, no immediate action occurs. The greater part of the oil floats over the surface of the acid, and, if the former be free from adulteration, no change of color takes place within several hours in either; but after the lapse of three or four days crystals of benzoic acid will begin to be formed from the oxidation of the hyduret of benzoyle by the nitric acid, and these will increase in quantity until the whole becomes a solid mass of crystals, which will gradually assume a bright emerald green color. This reaction is very characteristic. If spirit be present in the oil to the extent of eight or ten per cent., the acid, after a few minutes, will begin to react upon this, and a violent effervescence will shortly ensue, accompanied by the disengagement of nitrous vapors.

By using strong nitric acid, of specific gravity not less than 1.5, the presence of a very minute quantity of spirit may be detected. The pure oil, when mixed with an equal volume of this strong acid, forms a clear and uniform mixture, from which nothing separates, and which undergoes but a very slight change of color and no other visible alteration. The presence of two or three per cent. Of spirit, however, is sufficient to cause a violent reaction and the disengagement of nitrous vapors.

After trying several other reagents, the foregoing were those which were found to afford the most satisfactory results, and appeared to be conclusive with regard to those adulterations, likely to be practised.—*pharmaceutical journal, london.*

ON HOFFMAN'S ANODYNE LIQUOR.

BY WILLIAM PROCTER, JR.

Perhaps in no preparation in general use does the practice of manufacturers, and the requirements of pharmacopœial authorities, more widely differ than in the compound spirit of ether, universally known as hoffman's anodyne liquor. According to the united states and london pharmacopœias it consists of three fluid drachms of heavy oil of wine (oleum ethereum, U. S. P.,) dissolved in a mixture of eight fluid ounces of ether and sixteen fluid ounces of alcohol. The edinburgh pharmacopœia has only the simple spirit of ether, without the oil of wine, whilst the dublin pharmacopœia of 1850 under the name of spiritus æthereus oleosus, gives the following formula, which includes the preparation of the oil of wine and its subsequent solution, to make the anodyne:—mix a pint of alcohol and a pint and a half of oil of vitriol in a glass matrass, adapt a liebig's condenser, and by heat distil until a black froth rises. Separate the lighter etherial liquid in the receiver, expose it for 24 hours in a capsule, wash the residual oil with water, and dissolve it in a mixture of five fluid ounces of ether, and ten fluid ounces of alcohol. In france, hoffman's anodyne consists of equal parts of ether and alcohol, without oil of wine.

Owing to the careless or intentionally mystified manner of expressing himself, it is impossible now to ascertain whether the original preparation of hoffman (published in 1732) was constant in its strength, as now recommended by the pharmacopœia. Beaumé, (as quoted in macquer's chem. Dict., london, 1771,) says, in speaking of the rectification of sulphuric ether, "by distilling the liquor in the first receiver, together with a very small quantity of oil of tartar, by a very gentle heat of a lamp furnace, about two pounds and four ounces of pure ether may be obtained; and afterwards, when a new receiver is adapted, and a stronger heat applied, from eight to ten ounces of aromatic liquor, which makes a good *anodyne mineral liquor of hoffman*, will be distilled."

The third edition of lewis' dispensatory, published at dublin, 1768, has the following formula for this preparation, which appears to be what the apothecaries of that day employed:—

"hoffman's mineral anodyne liquor."

Into half a pound of concentrated oil of vitriol, placed in a large glass retort, pour by little and little, through a long stemmed funnel, one pint and a half of highly rectified spirit of wine. Stop the mouth of the retort, digest for some days, and then distil with a very gentle heat. At first a fragrant spirit of wine will arise; and after it a more fragrant volatile spirit, to be caught in a fresh receiver. The receiver being again changed, a sulphurous, volatile, acid phlegm comes over, and at length a *sweet oil of vitriol*, which should be immediately separated, lest it be absorbed by the phlegm. Mix the first and second spirits together, and in [every] two ounces of this mixture dissolve twelve drops of the sweet oil. If the liquor has any sulphurous smell, re-distil it from a little salt of tartar.

"whether this is the exact preparation, so much recommended and so often prescribed by hoffman as an anodyne and anti-spasmodic, we cannot determine. We learn from his own writings that his anodyne liquor was composed of the dulcified spirit of vitriol, [crude ether] and the aromatic oil which rises after it; but not in what proportions he mixed them together. The college of wirtemburg seems to think that all the oil was mixed with all the spirit obtained in one operation without regard to the precise quantities."

The product of this recipe must have been analogous to the present officinal spirit, the formula for which is evidently modeled after it. The great excess of alcohol distills over first, until the boiling point rises to the ether producing temperature, when ether is obtained, and finally the sulphurous oily product. The recipe gives no direction to isolate the oil of wine before measuring it, which is perhaps less necessary, as the ethereal part of the distillate is removed previously to the production of the oil which is found in the receiver in globules, and not in solution.

The process now adopted by the manufacturers in this city, avoids the isolation of the oil of wine, and from the nature of the conditions the product is liable to vary in the proportions of its ingredients, not only in different laboratories, but at different operations in the same laboratory. In the preparation of ether it is usual in this city to push the process as far as possible, as long as the residue is not so concentrated as to eliminate much permanent gas. In the rectification of this first crude product, the distillate is reserved as rectified ether as long as its specific gravity marks 54° beaumé, or there about. By continuing the process the product is found to consist of ether, alcohol and water, impregnated with oil of wine. Every one who has made ether, knows how very liable the product is to vary with an ill regulated heat; on the one hand unaltered alcohol will pass over, if the temperature is too low, whilst too great a heat, especially towards the last of the process, will favor the formation of oil of wine and sulphurous acid. This last distillate, therefore, will vary in composition, and it is from this that hoffman's anodyne is made in some of the best of our laboratories. *There is no known practicable method of ascertaining the per centage of heavy oil of wine in this liquid.* The means used by the manufacturer are founded on the sensible properties of an arbitrary standard specimen of hoffman's anodyne previously made, and on the degree of opalesence or milkiness it produces when added to a certain measure of water.—this milkiness is occasioned by the oil of wine present; but experience has shown that the degree of milkiness is not strictly in proportion to the quantity of oil present, the relative proportion of ether and alcohol, and perhaps water present in the anodyne liquid has a marked influence on the phenomenon; if too much alcohol, the milkiness is not produced, or but partially; if too much ether, oily globules separate and float with but moderate opalescence. In converting this second etherial distillate into commercial hoffman's anodyne, the operator has to make several essays, sometimes adding water, sometimes alcohol or ether, until the taste, the smell, and the opalescence agree, as nearly as can be approached, with his standard specimen. In the process of rectification it is probable that at least a part of the heavy oil of wine is decomposed with the production of the light oil or etherole, and that the commercial hoffman's anodyne differs in this respect, as well as in containing a much smaller proportion of oil of wine, from that of the pharmacopœia.

To get a better idea of the preparation in use here, authentic specimens were obtained from four of our largest manufacturing chemists, and compared with compound spirit of ether made for the occasion strictly according to the united states pharmacopœia. Their density was carefully taken with the 1000 grs. Bottle.

	Specific at 60° f.	gravity
A, wetherill & brothers,	.8925	
B, smith, pemberton & co.	.8723	
C, rosengarten & dennis,	.8495	
D, powers & weightman,	.8394	
E, u. S. Pharmacopœia	.8151	

Equal measures of each specimen and distilled water were mixed together; they all produced opaque milky liquids; globules of oil of wine soon separated from the mixture with e, and floated on the surface, while the liquid gradually lost its opacity as more of the oil arose. The mixture with d became less opaque by standing, a small portion of oil rising to the surface. The mixture with a, b and c retained their opacity without apparent separation of oil of wine, a being the most so.

A was the mildest and least repulsive to the taste, because least ethereal. C was the next least ethereal, but had pungency not arising from ether. B was more ethereal than the preceding, notwithstanding its greater specific gravity. D was yet more charged with ether. E presented sensible properties differing from all the others, being more ethereal and aromatic, but without a peculiar taste noticeable in the other specimens, more especially in c.

When 2½ fluid drachms of each specimen was shaken in graduated tubes with 60 grains of carbonate of potassa, they were de-hydrated somewhat in the ratio of their specific gravities. A and b dissolved the salt readily by a few minutes' agitation, and the separated aqueous alkaline solution equalled a third of the bulk of the mixture. In c and d only about half of the salt was dissolved, whilst in e the salt was merely rendered pasty.

To get an idea of the proportion of ether present in these specimens, a solution of dry chloride of calcium in an equal weight of water, was made. Five parts of this solution was mixed with three parts of each of specimens of hoffman's anodyne, in tall tubular vials, corked, well agitated and allowed to stand for twelve hours. In a, b and c, no separation of ether occurred, but in each of them a few globules arose to the surface, consisting chiefly of light oil of wine. In d a stratum of ether holding oil of wine in solution, equal to one seventh of the bulk of the spirit used, or nearly half a part. Whilst in e the super-stratum of ether equalled one-third of the spirit used, and had a light yellow color, due to the oil of wine.

These data will give an approximative idea of their compositions; it would appear that a was chiefly alcohol and water, with but little ether; that b contained almost as much water as a, but less alcohol and more ether; that c contained much less water than a or b, but less ether and more alcohol than b, and more ether and less alcohol than a; that d contained rather more water than c, but more ether and less alcohol than either of the preceding; and lastly that e contains more ether, and less alcohol and water than either of the others.

In regard to the proportion of ethereal oil, the experiments give no positive clue. It would appear that b and d contained the most among the commercial specimens, and that d approaches nearest the composition of the officinal spirit, yet all of them when compared with the officinal are deficient in this ingredient.

It must be apparent from these results, that the opacity of a mixture of hoffman's anodyne and water, is no index of the proportion of oil of wine the former contains, that property being dependent apparently on the state of combination in which the oil exists, nor would we pronounce on the medicinal value of the specimens, a task belonging to the physician. Whatever curative reputation the compound spirit of ether may have earned, certainly belongs to the commercial spirit, and not to that of the pharmacopœia, which is not to be had in the shops.

The exact nature of the liquid left after the rectification of ether is an inquiry well worthy of further investigation. The alcohol of commerce is not a homogenous substance. Besides water, it contains odoriferous oily matter, produced in the original fermentation, and which is not wholly removed in the rectification of whiskey. This matter, modified by the action of sulphuric acid and heat, with the volatile substances generated during the ether process, are contained in it. It may also be that the ether in this residue is more intimately combined with water than in a mere mixture of water, alcohol, and ether of the same strength, as suggested to me by mr. Pemberton.

The question very naturally arises, why do not the manufacturers prepare the officinal hoffman's anodyne, or why do they not furnish the ethereal oil of the pharmacopœia, that the apothecary may make it himself by simple mixing? There are several reasons. 1st, the apothecary, the physician, and to a large extent the consumer, have become accustomed to the present commercial preparation, and the majority, both of apothecaries and physicians, would reject the true officinal spirit, if presented to them, as not correctly made; 2d, druggists, as a general rule, would refuse to pay the greatly increased price, absolutely required to remunerate the manufacturer, for the greater consumption of time and materials, and increased skill and risk in manipulation. Having, on several occasions, prepared the officinal oil of wine and hoffman's anodyne, i can corroborate the statements of mr. Kent, at p. 255, relative to the small yield, and consequent costliness of officinal heavy oil of wine. The so-called oil of wine, which is imported into this city from england, and which is sometimes employed for making the officinal spirit, is an ethereal solution of etherole, one specimen yielding only seven per cent. Of it. And 3d, in the preparation of ether, the residue left in the still after the rectification of the ether above 54° beaumé, must either be thrown away, or converted to the only use to which it can be applied with advantage, viz., hoffman's anodyne. It is for this reason that the price of the commercial "anodyne" is so low, being about fifteen cents per pound.

It may become a question in the next revision of the pharmacopœia, whether it would not be better to reconstruct the formula for compound spirit of ether, somewhat on the plan of the manufacturers, or that quoted at page 213, from lewis's dispensatory, so as to render it more practicable and likely to be followed. Of course it should be done with due consideration of the difficulties involved in the production of a spirit of uniform strength.—*american journal of pharmacy.*

ON GUTTA TABAN.

BY BERTHOLD SEEMANN.

The taban (*isonandra gutta*, hook.), which was formerly so plentiful [in singapore], has long since been extinct. A few isolated trees may here and there occur, but they are very scarce, and i have not been able to obtain even the sight of one. Several of the white residents keep in their gardens as a curiosity, a plant or two, but they grow very slowly. It must ever be an object of regret, that on the first introduction of the taban gum, its proper name was not promulgated. Now everybody in europe and america speaks of gutta percha, when, in fact, all the time they mean the gutta taban. The substance termed by the malays "gutta percha" is not the produce of the *isonandra gutta*, hook., but that of a botanically unknown tree, a species of *ficus*, i am told. The confusion of these two names has become a popular error—an error which science will have to rectify.

The exportation of the indigenous gutta taban from singapore commenced in 1844, but as early as the end of 1847, all, or at least most, of the trees had been exterminated. That at present shipped from the place, is brought in coasting vessels from the different ports of borneo, sumatra, the malayan peninsula, and jahore archipelago.17 the difference existing in its appearance and property is owing to the intermixture of gutta percha, jelotong, gegrek, litchu, and other inferior guttas, made by the natives in order to increase the weight.—though far from being extinct in the indian archipelago, gutta taban will every year be more difficult to obtain, as the coast region is said to be pretty well cleared, and a long transport from the interior must, by augmenting the labor, increase the value of the article.

---

17 "the total export of gutta taban from singapore has beeni

In 1844   1 picul

In 1845	169 picul
In 1846	5,364 picul
In 1847	9,296 picul
In 1848 to the 1st of july	6,768 picul
Total	21,598 piculs.

Valued at 274,190 spanish dollars. About 270,000 trees have probably been felled during the three and a half years that the trade has existed, and the value of each tree has thus on an average, been about a dollar."—j. R. Logan, *"on the range of the gutta taban collectors, and present amount of import into singapore."* Mr. Logan has promised an article on the various substances intermixed with the taban, a subject of the highest interest; but he has hitherto disappointed his readers.

A few months after the publication of your first account of the plant, in january, 1847, an article on the same subject appeared in the *journal of the indian archipelago*, by one of its most able contributors, dr. T. Oxley. As that article contains many statements not contained in yours, and as it may possibly have escaped your notice, i shall make a few extracts from it.

"the gutta taban tree belongs to the natural order *sapotaceæ*, but differs so much from all described genera, that i am inclined to consider it a new one. I shall, therefore, endeavor to give its general character, leaving the honor of naming it to a more competent botanist, especially as, from want of complete specimens, i have not quite satisfied myself regarding the stamens and fruit.

"the tree is from sixty to seventy feet high, from two to three feet in diameter. In its general aspect it resembles the durian (*durio zibethinus*, linn.), so much so as to strike the most superficial observer. The leaves are alternate, obovate-lanceolate, entire, coriaceous, their upper surface is of a pale green and their under surface covered with a close, short, reddish-brown hair. The flowers are axillary, from one to three in the axils, supported on short curved pedicels, and numerous along the extremities of the branches. The calyx is inferior, persistent coriaceous, divided into six sepals, which are arranged in double series. The corolla is monopetalous, hypogenous, and divided, like the calyx, into six acuminate segments. The stamens, inserted into the throat of the corolla, are in a single series, and variable in number, but to the best of my observation, their normal number is twelve; they are most generally all fertile. The anthers are supported on slender bent filaments, and open by two lateral pores. The ovary is superior, terminated by a long single style, and six-celled; the cells are monospermous. The fruit is unknown to me.

"only a short time ago the taban tree was tolerably abundant on the island of singapore, but already, (middle of 1847) all the large timber has been felled. Its geographical range, however, appears to be considerable, it being found all up the malayan peninsula, as far as penang, where i have ascertained it to be plentiful. Its favorite localities are the alluvial tracts on the foot of hills, where it forms the principal portion of the jungle.

"the quantity of solid gutta obtained from each tree varies from five to twenty catties, so that, taking the average of ten catties, which is a tolerably liberal one, it will require the destruction of ten trees to produce one picul. Now, the quantity exported from singapore to europe, from the 1st of january, 1845, to the middle of 1847, amounted to 6,918 piculs, to obtain which, 69,180 trees must have been sacrificed! How much better would it be to adopt the method of tapping the tree practised by the burmese, in obtaining the caoutchouc, than to continue the present process of extermination."18

18 t. Oxley, in the *journal of the indian archipelago*, vol. 1, p. 22–30.

A mercantile house in singapore lately received from manilla a gum which was supposed by those who sent it to be gutta taban, but proved a different substance. It was accompanied by specimens of the tree producing it, and a note stating that the gum abounded in the philippine islands. As it will probably make its appearance in england, and perhaps become of some importance, i may add that those specimens presented to me by the merchant, belong to the genus *ficus*; but whether to a new or an already described species, want of books prevented me from determining.—*hooker's jour. Of botany.*

ON GAMBIR.

BY BERTHOLD SEEMAN.

Black pepper (*piper nigrum*, linn.) And gambir (*uncaria gambir*, roxb.) Are grown in great quantities [in singapore], and exclusively by the chinese, for both these articles are so exceedingly cheap, that europeans have not deemed it worth their while to engage in the speculation. Pepper and gambir plantations are always combined, because the refuse of the gambir leaves serve as an excellent manure for the pepper; and moreover, what is of equal, if not greater importance, kills the lalang, (*andropogon caricosus*, linn.), a plant which, like the couch-grass (*triticum repens*, linn.), spreads with astonishing rapidity over the fields, growing so close together and so high, that within a short spate of time valuable plantations are rendered useless, and many have to be given up from the utter impossibility of freeing the ground from this weed.

The process by which gambir is extracted and prepared is simple. The leaves are boiled in water, until all their astringent property is extracted. The decoction is then poured into another vessel, in which it becomes inspissated, and, when nearly dry, is cut in small square pieces, and thus brought into the market. M'culloch states that sago is used in thickening it. This, however, at least in singapore, is not the case; but, instead of sago, a piece of wood is dipped into the vessel, by which the desired effect is produced. It must, indeed, be an extraordinary substance, the mere dipping of which into the fluid can cause it to become a thickened mass. I was very eager to obtain a piece of this wood; unluckily, the chinaman whose laboratory i visited, could not be persuaded to part with his, and a friend of mine, who was exerting himself to procure a sample, had not succeeded at the time of the herald's departure: he promised however, to send it to england, accompanied by the malayan name, and specimens of the tree.—*hooker's journal of botany.*

ON THE GALBANUM PLANT.

BY F. A. BUSHE.

The author states, that in his travels in persia he discovered the plant which yields galbanum. In june, 1848, he found it on the declivities of the demawend. It is a ferula, from the stalks of which a liquid issues abundantly, by the odor and nature of which he immediately recognised galbanum, and his guides assured him, moreover, that galbanum is gathered from this plant. The author has not yet distinctly determined the plant. It appears to differ from *ferula erubescens* (*annales des sciences*, iii., sér. 1844, p. 316,) only by the absence of commissural vitæ; but as neither aucher-eloy, nor kotschy, who have both collected the ferula erubescens, make any mention of its yielding galbanum, the author is in doubt whether his plant be the same, or a variety of it. Don's genus galbanum (trib. Sibrinæ) and lindley's opaïdia (trib. Smyrneæ) do not agree with the plant seen by bushe, unless that both of these authors have made their descriptions from imperfect fruits, or that there exist other plants which yield galbanum.—the plant which bushe describes is called in some parts of persia, *khassuch*, (not *kasneh*, which means cichor intybus, nor gäshnis, which is coriand. Sativum), and appears to be confined to certain districts of persia. In the whole large district of the elburs-chain, from the south-east angle to the south-west angle of the caspian sea, it is only found in the neighborhood of the demawend; but here at an elevation of from 4000 to 8000 feet, and even on the declivity of the top of the demawend. It exists neither on the mountains of talysch, nor in the districts of karadagh and tabris. It is said to re-appear on the mount alwend, near hamadan, and in the neighborhood of the great salt desert. Near hamadan aucher-eloy has gathered his ferula erubescene, and this supports the supposition that the author's plant is the same. In the salt desert itself bushe did not meet with it again. The inhabitants of the demawend collect the gum resin, which issues spontaneously from the lower part of the stalk; they do not make incisions in the plant; but it is not at this place that the galbanum is collected for commercial purposes. When fresh, the gum resin is white like milk, liquid, and somewhat glutinous. In the air it soon becomes yellow, elastic, and finally solid. The odor is rather strong, unpleasant, and similar to that of our commercial galbanum.—*central blatt*, für 1852, no. Xiii.

EDITORIAL.

THE PREVENTION AND CURE OF MANY CHRONIC DISEASES BY MOVEMENTS.

An exposition of the principles and practice of these movements, for the correction of the tendencies to disease in infancy, childhood and youth, and for the cure of many morbid affections of adults. By m. Roth, m. D., london, 1851.

Open quackery was at one time contented with the market-place and the stage; its merits and achievements were announced only by the lungs of its professors and their assistants. We have changed all that. Quackery has improved with the age. It has got possession of the newspapers, and forces its way in the pulpit; it has its colleges and graduates, it edits journals and writes books; but it has changed its form, not its spirit; at bottom it is as shameless, and lying and rediculous as ever. While its essence is eternal its form is constantly changing. A variety springs up, flourishes, attains its maturity, then dies away, to be replaced by another, or to be revived in a distant country or a future generation. The facilities of intercommunication afforded by railroad and steam vessels yield the same advantage to imposture and credulity, that they give to science and truth. We import nonsense and humbug as well as silks and dry goods. But as was observed on another occasion, home manufacture has sprung up, and we have become exporters as well as importers. Spiritual knocking are set off against mesmerism; thompsonianism is sent in exchange for hygeia; native sarsaparillas have driven the foreign from the market; mormonism goes a long way to balance homeopathy, while the "great harmonican," in size, in pretension and in absurdity, is scarcely to be rivalled any where in the present age.

The newest delusion that pretends to be a system, kinesipathy, is, in the country of its origin, already several years old. It comes to us from sweden, and recommends the treatment of diseases by means of various exercises, and above all, blows on different parts of the body. All these are set forth with the greatest gravity, and defined and commented on with as much precision as if the author was bringing forward a national pharmacopœia. In the treatment of disease the motives, positions, and blows, are varied in the strangest, and often most ludicrous manner. Witness the following *prescription* for gonorrhea, which is complete except as the author states "some movements depending on particular circumstances."

1. "percussion on the sacrum in the stride standing position.

2. "transversal chopping on the neck in the sitting position.

3. "pressure above the os pubis in the lying position, with elevated back, while the separated and bent legs are drawn towards the abdomen. Vibration of the perineum, in the same position."

"the treatment begins with percussing the sacrum, in the stride standing position, which in the first day or two not only allays and relieves the more violent inflammation and copious secretion, but also changes the whole state of the disease in such a manner, that the following treatment by movements, (different according to the state of the patient,) produces an increased flow of arterial blood in the upper extremities, and the cure is very much accelerated. In the first stage, during which only moderate stitching pains, tension, and little secretion appears; the percussion on the sacrum alone is sufficient, if repeated three or four times daily. If the symptoms become more violent, and accompanied by chordee and pain during urinating, &c., then other movements are necessary, then make use of the transversal chopping of the neck, which acts strongly against the chordee, and of the pressure above the os pubis in the above mentioned lying position, which increases the venous absorption of the bladder and sexual organs, by its effect on the excited nerves of these parts. In the second period if the urinating is very difficult, the perineum swollen and painful, the discharge mixed with blood, and fever is present, then a more general treatment is necessary. To increase the more local absorption in the urethra, vibrations along the whole tract of the perineum from before backward are employed."

That percussion on the sacrum has long been known as a remedial measure in moral complaints we are perfectly aware, but that it was to become an article of materia medica is something new under the sun!

Kinesipathy has not yet, we believe, been formally introduced into the united states, but we hear that a new set of quacks, who call themselves psychologists, have adopted something from its rules, and are employing "percussions and flagellations" as one of their means for the cure of the various ills that flesh is heir too.

After all some partial truth, long well known and acted on by the profession, as is the case in most successful quackeries, underlies kinesipathy. Exercise and stimulation of the external surface, are in themselves exceedingly beneficial, and under the influence of a charlatan, patients will submit to a discipline, which if directed by a physician would never receive more than momentary attention.

PHARMACY IN RICHMOND.

—we are glad to see the following call to the apothecaries of richmond, in the july number of the american journal of pharmacy, and we hope that the example will be imitated in all our towns, in which the number of pharmaceutists is sufficient to form a society. Mutual association is the best means of promoting the true interests and standing of the profession.

"the undersigned, believing that by friendly co-operation among themselves, their respectability will be increased; their standing in the community will become more elevated, faults in their profession be remedied, evils to which they are now subjected be removed; that their art may be more systematized, and better regulated; a more friendly feeling towards each other be excited amongst them, their mutual interests advanced, and the public good promoted; do most earnestly call upon their brethren, engaged in pharmaceutical pursuits, to meet at the gentlemen's parlor, exchange hotel, on friday evening, 11th inst., at 8 o'clock, for the purpose of considering the advantages that would result to all of them, from the formation of some organized association, that would have for its object the above named desirable ends; as well as to encourage among themselves mutual improvement in the knowledge so necessary to a proper discharge of those duties, (both to themselves and the public,) which their situations as men occupying positions among the most responsible in life, impose upon them.

As the organization which it is now proposed to form, would contemplate the good of all its members, it is most earnestly hoped that all the druggists and apothecaries who feel any interest in this important subject, will cordially unite their intelligence and talents in an effort to accomplish the above named ends, and that the proper preliminary steps will be taken for the formation of a society of the apothecaries in this city, which will prove beneficial to its members, an honor to their profession, and a credit to the city of richmond."

Andrew leslie,

S. M. Zachrisson,

Purcell, ladd & co.,

Seabrook & reeve,

Adie & gray,

Peyton, johnston & bro.,

H. Blair,

Chas. Millspaugh,

Alex. Duval.

Richmond, june 8th, 1852.

SUPPOSITORIES OF BUTTER OF CACAO.

—butter of cacao has of late been largely employed in the formation of suppositories, for which it is admirably adapted, by its consistence, and by the facility with which it becomes liquid at the temperature of the body. Some times a good deal of difficulty is encountered in incorporating it with laudanum, chloroform, extracts and solutions. In such cases m. Stanislas martin recommends that the butter be first moulded in the desired form, and that then a cavity be formed in it, by means of an iron wire slightly warmed, sufficiently large to contain the prescribed medicine. The orifice can then be closed with a thin layer of the butter of cacao, formed by rubbing a morsel of it upon an iron spatula, or the blade of a knife slightly warmed in a spirit lamp.

A number of the suppositories thus prepared beforehand, can be preserved in envelopes which serve them for a mould, these being removed only when they are about to be used.

Delegates to the convention for 1852.

At a meeting of the college of pharmacy of the city of new york, held june 28th, messrs. George d. Coggesshall, william hegeman and l. S. Haskell, were elected delegates from this college to the national pharmaceutical convention, to meet at philadelphia, on the first monday in october next. It was resolved that in case of any disability of either of their number to attend, the remaining delegates should be authorised to fill the vacancy.

The re-issue of president guthrie's official call for the meeting of the convention was expected in time for this number of the journal, but has not been received. It will doubtless appear in our next with a further notice of this important subject.

AMOUNT OF LOSS IN POWDERING VARIOUS DRUGS.

The following results are from the mill returns of a drug house in this city. They show the actual loss incurred in powdering these different articles, and are, so far, of service by indicating the practical loss arising from the process.

As the per centage of loss varies very much with the quantity subjected to the process, *ceteris paribus*, the quantities of each parcel are also given.

	Quantity lbs.	Percentage of loss	Quantity lbs.	Percentage of loss	Quantity lbs.	Percentage of loss	Quantity lbs.	Percentage of loss
SALTS, CRYSTALINE SUBSTANCES. &c.								
Acid. Tartaric.	556	1.08	1426	1.61	723	1.38	256	4.95
	554	1.44						
Cobalt (Arsenic),	122	1.63						
Aluminæ & Potassæ Sulph.	74	5.40	49	6.12				
Ammoniæ Muriat.	202	8.41						
Potassæ Nitrat.	500	3.98	190	2.36	500	1.80	90	3.06
	300	8.17						
———— Sulphat.	63	1.59	98	3.06				
———— Bitartrat.	1166	.43	2121	.47	1007	.49	1115	.44
	1115	.41	1160	.52	1116	.44	2650	.37
	1068	.47	1163	.43	1155	.43		
Sodæ Biborat.	110	20.91	50	10.00				
Soap, Olive Oil, white,	62	33.33						
VEGETABLE SUBSTANCES, BARKS.								
Canella Alba,	67	4.48	50	4.04				
Cassia,	30	5.00	74	5.40				
Cinchona Maracaibo,	165	3.94	174	4.25	921	4.56		
Cinchona Flava, (Calisaya)	30	5.00	47	4.25	40	5.00		
———— Rubra,	44	4.54	160	1.03	39	5.08	96	4.66

Mezerion,	32	7.81						
Myrica Cerifera,	85	3.53	92	4.34				
Prinos vertlcill.	24	4.16						
Prunus Virginian.	50	4.00						
BERRIES.								
Capsicum,	166	3.67	95	3.15	64	4.69	80	3.75
Cubeba,	68	4.32	50	4.00	79	3.77	54	3.70
	92	3.26						
GUMS AND RESINS.								
Aloes Soct,	220	7.27	320	5.23				
Acacia,	225	4.00	217	3.64	121	4.13	75	4.69
	64	3.12	93	3.76	64	3.12		
Catechu,	70	4.28	71	4.89				
Euphorbium,	52	3.84						
Gambogia,	31	4.84	38	3.89				
Kino,	50	4.00	44	3.41	44	3.40		
Mastiche,	15	8.47						
Myrrha,	117	4.27	35	5.71	5.69			
Opium,	70	7.14	75	6.66	100	5.00		
	50	6.00	61	8.94	25	6.00	95	8.42
	81	4.93	63	6.72	100	7.25	75	6.00
	131	6.46	62	6.78	27	8.25	155	5.63
Sanguis Draconis,	10	5.00						
Scammonium Lachrym,	29	6.89	9	8.33	14	3.57		
	45	4.44	35	2.86				
Tragacantha,	30	5.00	35	4.28				
HERBS.								
Aconite,	38	5.26						
Cicuta,	35	5.71						
Digitalis,	47	4.25	32	4.34	28	3.57		
Lobelia,	28	4.38	34	4.61				
Hyoscyamus,	40	8.75						
FLOWERS.								
Arnica,	17	5.88						
Caryophyllus,	28	5.36	55	2.72	50	4.00		
Humulus,	268	4.10	195	5.12	222	3.80	252	3.57
	218	4.11	193	4.14				
FRUIT.								
Colocynth.[19]	26	65.38	55	69.09				
LEAVES.								
Buchu,	104	.96						
Senna Alex.	41	3.61	26	5.66				
Senna Indic.	50	3.96						
Uva Ursi,	42	4.70	50	4.00				
ROOTS.								
Calamus,	27	7.41						
Cimicifuga Racemosa,	69	4.34						
Colomba,	194	4.13	95	2.52	79	3.79	94	4.25
Cucuma, ground,	650	3.08						
Gentiana, ground,	227	2.20	280	2.50	149	2.68		
——— powdered,	72	4.17	71	4.22				
Glyrrh	156	3.84	145	4.13	70	4.11	313	4.15
Helleborus,	38	4.31						
Hydrastis canad.	37	5.40	50	5.00				

Ictodes Fœtidus,	25	4.00							
Inula,	50	4.00							
Ipecac.	99	4.44	80	3.75	109	4.13	73	4.76
	96	4.17	321	3.42				
Iris Flor.	232	3.02	138	3.62				
Jalap,	141	4.52	331	3.76	193	4.39	201	4.23
	271	3.13						
Rheum Indic.	96	4.16	78	3.84	75	4.00	40	3.75
	96	4.14	87	3.44	98	3.57	314	4.46
———— Russicum,	28	3.57	63	4.76	30	4.17		
Sanguinaria,	50	3.96						
Salep,	67	6.66	25	4.00				
Scilla,	27	11.11	81	6.17	55	8.18	40	13.12
	30	16.66						
Senega,	59	5.08						
Serpentara,	45	4.44						
Spigelia Marilan.	52	4.76						
Valeriana,	47	4.24						
Zingib. Jam.	114	4.37	58	5.17	115	4.00		
SEEDS.								
Anisum,	58	4.27	102	2.94				
Cardamomum,[20]	50	26.00	61	4.92				
Colchicum,	61	4.09	37	4.00				
Coriandrum,	99	2.02						
Linum, ground,	533	.93	.81					
Lobelia,	67	7.46						
Nux Vomica,	100	3.00	52	3.84	66	4.54		
SUNDRIES.								
Cantharis,	68	4.41	68	4.41	65	3.82	112	3.57
	39	3.79	41	4.88	53	6.00	42	3.57
Ext. Colocynth. Comp.	33	4.57						
Ext. Glyyrrh.	50	4.08	200	3.50				
Ext. Jalap,	20	4.86						
Galla,	70	4.21	73	4.11	28	5.26	56	3.54
Secale Cornut.	31	4.79	29	5.08	30	3.33		

[19] this includes loss of seeds.

[20] of this 21.00 is loss in hulls.

From the above results the following table, showing the average loss on each article, has been calculated:—

Average
per centage
of loss.

Salts, crystaline
substances, &c.

Acid, tartaric   1.50

Cobalt (arsenic)	1.63
Aluminæ et potassæ, sulphat. (calcined)	5.76
Ammoniæ muriat.	8.41
Potassæ nitrat.	2.80
———— sulphat.	2.37
———— bi-tartrat.	.45
Sodæ bi-borat.	15.45
Soap, olive oil, white	33.33

Vegetable substances.
Barks.

Cannella alba	4.26
Cassia	5.20
Cinchona maracaibo	4.25
———— flava (calisaya)	4.75
———— rubra	4.58
Mezerion	7.81
Myrica cerifera	3.98
Prinos verticill.	4.16
Prunus virginian.	4.00

Berries.

Capsicum	3.81
Cubeba	3.81

Gums and resins.

Aloes soct.	6.25
Acacia	3.78
Catechu	4.58
Euphorbium	3.84
Gambogia	4.36
Kino	3.60
Mastiche	8.47
Myrrha	3.15
Opium	6.61
Sanguis draconis	5.00
Scammonium lachrym	5.22
Tragacantha	4.64
Spegelia mariland.	4.76

Herbs.

Aconite	5.26
Cicuta	5.71
Digitalis	4.04
Lobelia	4.49
Hyosciamus	8.75

Flowers.

Arnica	5.88

Caryoph.	4.03
Humulus	4.14
Fruit.	
Colocynth.	67.23
Leaves.	
Buchu	.96
Senna alex.	4.63
——— ind.	3.96
Uva ursi	4.35
Roots.	
Calamus	7.41
Cimicituga racemosa	4.34
Colomba	3.47
Curcuma ground,	3.08
Gentian. Ground,	2.46
——— powdered	2.20
Glyyrrh.	4.06
Helleborus	4.31
Hydrastis canad.	5.20
Iclodes fœtidus	4.00
Inula	4.00
Ipecacuanha	4.10

Iris flor.	3.34
Jalap	4.00
Rheum indicum	3.91
———— russic.	4.17
Sanguinaria	3.96
Salep	3.84
Scilla	9.43
Senega	5.08
Serpentaria	4.44
Lobelia	7.46
Valerian.	4.24
Zingib. Jam.	4.51

Seeds.

Anisum	3.60
Cardamom.	4.92
Colchicum	4.05
Coriandrum	2.02
Linum (ground,)	.87
Nux vomica	3.79

Sundries.

Cantharis.	4.31
Ext. Coloc. Comp.	4.54

Ext. Glyyrrh.	6.25
Ext. Jalap	4.87
Galla	4.34
Secale cornutum	4.39

<hr size=0 width="100%" align=center>

ON THE PREPARATIONS OF IRON USED IN MEDICINE.

BY HENRY WURTZ.

The preparations of iron being among the most important articles of the pharmacopœia, it is surprising that so little attention is paid by many druggists and pharmaceutists to the preparation and preservation of these articles in a pure state. The greater part of the preparations of iron to be found in the shops are far from having the chemical composition indicated by their labels, and in fact, few of the formulas given in any of the pharmacopœias for preparations of iron, are capable of giving even tolerably pure products.

If there is any difference in a therapeutical point of view, between compounds of the protoxide and compounds of the peroxide of iron, and if any value is to be attached to definite composition in medicines, enabling physicians to administer *known quantities* to their patients, this state of affairs should not exist. Persons who handle the compounds of protoxide of iron, should be aware of the fact that few substances are more speedily and completely destroyed than these by the action of moist air; thus, one hundred parts of the *carbonate of iron*, require less than seven parts of oxygen for complete conversion into *sesquioxide of iron*, and one hundred parts of pure *copperas* require less than *three* parts of the same element to effect a like change in all the protoxide of iron which it contains.

As these protoxide of iron compounds, however, oxydate themselves only in the presence of water, the mode of preservation which i would propose, is very simple: it is only necessary to dry them perfectly and to introduce into the vessels in which they are to be preserved, a few small lumps of *quicklime*, which will keep the air in the interior of the vessel continually dry. To prevent any contamination of the preparation by direct contact with the lime, the latter must be securely folded in one or two thicknesses of filtering paper.

The iodide of iron and the carbonate, phosphate, arseniate, lactate and citrate of protoxide of iron may be preserved in this way, also the anhydrous sulphate (ferri sulphas siccatum), but it is evident that *crystallized* copperas would not retain a definite composition under these circumstances, because it would soon lose its crystal water. To preserve crystallized copperas, it is best to pulverize the crystals rather finely and dry the powder by repeatedly pressing strongly between folds of filtering paper, before putting up. Some have attempted to preserve the crystals under the surface of strong alcohol, but having tried this plan i must report unfavorably, for although the copperas remained for a while intact, yet, on examination after a considerable lapse of time, a large proportion of sesquioxide of iron was found. In fact, this result was to be anticipated in consideration of the well-known fact that strong alcohol has itself an attraction for oxygen, and always absorbs a certain amount of it when exposed to the air, serving thus merely as a medium for transmitting oxygen to any copperas which may be immersed in it.

I think it may be confidently stated that none of the protoxide compounds of iron should be kept in solution, either in water or alcohol, for medical purposes, unless in vessels hermetically closed. Some say, notwithstanding, that *iodide of iron* in solution may be preserved by keeping in it a piece of metallic iron, a deposite being formed, however, in the liquid which is supposed to be nothing more than sesquioxide of iron, but in which i strongly suspect the presence of a *subiodide of iron*, and consequent abstraction of iodine from the solution. Of course, however, this question can only be settled by a chemical examination of the deposit alluded to.

The sulphate of iron is the starting point in preparing all the compounds of iron which are used in medicine, and it is important therefore, to know how to separate easily the impurities which are contingent to this extremely cheap article of commerce. The impurities which commercial copperas most frequently contains are more or less sulphate of sesquioxide, together with a little sesquichloride of iron, and more rarely, traces of the sulphate of copperas, manganese, alumina and lime A small addition of *oxide of silver* to the solution will precipitate all chlorine present, and subsequent digestion for a few minutes with *carbonate of baryta* will remove every trace of sulphate of sesquioxide of iron, and of alumina. Copper may, of course, be removed by immersion of metallic iron. Traces of lime may be separated by recrystallization, but if traces of *manganese* are present, as is sometimes the case, i, know no way by which it can be separated. I am not aware, however, that the presence of such a trace of manganese in a preparation of iron would impair its therapeutical value. Another method of getting rid of the sulphate of sesquioxide is to acidulate the solution with sulphuric acid and, agitate with some pulverized *protosulphide of iron*, which will reduce the sesquioxide to protoxide.

When a solution of pure sulphate of protoxide of iron, free from sesquioxide, merely is required for preparing the carbonate or other insoluble protocompound, the method with carbonate of baryta is to be preferred, and in some rare cases when the presence of sulphate of lime in the solution of copperas obtained is of no importance, carbonate of lime may be substituted for carbonate of baryta, and will accomplish the same object.

When a solution of pure protosulphate of iron thus obtained is used for the preparation of carbonate of iron, care must be taken to use for precipitating, a solution of carbonate of soda which is free from silica, phosphoric acid, etc., which if present would surely go down with the precipitate. The precipitated carbonate should be washed with water which has been freed from *air* by previous boiling and better with water which is still boiling hot, dried as quickly as possible, first by pressure between folds of paper and then in a water bath, and preserved in well closed vessels containing lumps of quicklime as recommended above.

The formulas given in the pharmacopœias for the preparation of the sesquioxide of iron, which besides being employed as a remedy itself, is used in preparing all the other sesquicompounds of iron used in pharmacy, appear to be open to great objection on the ground of affording, instead of a pure sesquioxide of iron, an *indefinite mixture* of sesquioxide with carbonate of the protoxide. No necessity whatever exists for this; the following *modus operandi*, besides being much less troublesome in its execution than those given by the pharmacopœias, will furnish a product of constant composition, being an anhydrous sesquioxide of iron free from protoxide, and either chemically pure or very nearly so. The materials required are, five parts of commercial copperas which has been recrystallized once or twice, six parts of crystallized pure carbonate of soda, (na o, c o^2 + 10 ho) or two parts of dry carbonate of soda, and one part of nitrate of soda. (chili saltpetre). The carbonate and nitrate of soda are dissolved together in one portion of hot water and the copperas in another portion, and the two solutions, after filtrating mixed together, evaporated to dryness and the dry mass exposed to the lowest possible red heat for a few minutes. On pouring water upon the mass thus obtained, sulphate of soda and nitrate of soda dissolve and sesquioxide of iron separates as a heavy powder very easily washed by decantation. When thoroughly washed and dried it appears as a dark reddish brown *perfectly impalpable* powder, which is perfectly and easily soluble in dilute acids, and even in acetic acid and the composition of which is fe^2 o^3.

One great advantage of this process, is an avoidance of the immense tedium of *washing the precipitates* obtained in the ordinary processes.

I have but one more suggestion to make with regard to preparations of iron, and that is in the preparation of *ferri pulvis* or powder of iron by reduction of the sesquioxide— to propose the substitution of common coal gas as a reducing agent for the hydrogen gas directed by all the formulas, the former being obviously so vastly more convenient and far less expensive.

NOTE ON THE PREPARATION OF BESTUCHEFF'S TINCTURE.

BY FR. MAŸER.

Pure sesqui-chloride and poto-chloride of iron are unknown to the pharmacopœia of the united states, a fact which seems strange to a german pharmaceutist, since they are met with in every german dispensatory, and require great care for their proper preparation.

The american pharmacopœia indeed recognizes a tincture of chloride of iron, prepared by dissolving the sub-carbonate (sesqui oxide) of iron in hydrochloric acid, and adding alcohol. This tincture would be rejected throughout germany, since they endeavor there to obtain the preparations of perchloride of iron free from any traces of sesqui-chloride, while those of the sesqui-chloride should contain no admixture of the proto salt. This shows the practical character of the american pharmacopœia, which does not demand of the apothecary a purity of preparation which it is next to impossible to meet.

While making this acknowledgment, a good formula for the preparation of sesqui-chloride of iron still remains desirable.—this drug too, is sometimes used in american practice, as may be seen from the "notes on pharmacy," by mr. Benjamin canavan, in the may number of the *new york journal of pharmacy*. Mr. Canavan has given one of the oldest formulæ from the austrian pharmacopœia of 1820, as found in the *pharmacopie universelle* by jourdan. This formula directs us to dissolve the iron in a kind of aqua regia, and then to evaporate the superfluous acid by means of a sand bath. The sesqui-chloride thus obtained is employed in the preparation of "bestucheff's tincture," by dissolving one ounce of it in an ounce of water, adding twelve ounces of ether and agitating, then decanting the ethereal solution, and finally mixing it with four times its bulk of alcohol.

Having had frequent occasion to prepare this tincture as well in germany as in this city, it may not be unsuitable if i give here the formula for its preparation, which seems to me the most convenient, as well as my reasons for thinking so.

The sesqui-chloride of iron may be obtained in a pure and neutral state, by passing a current of chlorine gas through a solution of proto-chloride of iron, until a solution of the red ferrocyanide of potassium of gmelin no longer produces a blue precipitate, and then evaporating the solution by means of a water bath. In this manner the salt can readily be obtained in a crystalline form. One ounce of the crystals thus obtained is to be dissolved in twelve ounces of ether, if we retain the alleged proportions, mixed with four times its bulk of alcohol, and finally bleached by exposing it to the direct light of the sun.

The prussian pharmacopœia of 1846 gives the following proportions:—one drachm of the sesqui-chloride of iron, or two drachms of the aqueous solution, one fluid ounce of ether, and three fluid ounces of alcohol.

Here we have to notice,—1st, that it is preferable to take ether and alcohol by weight rather than by measure, since their volume is very much influenced by the temperature, which may range from 32° to 60° or 80.°

2nd, that the sesqui-chloride, prepared with nitro-nuriatic acid, is not so easy to obtain in crystals, in consequence of the adhering nitro-nuriatic acid, which is always retained in small quantities. On the other hand, by drying the salt you will, in almost every case, spoil a quantity of it by driving off too much of the acid.

3rd, that the sesqui-chloride of iron, if in crystals, is easily and wholly soluble in ether, while the aqueous solution of it is but partially so, a portion being decomposed, as is evidenced by the solution becoming muddy. The ethereal solution, if prepared in the last mentioned manner, must be of uncertain strength, which is avoided by the first.

In europe bestucheff's tincture is much used by physicians. It sometimes agrees better in the bleached state, sometimes when colored. When first prepared the tincture has a yellow hue, which it loses by exposure to the light of the sun. If, after it has thus been bleached, it is placed in a dark closet, it again becomes yellowish, though the color is not so deep as at first.

ON SOCOTRINE ALOE JUICE, OR LIQUID SOCOTRINE ALOES.

BY JONATHAN PEREIRA, M. D., F. R. S.,
(PHYSICIAN TO THE LONDON HOSPITAL.)

It has long been known that the socotrine aloes imported into england varies considerably in its consistency, and is sometimes met with in a soft or semi-fluid state. Frequently, on opening a package of this sort of aloes, the interior is found to be quite soft, while the exterior is firm and hard. In general this arises from insufficient evaporation of the aloe juice.

In the third edition of my *elements of materia medica*, (vol. Ii., part 1, p. 1077, published in 1850,) i have briefly referred to a soft or semi-liquid socotrine aloes, which had a bright or palm-oil yellow color and odor. At that time i had but little opportunity of investigating this very interesting drug; but a large importation of it having recently taken place, i have more fully examined it, and, as it appears to me to be the raw or unboiled juice of the plant yielding what is known in commerce as socotrine aloes, i propose to distinguish it from the ordinary soft socotrine aloes by the name of *"socotrine aloe juice."*

Messrs. Horner, the holders of the whole of the present importation of this juice, inform me that it was purchased of the arabs up the red sea, by a merchant, who was assured by the venders that it was very fine aloe juice, and had not been boiled or otherwise altered. It was imported into london by way of madras, in casks each containing six cwt. I am informed that the contents of some of the packages have undergone decomposition during the voyage.

Its consistence is that of treacle or very thin honey; its color deep orange or palm oil yellow; its odor powerful, fragrant, and resembling that of fine socotrine aloes. By standing it separates into two parts,—an inferior, paler colored, opaque, finely granular portion and a superior, darker colored, transparent liquid. The latter forms, however, a very small portion of the whole mass.

When the granular portion is submitted to microscopic examination, it is found that the opacity and granular appearance arise from myriads of beautiful prismatic crystals. If a temperature of 132° fah. Be applied to the juice these crystals melt or dissolve, and the juice becomes deep red and transparent; and when the liquid becomes cold it retains its transparency, and does not deposit any crystals. By evaporation the juice yields a solid, transparent extract, having all the characters of fine socotrine aloes, in which no traces of crystalline texture can be discovered. Mr. Jacob bell has ascertained that 14 LBS. Of the juice yield 8lbs. 12ozs. Of solid extract, or $62\frac{1}{2}$ per cent. When the juice is mixed with cold distilled water, it becomes opaque yellow, and renders the water turbid, but is not miscible with it. If, however, heat be applied, the juice dissolves in the water, forming an almost clear, rich red liquid. As the solution cools, it at first becomes turbid, owing to the separation of an opaque yellow precipitate, which, apparently, is the crystalline principle in an amorphous form. This gradually separates from the liquid and collects as a clear resiniform mass (commonly called the *resin* of aloes) at the bottom of the vessel, leaving the supernatant liquid tolerably clear. If the juice be shaken up with rectified spirit of wine, an uniform clear mixture is obtained, from which numerous yellow crystals rapidly fall to the bottom of the liquid. Similar results are obtained when we mix the juice with equal parts of rectified spirit of wine and water.

This crystalline constituent of socotrine aloes is doubtless, either the *aloin*21 described by messrs. T. & h. Smith, of edinburgh, and by dr. Stenhouse, or a principle closely allied to it.

Dr. Stenhouse, to whom i have given a sample of it, is now engaged in its investigation; and in a letter which i have received from him, he says that though he has not been able to get the aloin ready for analysis, yet from the experiments he has already made with it, he has scarcely a doubt that it will be found identical with that formerly obtained from barbados aloes. It forms, he adds, a precisely similar combination with bromine, and, in short, agrees with it in every particular; i shall, therefore, provisionally term this crystalline principle the *aloin of socotrine aloes*. On comparing it with a fine specimen of aloin, kindly presented to me by messrs. Smith, i find its crystals smaller and more tapering—the summits of the crystals being more acute.

21 see new york journal of pharmacy, no. Vi. Page 177.

In drying, the crystals of the socotrine aloin have a strong tendency to break up; so that crystals which in the moist state are moderately large and regular, become small and pulverulent when dry. Like the aloin crystals of messrs. Smith, the aloin crystals of socotrine aloes, strongly doubly refract and depolarize light, and are, therefore, beautiful objects when viewed by the polarizing microscope.

The crystals of aloin contained in socotrine aloe juice cannot be confounded with the crystals of oxalate and phosphate of lime found in the juices of various plants, and which are called by botanists *raphides*. The appearance under the microscope of the former is very different from that of the latter. Moreover, the ready fusibility, solubility, and complete combustibility of aloin crystals easily distinguish them from the calcareous salts just referred to. On platinum foil the aloin burns without leaving any residue, except such as may arise from the presence of traces of some foreign matter.

Aloin may be readily obtained from the juice by mixing the latter with spirit (either rectified or proof,) and collecting and drying the precipitate. When procured in this way it appears to the naked eye like a yellow powder; but when examined by the microscope it is found to consist of minute fragments of crystals.

The tincture from which the aloin has been separated, yields by distillation a spirit having the fragrant odor of the juice; showing that the latter contains some volatile odorous principle. By evaporation the tincture yields a resiniform extract.

In the first edition of my *elements of materia medica*, published 1840, i have stated, that by digesting hepatic aloes in rectified spirit of wine, a yellowish granular powder is obtained which is insoluble in [cold] water, alcohol, ether, and dilute sulphuric acid, but is readily soluble in a solution of caustic potash, forming a red colored liquid. The powder like residue here referred to, is identical with the aloin of socotrine aloes. When examined by the microscope, it is perceived to consist of very minute prismatic crystals, which depolarize polarized light like the larger crystals of aloin above referred to. I think, therefore, that it may be safely inferred that hepatic aloes has been prepared without the employment of artificial heat, and that its opacity is due to the presence of minute crystals of aloin.

When socotrine aloes is digested in rectified spirit, an insoluble portion is also obtained; but its color, instead of being yellow, as in hepatic aloes, is dark brown. On submitting this dark brown insoluble portion to microscopic examination, i find that it contains depolarizing crystals.

Artificial socotrine aloes (prepared by evaporating this aloe juice) also yields, when digested in rectified spirit, a dark brown insoluble portion.

I think, therefore, that socotrine aloes differs from hepatic aloes in the circumstance of its having been prepared by the aid of artificial heat; by which its aloin constituent has become altered. This inference is further substantiated by the fact, that after it has been melted, hepatic aloes is found to have acquired the clearness and transparency of the socotrine sort.

The clear supernatant portion of aloe juice, from which the above crystals have subsided, would probably also yield, by spontaneous evaporation, an extract resembling, or identical with, socotrine aloes.

That socotrine and hepatic aloes were obtained from the same plant, and were not different species of aloes, i have long suspected; and in the first edition of my work on materia medica, published in 1840, i have observed that "the similarity of the odor of socotrine and hepatic aloes leads to the suspicion that they are obtained from the same plant; and which is further confirmed by the two being sometimes brought over intermixed, the socotrine occasionally forming a vein in a cask of the hepatic aloes."

The intermixture of the two sorts of aloes in the same cask might be explained by supposing that the consolidation of the clear portion of the juice has produced the so-called socotrine aloes; while the opaque aloin containing portion of juice has yielded what is termed hepatic aloes.

In the third edition of my work above alluded to, i have stated that the name of *opaque liver-colored socotrine aloes* might with propriety be applied to hepatic aloes. But until the present time i have been unable to offer a plausible explanation of the cause of the difference in these two commercial kinds of aloes.

From the preceding remarks i think we may infer:

1. That *aloin* pre-exists in a crystalline form in the juice of socotrine aloes.

2. That the substance which deposits as a decoction of socotrine aloes cools, and which is usually termed the *resin* or the *resinoid* of socotrine aloes, is the aloin in a modified state.

3. That hepatic aloes[22] is the juice of the socotrine aloes plant which has been solified without the aid of artificial heat.

4. That hepatic aloes owes its opacity to the presence of minute crystals of aloin.

5. That the juice of socotrine aloes yields, when evaporated by artificial heat, an extract possessing all the properties of commercial socotrine aloes.—*pharm. Journ. April, 1852.*

---

22 by the term *"hepatic aloes"* i mean the opaque liver-colored aloes imported into england from the east indies (usually from bombay). This sort of aloes is very different from the *hepatic barbadoes aloes*, which formerly appears to have been exclusively called "hepatic aloes."

THE CHEMICAL COMPOSITION OF COD-LIVER OIL.

BY DR. H. L. WINCKLER.

Of all the drugs which have been introduced into medical practice within the last ten years, none has excited so much attention, and has met with so favorable a reception, as cod-liver oil. To what principles its peculiar properties are to be referred, has not yet been ascertained. By some they have been attributed to the presence of a small quantity of iodine; but this has not proved a satisfactory explanation. Many chemists have endeavoured to solve this problem, but without success.—amongst others, dr. De jongh, who attributed its virtue to gaduin—a new principle which he had discovered in the oil, with the usual fatty acids, and some of the constituents of bile, and traces of iodine and bromine.

The results of my researches are different, in an important degree. According to my experience, cod-liver oil is *an organic whole* of a peculiar character, differing in its chemical composition from any of the fat oils which have been heretofore applied to medical purposes.

The evidences for this conclusion are the following:—

1. When the clear, pale cod-liver oil is saponified with potash, and the resulting soap treated with tartaric acid, oleic and margaric acids are obtained.

2. When a mixture of six parts of caustic potash, twenty-four parts of distilled water, and twenty-four parts of cod-liver oil, after being allowed to remain at an ordinary temperature, and often shaken, and finally diluted with twenty-four parts of distilled water, is distilled, a distillate is obtained, which possesses an intense odor of cod-liver oil, and contains an appreciable quantity of a peculiar organic compound, namely, oxide of propyl.

3. When nine parts of cod-liver oil are saponified with five parts of oxide of lead, with the necessary quantity of distilled water, in a porcelain vessel, by the heat of a water

bath, the oil is decomposed into oleic and margaric acids, and a new acid propylic acid. The chief part of this acid combines, like the oleic and margaric acids, with the oxide of lead, as it appears, to form a basic compound; and another lead salt, probably an acid one, can be washed out of the plaister with distilled water. It is worthy of remark, that no glycerine is formed in this process. The plaister smells of train oil and herrings; and when it is exposed in a thin layer to the action of the atmosphere in a water bath, it becomes colored dark brown, after the evaporation of the water; and by the same means it loses its penetrating odor. The cause of the coloring is due to the strong disposition which the salts of propylic acid possess to oxidize, and consequently, to become brown. When the solution of the acid propylate of lead is treated with sulphuretted hydrogen, after the separation of the sulphuret of lead, is obtained an entirely colorless and strongly acid reacting solution, which by evaporation in a water bath, becomes by degrees colored. At the commencement of the last part of the operation it loses its penetrating odor, and at last leaves a dark brown residue. Exactly in the same manner, the watery solutions of neutral propylates of barytes and ammonia behave themselves. The neutral, colorless, and undecomposed ammoniacal salt smells of herrings; and the baryta salt, as concentrated decoction of meat.

4. When the before-described (no. 2) solution of cod-liver oil soap is thrown into a capacious distillery apparatus, with the addition of caustic lime and chloride of ammonium, (in the proportion of six drachms of caustic potash, three ounces of cod-liver oil, six ounces of water, six ounces of fresh burnt lime, and one drachm of chloride of ammonium,) with the precaution, that the mixture of lime and chloride of ammonium be not added until the soap is formed in the retort, so that it may penetrate thoroughly the mass, and the distillation proceeded with by means of a gentle heat, as the formation of hydrate of lime evolves considerable heat, there distils rather quickly a clear, watery fluid, over which is a concentrated solution of propylamin free from ammonia. By saturating this solution with diluted sulphuric acid, and adding alcohol, sulphate of propylamin readily crystallizes out of it.

This simple experiment serves to prove, with certainty, that cod-liver oil contains oxide of propyl. The propylamin thus obtained possesses all the properties of that obtained from the pickle of herrings, or ergot of rye.

Cod-liver oil by saponification with potash, is separated into oleic and margaric acids, and *oxide of propyl*; and with oxide of lead, into oleic and margaric acids, and propylic acid—a higher result of the oxidation of propyl—and gives by either process of saponification no *hydrate of the oxide of glycyl*. The glycyl (c_6 h_3) is in this oil replaced by propyl (c_6 h_7). Only in cod-liver oil are the conditions offered for the formation of propylamin (n h_2 c_6 h_7), by the presence of ammonia, as all the fat oils employed in medicine are free from this substance; therefore none of these oils can be substituted for cod-liver oil.

[should this research of winckler, as to the existence of the hydrate of the oxide of propyl in combination with the fatty acids in cod-liver oil, be confirmed, it will establish an important fact in chemistry, and may explain the therapeutic action of that remedy which has heretofore puzzled both chemists and physicians. The combinations of the radical propyl have been previously only known as artificial productions; therefore wincklers's experiments, if true, show that they exist in nature, or, in other words, that they are educts, and not products, from cod-liver oil. Moreover, the presence of oxide of propyl, and the absence of oxide of glycyl in cod-liver oil, will enable chemists to distinguish by tests, with certainty, this oil from other fatty oils.]—*annals of pharmacy, june, 1852.*

GUARANA.

COMMUNICATED BY D. RITCHIE, SURGEON, R. N.

A medicinal substance named guaraná was presented to me about two years ago by a brazilian. The virtues which he asserted that it possessed induced me to employ it as a remedy in several troublesome and obstinate cases of disease. The consequent benefit was so decided, that i was convinced of the great value it possessed as a remedial agent. This conviction, with the belief that it was still unknown, impelled me to bring the subject under the notice of the *profession* in this country. A short account of it was therefore transmitted to the editor of the "edinburgh monthly medical journal," who forthwith submitted it to professor christison. To the kindness and extensive acquirements of this gentleman i am indebted for the information, that the subject had already engaged the attention, of the brothers martius in germany, and several french writers. It was a matter of satisfaction to me to find that the opinions i had expressed regarding the great prospective importance of this substance were fully borne out by all those who have diligently examined it.

As a knowledge of the properties and uses of guaraná appears to be still little diffused in this country, i shall consider that i am performing an acceptable service to the medical profession in placing before it an abstract of the more important facts that are known regarding this substance. Public attention was first directed to it by m. Gassicourt in 1817, (journal de pharmac., tom. Iii., p. 259); but the merit of discovering the source whence it is derived, and of furnishing a more complete description of it, belongs to von martius, in the year 1826, (reise, vol. Ii., p. 1061, *et seq.*)

The term guaraná is derived from the name of a tribe of indians, who are dispersed between the rivers parama and uruguay, by whom it is very commonly used as a condiment or medicine. It is, however, more extensively prepared for commercial purposes by the mauhés, an indian tribe in the province of tapajoz. It is, according to martius, prepared from the seeds of the paullinia sorbilis, a species belonging to the natural family sapindaceæ. The characters of the species are:—glabra, caule erecto angulato, foliis pinnatis bijugis, foliolis oblongis, remote sinuato-obtuse-dentatis, lateralibus basi rotundatis, extimo basi cuneato, petiolo nudo angnlato, racemis pubescentibus·erectis, capsulis pyriformibus apteris rostratis, valvulis intus villosis. The seeds, which ripen in the month of october and november, are collected, taken out of their capsules, and exposed to the sun, so as to dry the arillus in which they are enveloped, that it may be more readily rubbed off by the fingers. They are now thrown upon a stone, or into a stone mortar, and reduced to powder, to which a little water is added, or which is exposed to the night dew, and then formed by kneading into a dough. In this condition it is mixed with a few of the seeds entire or contused, and divided into masses, weighing each about a pound, which are rolled into cylindrical or spherical forms. These are dried by the sun or by the fire, and become so hard as to be broken with difficulty. Their surface is uneven, brown, or sometimes black, from the smoke to which they have been subjected; their fractured surface is conchoidal, unequal, and resinoid; color reddish brown, resembling chocolate. This is the guaraná, and in this condition, or reduced to powder, it is kept for use or carried to market. The museum of the edinburgh college of physicians contains a specimen of it in each of these forms. As it is liable to be adulterated with cocoa or mandioca flour, it is of great importance to be aware that the genuine article is distinguished by its greater hardness and density, and that, when powdered, it does not assume a white color, but a grayish-red tint.

A chemical analysis of this substance was first made by theodore martius, in 1826, (buchner's repert. De pharm. Xxxi., 1829, p. 370). He found it to consist of a matter (tannin?) Which iron precipitated green, resin, a fat green oil, gum, starch, vegetable fibre, and a white, bitter, crystalline product, to which the efficacy of the medicine was principally owing, and which he called guaranine. This he believed to be distinct from, but allied to, theine and caffeine, and to possess the following elementary constituents:—c_8, h_{10}, o_2, n_4.

Another very careful analysis of guaraná was made in the year 1840, by mm. Berthemot and dechastélus, (journal de pharmacie, tom. Xxvi., p. 518, *et seq.*), which varies in some degree from the preceding. They found the matter, which was considered to be resin by martius, a combination of tannin with guaranine, existing in a form insoluble in water or ether. They also determined the perfect identity of the crystalline matter with caffeine. It is found to exist in a much larger proportion in the fruits of the paullinia than in any of the plants from which it has hitherto been extracted. Alcohol is the only agent which completely removes it from the guaraná. To this solution the addition of lime or hydrated oxide of lead gives, on the one hand, the insoluble tannates, and on the other, the crystalline matter.

The medicinal virtues of this substance have been attentively examined by theodore martius, (op. Cit.), and more particularly by dr. Gavrelle (sur une nouvelle substance médicinale, etc.: paris, 1840), who employed it very often while in brazil, as physician to don pedro, and afterwards in france. By both it is considered a valuable remedy, and an important addition to the materia medica. By the vulgar it is held to be stomachic, antifebrile, and aphrodisiac; is used in dysentery, diarrhœa, retention of urine, and various other affections. It stimulates, and at the same time soothes, the gastric system of nerves. It reduces the excited sensibility of the cœliac plexus, thereby diminishing febrile action, and strengthening the stomach and intestines, particularly restraining excessive mucous discharges, increasing the action of the heart and the arteries, and promoting diaphoresis. It is therefore indicated as a valuable remedy in fevers, or reduced vital power resulting from cold or prolonged wetness, grief, to great muscular exertion, depression of spirits, long watching, and also in colic, flatulence, anorexia, nervous hemicrania, or in a dry condition of the skin. It is contra-indicated in a plethoric or loaded condition of the abdominal viscera, and when there exists determination of blood to the head. It is said to increase the venereal appetite, but to diminish the fecundating power.

In cases where irritation of the urethra or urinary bladder succeed venereal or attend organic disease, it exerts a most salutary effect in soothing the irritability of the mucous membrane, relieving the nervous prostration which accompanies these affections, and exalting vital power. Unlike the disagreeable remedies which are generally, and often without success, employed in these affections, it is taken with pleasure, and with an amount of success which, as far as my experience extends, is universal.

If we examine guaraná according to its chemical characters, it must be guarded as a most valuable substance, from its possessing in so great a proportion that important nitrogenous principle guaranine. This, if not identical with caffeine, is at least analagous to it, and to theine, and theobromine,—all important elements of food and grateful stimulents. From its chemical constitution, then, we may predict with great certainty its physiological action being powerfully tonic; but in the combination in which it is found, experience indicates that it possesses conjoined more valuable properties than belong to the simple tonics. Its power of correcting generally the discharges, and restoring the normal vitality of the mucous membranes, must be viewed as one of these.

Guarana, in the state of powder, is exhibited in doses of

3

J, three or four times daily, mixed with water and sugar, or with syrup and mucilage, conjoined with an aromatic, as cinnamon, vanilla, or chocolate. A convenient form is that of extract, obtained by treating the guaraná with alcohol, and evaporating to the consistence of pills. This may be exhibited in the form of solution or pills. The brazilians, however, use the powder with sugar and water alone, and consider this draught grateful and refreshing.— *monthly jour. Of medical science, may, 1852.*

COLORED FIRES FOR PYROTECHNICAL PURPOSES.

Erdmann, in the last number of his journal, gives the following formulæ for preparing colored fires, which he has proved and found to answer the purpose intended admirably. He particularly enjoins the caution that the ingredients, after being powdered in a mortar *separately*, should be mixed with the hand, as dangerous explosions would inevitably follow from the ingredients being rubbed together with any hard substance.

Red.

	Parts.
Chlorate of potash,	61
Sulphur,	16
Carbonate of strontia,	23

Purple red.

	Parts.
Chlorate of potash,	61
Sulphur,	16
Chalk,	23

Rose red.

	Parts.
Chlorate of potash,	61
Sulphur,	16
Chloride of calcium,	23

Orange red.

	Parts.
Chlorate of potash,	52

| Sulphur, | 14 |
| Chalk, | 34 |

Yellow, no. 1.

	Parts.
Chlorate of potash,	61
Sulphur,	16
Dried soda,	23

Yellow, no. 2.

	Parts.
Saltpetre,	50
Sulphur,	16
Dried soda,	20
Gunpowder,	14

Yellow, no. 3.

	Parts.
Saltpetre,	61
Sulphur,	$17\frac{1}{2}$
Dried soda,	20
Charcoal,	$1\frac{1}{2}$

Light blue.

	Parts.
Chlorate of potash,	61
Sulphur,	16

Burnt alum,   23

Dark blue.

	Parts.
Chlorate of potash,	60
Sulphur,	16
Carbonate of copper,	12
Burnt alum,	12

  Sulphate of potash and ammonio-
sulphate of copper may be added
to render the color more intense.

Dark violet.

	Parts.
Chlorate of potash,	60
Sulphur,	16
Carbonate of potash,	12
Burnt alum,	12

Light violet.

	Parts.
Chlorate of potash,	54
Sulphur,	14
Carbonate of potash,	16
Burnt alum,	16

Green,

                                                     Parts.

Chlorate of potash,	73
Sulphur,	17
Boracic acid,	19

Light green.

	Parts.
Chlorate of potash,	60
Sulphur,	16
Carbonate of barytes,	24

For theatrical purposes.

White, no. 1.

	Parts.
Saltpetre,	64
Sulphur,	21
Gunpowder,	15

White, no. 2.

	Parts.
Saltpetre,	64
Sulphur,	22
Charcoal,	2

Red.

	Parts.
Nitrate of strontia,	56
Sulphur,	24

Chlorate of potash,	20

Green.

	Parts.
Nitrate of barytes,	60
Sulphur,	22
Chlorate of potash,	18

Rose.

	Parts.
Sulphur,	20
Saltpetre,	32
Chlorate of potash,	27
Chalk,	20
Charcoal,	1

Blue.

	Parts.
Saltpetre,	27
Chlorate of potash,	28
Sulphur,	15
Sulphate of potash,	15
Ammonio-sulphate of copper,	15

<hr size=0 width="100%" align=center>

EXTRACTUM LOBELIÆ FLUIDUM.

BY WILLIAM PROCTER, JR.

Having had occasion to prepare a fluid extract of lobelia at the solicitation of a druggist, the following process was employed, which is based on the fact, that in the presence of an excess of acid, the lobelina of the natural salt which gives activity to the drug, is not decomposed and destroyed by the heat used, as explained on a former occasion, (vol. Xix. Page 108 of this journal.)

Take of lobelia (the plant,) finely bruised, eight ounces, (troy)

Acetic acid	One fluid ounce.
Diluted alcohol	Three pints.
Alcohol	Six fluid ounces.

Macerate the lobelia in a pint and a half of the diluted alcohol, previously mixed with the acetic acid, for twenty-four hours; introduce the mixture into an earthen displacer, pour on slowly the remainder of the diluted alcohol, and afterwards water until three pints of tincture are obtained; evaporate this in a water bath to ten fluid ounces, strain, add the alcohol and, when mixed, filter through paper.

Each teaspoonful of this preparation is equal to half a fluid ounce of the tincture. It may be employed advantageously to make a syrup of lobelia, by adding two fluid ounces of the fluid extract, to ten fluid ounces of simple syrup, and mixing. Syrup of lobelia is an eligible preparation for prescription use, in cases where lobelia is indicated as an expectorant.—*american journal of pharmacy*.

NEW METHOD FOR PREPARING AND EXHIBITING PROTIODIDE OF IRON.

BY M. H. BONNEWYN.

Several methods have been proposed for the preparation and exhibition of protiodide of iron, all of which are, as far as i am acquainted with them, subject to many inconveniences and objections. It is on this account that i offer to my fellow-laborers a new method, which both on account of its uniformity of action and facility of administration, deserves to be adopted universally.

Every practical man knows that all preparations of protiodide of iron are bad, for instance, syrupus ferri iodidi is a medicine which is generally disliked, and in some individuals causes nausea and even vomiting. The pilulæ ferri iodidi likewise disagree with some constitutions, and when they seem to agree, they never produce the same regular effects even if prepared at the same labratory. According to trials made by an experienced physician, who has administered the protiodide, prepared according to my method, i am assured that this remedy prepared by a double decomposition in the stomachs of the patients, has always agreed with them, and produced more constant and salutary effects. It is already a well-known fact, that the iodide of iron in its incipient state is better assimilated by the organs.

NO. 1. Dissolve one gramme of iodide potassium in 300 grammes of water. NO. 2. Take sulphate of iron 1½ grammes; make a powder and divide into eighteen equal parts. Dissolve one of the powders in a large table-spoonful of sugared water before swallowing it; take immediately afterwars, one table-spoonful of the solution.

It is evident that by this operation, each time their is produced in the stomach one grain, or about five centigrammes of iodide of iron in its incipient state.

Although these proportions do not correspond absolutely, but only approximately with their chemical equivalents, nevertheless, their effects answer fully the purposes both of the chemist, and physician.—*annals of pharmacy and practical chemistry.*

TANNATE OF ZINC.

—the preparation announced of late, under the name of the salt of barnit, as infallible against gonorrhœra when used as an injection, is, according to the analysis of m. Chevalier, a tannate of zinc. This salt which is soluble, may be prepared by saturating a solution of tannic acid with freshly precipitated and moist oxide of zinc, filtering and evaporating in a water bath.

EDITORIAL.

THE CONVENTION.

—we cheerfully give place to the following *notice* from dr. Guthrie, in regard to the approaching meeting of the pharmaceutical convention. We regret to learn that the time appointed, is not the most convenient one for many of the delegates whom we may expect from the south. It is too late, however, to change the time of meeting, were there any authority by which such change could be made. In view of the importance of the object, we hope that there may be a full attendance on the part of the delegates, even at the cost of some personal sacrifice. If the whole country be represented, a time can then be chosen for a future meeting which will suit a majority of those present:—

"notice.—the annual meeting of the u. S. Pharmaceutical convention, will take place in philadelphia, on wednesday, the 6th of october next.

It being a matter of much importance that this meeting should number as many of our druggists and chemists as possible, i deem it proper to suggest that not only all regularly incorporated and unincorporated associations of this kind should see that they are fully represented, but that where no associations exist as yet, the apothecaries should send one or more of their number as delegates to the convention,—such will, no doubt, be cheerfully admitted to seats in the convention.

This meeting it is to be hoped, will either take the necessary steps to the formation of a regular and permanent national organization, or possibly effect such organization during its sittings.

We trust all who feel an interest in this important subject, will remember the time and place, and give us their assistance in person or by delegate.

C. B. Guthrie, *president of convention.*

The american journal of pharmacy.

—the editor of the american journal of pharmacy, has done much to raise the standard of american pharmacy. He has a solid reputation founded on large knowledge and great industry. It is with pleasure then that we observe the attention he bestows upon our journal. He has taken, however, rather an unusual course, in animadverting separately upon most of the directly practical articles that have appeared in our pages, and his criticisms have given rise to some reclamations on the part of our contributors, which we subjoin:—

Comments on "comments."—the american journal of pharmacy (philiadelphia), for july, contains "pharmaceutical notices, being extracts from various articles in the new york journal of pharmacy, with comments by the editor," in which our friend procter, criticises, rather severely, some of the pharmaceutical formulæ and suggestions that have been offered in this journal. With full respect for the great acquirements and high character as a practical pharmaceutist, to which my friend procter is justly entitled, i should have been glad if the articles, upon which he comments, had met his approval; and i know of no one that i would rather should set me right, if anything that i have offered does not find acceptance with him. With the greater part of his comments, i do not think there is occasion for controversy,—matters of fact readers can judge for themselves, and it certainly is of little consequence, who may be found in error, compared with the elucidation of truth.

In respect to the *consistence* of syrup of gum arabic, he is probably nearer right, (during this hot weather, at any rate) than i was, and still, i think he is not right. My experience with the present officinal formula, had been in the cold season, when i found the syrup decidedly too thick for convenient use, especially by itself; a large proportion of it crystallized in the temperature of the shop, and the mouth and neck of the bottle choked up with candied syrup every two or three times it was used. I had found the former syrup to answer very well in regard to consistence and flavor, though, it certainly could not be considered permanent; it had to be made in small quantities and frequently; indeed, i do not suppose that any liquid combination of gum, sugar and water only, can be made of a permanent character. Since reading mr. Procter's comments, i have made this syrup again by the present formula, and it does keep decidedly better at this season, than that made in the other proportions, yet not perfectly; and there is considerable crystallization, even in the very hot weather we have had lately. I infer that syrup which crystallizes at this season, has an excess of sugar in it, the crystals formed tending further to reduce the remaining syrup, and thus sooner promote acidity than if a proportion of sugar had been used which could remain in solution. Perhaps, a medium between the two formulæ could be hit upon, in which the proper balance might be better attained.

In the formula offered for compound syrup of squill, in our journal for april, there is an error of four ounces in the quantity of honey, which should have been *twenty-two* ounces. Whether it was made by the printer or not cannot be ascertained, as "the *copy* has been destroyed." I had not noticed it until my attention was called to it by mr. Procter's comments. The quantity of sugar used by me in making this syrup was, for convenience, one pound avoirdupois weight; that of honey, one pound and a half, same weight. In transcribing the formula for a medical journal, i thought i must, per custom, render it in troy weights; so as 15 OZ. Troy are 200 grs. More than one pound av., i set down 15 OZ., and intended to set down 22 OZ. Of honey, as being only 60 grs. More than one pound and a half av. I think this addition of 4 OZ. Of honey will make the whole come up to mr. Procter's measure of "56 fluid ounces before the ebullition," &c., and a little over. The boiling can be continued only for a few minutes. I was formerly in the practice of boiling to three pints, and adding 48 grs. Tartar emetic, but finding that i had to evaporate more than half a pint, and judging that the strength of the resulting preparation was rather lessened than increased thereby, i concluded to stop at three and a half pints. As to the proportion of sugar and honey, they amount together to 2½ pounds av., which with two pints of an evaporated menstruum, containing the extractive matter soluble in diluted alcohol of 8 OZ. Of the roots, furnishes a syrup of good consistence. It may be observed, that solution of sugar in a menstruum so charged, is quite different from that in water. Perhaps, however, an equal amount of sugar with that of the honey, would be preferable. I can only say, that i employed the same quantity a number of times, but reduced it several years since, because it appeared to be too much for some reason, the particulars of which i do not recollect. And as this formula has always given me a satisfactory preparation, i have thought no more about it, until now. Or perhaps, it would be better to continue the evaporation to three pints, with the advantage of producing a more symmetrical result, corresponding, at the same time, with the quantity of the pharmacopœia. But, is not the officinal formula "almost as far out of the way" the *other* way? Forty-two oz. Of sugar in forty-eight fluid oz. Of syrup! Can such an amount remain in solution twenty-four hours at any ordinary temperature? If mine is an *"anomaly,"* is not this an *impossibility*, "in point of consistence"? In reference to the alcoholic objection, it may be remarked, that the evaporation in the case commented upon, is not "from 4 pints of tincture to 2 pints," but from 4¾ pints to 2 pints. The small portion of alcohol, that may remain after this evaporation and the continued heat to the end of the process, can scarcely be of serious consequence in the doses in which it is prescribed; it may have some influence in preserving the syrup, and also in promoting its medical action. Be all this as it may, so far as taste is a criterion, this preparation appears to be of at least double strength in the qualities of both roots, of the officinal syrup carefully made by the second process given,—the first being, as i suppose, with all apothecaries of the present day, "an obsolete idea."

G. D. C.

REMARKS ON THE COMMENTS MADE BY THE EDITOR OF THE PHILADELPHIA JOURNAL OF PHARMACY, ON SOME EXTRACTS FROM VARIOUS ORIGINAL ARTICLES, PUBLISHED IN THE NEW YORK JOURNAL OF PHARMACY

:—

After giving the formula for preparing stramonium ointment, as modified by e. Dupuy, the editor of our contemporary adds, "the objection to the officinal formula on the score of color, is hardly valid, and if it was so, it would be better to color it with extract of grass, than to substitute a preparation which will constantly vary in strength and appearance or with the age of the leaves. The officinal extract of stramonium, is easily incorporated with lard, and produces a brown colored ointment of comparatively uniform strength." We do not pretend to have furnished a formula vastly superior to that received in our officinal guide. But as we were writing for our locality chiefly, and knowing the general expectation and usage of furnishing stramonium ointment of a green color, we have given a formula which does furnish an ointment having a proper strength, requisite color, without the loss of time and material necessarily incurred in manufacturing a color ad hoc as suggested by w. Procter, jr., which from the contamination of the decomposed chlorophylle of the extract, would never compare favorably (notwithstanding all that useless waste of trouble,) so far as its appearance is concerned, with the far readier mode proposed for transforming at once by a few short manipulations the dry stramonium into an alcoholic extract and ointment without liability to alteration during the process. Respecting the keeping of both ointments, we can affirm that the one prepared by the modified formula, will keep as well if not better and longer, than the other, and as the color is a point of some importance for our public and practitioners, we are satisfied that it will be preferred on the score of economy of time as well as for its color, which is desirable at least within our circle of custom.

Emplastrum epispasticum with camphor and acetic acid.—mr. Procter, objects to the addition of acetic acid to the officinal blistering cerate, and seems to smile at the idea of fixing by it the volatile principle of the cantharis, which, by the way, he gratuitously makes the author to say is a neutral substance, when he says not a word about it. He quotes the authority of mr. Redwood, who in the pharmaceutical journal, october, 1841, speaks of acetic acid as not being a good solvent for cantharidine. The reason is, in all probability, from the fact of his using the london standard strength, which is but 1.48. For messrs. Lavini and sobrero, (memoire lu a l'academie des sciences de turin, 9 mars, 1845,) state that "concentrated acetic acid,, dissolves cantharidine, but more readily under the influence of heat." Respecting the volatility of cantharidine, these same chemists have stated in the same paper "that while manipulating with but 52 grammes of flies, for the researches they were making on cantharidine, one of them suffered from blisters produced on the face and lips, by the emanations from these insects." Besides their authority, soubeiran, in his traite de pharmacie, and dorvault in the officine, both state that cantharidine is a very volatile substance, even at ordinary temperature, and if that is, as it appears to be, the ease, what reliable information have we that only 1-30th of a grain was volatilized in the experiment mentioned by w. Procter, jr., made with 100 grs. Of powdered cantharides? Is it not very probable, that in removing the hygrometric water, much more was lost?

Whatever may be the changes which take place by the addition of acetic acid in a concentrated state, it is a fact, proved by experience, that the blistering plaster thus prepared, keeps better—that is, retains its power longer than the officinal one even exposed to the air in thin layers. As an example of the stability of this combination, we have *brown's cantharidine* which, to all appearance, is made from an etherial extract of cantharides additioned with concentrated acetic acid and incorporated in melted wax. We find such a mixture, although spread on paper and but imperfectly protected from the air, retaining for a long period its vesicating properties. Is this advantage produced by a simple acid saponification of the cerate, without reaction on the active principle, but that of protecting it from atmospheric influences? We think it probable that there is a modification taking place, both on the cantharis and other components of the cerate.

E, D.

THE RICHMOND PHARMACEUTICAL SOCIETY.

—a large number of the druggists and apothecaries of the city of richmond, held a meeting on the 11th of june for the purpose of forming a pharmaceutical society, and, having appointed a committee to draft a constitution and bye-laws, and to report to an adjourned meeting, on the 28th of the same month, assembled on that day, and adopted the constitution and bye-laws reported by the committee. The election of officers was postponed until the 6th of july.

At a full meeting of those who had signed the constitution, the following gentlemen were elected officers of the society, for the next twelve months, viz:—

President,	Alexander duval.
1st vice president,	James p. Purcell.
2nd vice president,	J. B. Wood.
Recording secretary,	Chas. Millspaugh.
Corresponding secretary,	S. M. Zachrisson.
Treasurer,	W. S. Beers.
Librarian,	John t. Gray.

After which, several nominations for members and associate members having been made, the society adjourned to monday, 13th instant, that the president might, during the recess, appoint the standing committees, as required by the constitution.

The society having assembled on the 13th instant, the following committees were reported:—

Committee on admission—j. Bum, john t. Gray, e. J. Pecot.

Committee on pharmaceutical ethics—o. A. Strecker, s. W. Zachrisson, a. Bodeker.

Committee of finance—peyton johnston, benjamin f. Ladd, edward mccarthy.

Committee on library—andrew leslie, james p Purcell, william m. Dade.

Executive committee—john purcell, w. S. Bum, r. R. Duval:—

After which, several nominations were made. Appropriations were placed at the disposal of the library committee for subscriptions to various periodicals, and for the purchase of books, after which, the meeting adjourned.

NEW YORK JOURNAL OF PHARMACY. SEPTEMBER, 1852.
ON THE OIL OF GRAIN SPIRIT, OR FUSEL OIL.

BY EDWARD N. KENT.

The oil of grain spirit, has recently attracted considerable attention from the fact of its being the basis of a number of artificial perfumes or essences, one of which has been extensively used under the name of banana or pear essence.

The crude oil, as is well known, consists principally of hydrated oxide of amyl, mixed with more or less alcohol, and small quantities of other substances, the nature of which is not generally known, though it has been asserted that œnanthic ether and œnanthic acid may be found among them. To obtain the latter articles was a desired object, and that which led to the subject of this paper.

Crude fusel oil, (or oil of grain spirit) when distilled in a glass retort, commences to pass over at about 190° fahrenheit, and a considerable portion is obtained below 212; which consists mostly of alcohol and water, with a small quantity of the hydrated oxide of amyl. By changing the receiver and continuing the operation to about 280°, a large product is obtained, consisting principally of hydrated oxide of amyl, but contaminated with a little alcohol and water, and a trace of less volatile oil, which may be found in larger quantity in the residue remaining in the retort. This residue is small, of an agreeable odor, and consists of several substances among which may be found, an oil having the intoxicating smell, but not the chemical properties of œnanthic ether, other than a similarity in its boiling point.

To obtain a more perfect separation of the substances contained in the crude oil, a small copper still was constructed, on the principal which is now so successfully used in the manufacture of high proof alcohol, and which proved highly useful for the above purpose. This still is so arranged, that the vapor which is evolved by the boiling liquid, passes through a series of bent tubes, each of which is connected with a return pipe for returning vapors less volatile than boiling water, back to the still. These tubes are enclosed in a copper funnel filled with cold water, which becomes heated as the operation proceeds, and finally boils; the less volatile vapors are thus prevented from passing over, and the alcohol and water are almost perfectly separated from the oil remaining in the still.—if the water is then drawn off from the vessel containing the serpentine tube, the distillation may be continued till it ceases spontaneously.

The product thus obtained, when rectified from a little dry caustic potash to remove coloring matter and acetic and valerianic acid, and again rectified from dry quick lime to remove water, gives pure hydrated oxide of amyl.

The residue left in the copper still is most easily obtained by distillation with water, containing a little carbonate of soda to neutralise the free acids contained in it. A small quantity of a yellow oil is thus obtained, having an agreeable vinous odor similar to œnanthic ether, but unlike that ether it yields fusel oil, instead of alcohol, when distilled repeatedly from caustic potash. It is consequently an *amyl* compound, while œnanthic ether is known to be the œnanthate of oxide of *ethyle*.

The residue remaining in the still after the above distillation with water, consists of acetic and valerianic acids in combination with the soda, and the solution holds in suspension a considerable quantity of byrated oxide of iron, which formerly existed in combination with the acids.

From the above statement it appears that crude fusel oil contains the following substances, viz:—

Alcohol,

Water,

Hydrated oxide of amyl,

Acetic acid,

Valerianic acid,

Oxide of iron.

And an amyl compound, analagous to œnanthic ether.

EASY METHOD TO MAKE HYPOSULPHITE OF SODA.

BY JOHN C. TALLON.

Happening to inquire the price of hyposulphite of soda of a wholesale druggist, it appeared to me that the cost of its production is *greatly* under the wholesale price, i therefore suggest to apothecaries who may wish to make it *pure*, for their own consumption, the following: through a saturated solution of sal soda (ascertained to be free from sulphate) pass sulphurous acid gas until a small quantity, taken out of the solution after agitation, on the end of a glass rod, gives a white precipitate with nitrate of silver; then put the solution into a beaker glass, and boil it with sulphur (about one-twentieth of the weight of the soda in solution) until a little of the liquid, put into a test glass, gives, with a few drops of hydrochloric acid, a precipitate of sulphur, and another portion with nitrate of silver a white precipitate, immediately turning yellow and then black, when the liquid is to be filtered and evaporated quickly, until the salt be crystallized quite dry. The crystals are to be put into a closely stopped bottle, and kept well secured from the atmosphere. The advantage of this process over the common one is that it can be made in the store without any annoyance from the stench of melted sulphur; it costs but little and does not require the *continued* attention of the operator.

709 greenwich street, new york, august 12, 1852.

NOTES IN PHARMACY, NO. 4.

BY BENJAMIN CANAVAN.

TINCTURA BESTUSCHEFFI.

—in the last number (8) of this journal, mr. Mayer, speaking of this preparation, says that the formula given by me in the may number, is the "oldest" from "the austrian pharmacopœia of 1820," and suggests, as an improvement, preparing the salt by passing through a solution of protochlor. Ferri, a current of chlorine, to the proper point of saturation. The formula i gave *is* the "oldest" and the *original*, for which reason i selected it, affording as it does *the* "bestuscheff's tincture," at one time so highly valued, and though i did not consider it very creditable to the scientific accuracy of its "fatherland," it is the one which "did the good." The advantages, seemingly, claimed by mr. Mayer for his process, is its affording a more certain preparation. This does not appear evident, as the resulting tincture will be the same, respectively, by whatever process, supposing equal care to be used in conducting it. It may be possible that a stronger solution is obtained, but that is not asserted, nor is it important, as that would concern the *dose*, not the effect of the medicine. The difference, aside from the identity of the preparation, appears to me to be that, in one case experiment will be necessary to ascertain the strength of the tincture, whilst in the other it can be determined more quickly by calculation, but the extra labor required in the process in the later case, more than counterbalances any superiority there may be in this respect. I have, however, no objection to make to mr. Mayer's process, which is a very *neat* way of making "ethereal tincture of sesquichloride of iron"; but, i think, those who desire to make "bestuscheff's tincture," will consider it more strictly accurate to adhere to the "oldest formula."

DECOMPOSED CHLOROFORM.

—a specimen of this article lately came into my possession, to which, i think it right to direct the attention of apothecaries, although, its villainous odor was so disagreeable and suffocating, as to render it almost impossible that it could be administered, still it may serve to teach the necessity of all those having to do with the article, exercising such increased care that so bad an article could not pass through their hands unnoticed; for what might be the consequences in such a case if the sensible properties of the article did not happen to be so repugnant? And as it is desirable, in a scientific point of view, to know everything about so important an agent, it is proper and necessary that anything unusual in its regard should be recorded. The article in question, was contained in a badly stopped bottle, and had leaked one-eighth of its quantity. On removing the cupping, an efflorescent crust was observed coating the upper surface of the lip of the bottle and contiguous stopper, of a whitish, partly yellowish-green appearance, having a caustic taste, and washing off readily with water but not with chloroform, and precipitating nitrate of silver; the precipitate being soluble in ammonia and not in nitric acid, leading me to infer from this and other circumstances, that this substance was, probably a hydrochlorate of ammonia. The neck of the bottle before the stopper was removed, presented a yellowish appearance from some colored substance being interposed between it and the stopper, a pretty constant accompaniment of this kind of decomposition, which should always be noted. On removing the stopper, fumes escaped having a most suffocating odor, causing the bottle to be withdrawn quickly from the nostril and giving with ammonia, the white fumes characteristic of hydrochloric acid gas. By exposure the peculiar odor disappeared, and the whole of the liquid passed off without leaving any residue, except a slight greasy appearance on the sides of the glass from which it was evaporated, which *was not* owing to sulphuric acid. The specific gravity was that of good chloroform, and sulphuric acid aoquired no color when agitated with a portion, and the reaction with litmus was strongly acid. The bottle having been emptied, the small portion which adhered to the glass, collecting in the bottom, assumed a yellowish appearance resembling common muriatic acid.

Not having leisure or means to make an elaborate examination, i handed some to one of our professors of chemistry, who will make an accurate analysis. In the meantime, i deemed it prudent to note these particulars. A large quantity of the article, made at the same time and by the same process, i have since learned, has been found to have undergone a similar change. The manufacturer, supposes the decomposition to have arisen in some way from the sulphuric acid used in the process after the manner of professor gregory, although every means was used to separate it and none could be detected in it when recently made; some, however, which was thus supposed to be free from acid, i found to slightly redden litmus, although the smell was remarkably fine; but it has been found i learn, that of two specimens of the article taken from the same bottle and *exposed to the light*, one underwent decomposition and the other not. It has occurred to me, that the surest way of separating the acid would be to distil the chloroform from it; but it should be remembered that the process of gregory, was intended to be adopted for smaller quantities for immediate use, and not for its manufacture on a large scale, to be kept.

SUPPOSITORIA.

—in the number of the *new york medical times* for december, 1851, i took occasion to mention the superiority of cacao butter, to the other excipients for the formation of suppositories, a means of medication which had *become almost obsolete*; not unlikely from the circumstance of their having been prepared with iritating substances which counteracted their intended effect. In the last (july) number of the *american journal of pharmacy*, (philadelphia,) mr. A. B. Taylor, (who has not, apparently, seen my little note,) gives several formulas for these, which require the cacao butter to be melted, in which state the medicament is incorporated with it, &c. I recur to the subject for the purpose of stating that i have not found it necessary to adopt this very troublesome and tedious, not to say inaccurate method. The article, at all seasons, becomes sufficiently plastic when "worked" in the mortar, or in very cold weather, with the addition of a drop or so of almond or other proper oil, to admit of being *rolled* with the spatula into form, the most convenient one for which i have found to be that of a cylinder about an inch long, weighing twenty grains, and fitting exactly the calibre of the instrument used for introducing them, which i generally use as a mould. The active ingredients used are mostly sulph. Morph. And extr. Opii aquos. The latter of which is superior to opium, of course, being *nearly* free from narcotine. *Vaginal suppositories* would be equally applicable and useful as anal ones.

EDITOR AMERICAN JOURNAL OF PHARMACY.

—professor proctor has done me the honor to notice, favorably, some trifles which i have found time to contribute to our journal, among others an observation concerning the supposed decomposition of fowler's solution, with respect to which he says he "does not understand where the garlicky odor came from, as it is only the *vapor* of metallic arsenic that possesses this peculiarity." I beg to assure the professor that the odor *came from the bottle*. The immediate cause of it is certainly *mist*-erious, though it is not impossible that among the intricacies of chemical action sufficient heat may have been evolved to act on how small soever a portion of the metal in a *nascent state* as to cause the peculiar odor. *Spontaneous combustion* taking place in a mass of the common mineral known as "cobalt," produces, unmistakeably, both vapor and the odor of arsenic, and i have heard of a ships' crew having been salivated by the vapor arising from a cargo of quicksilver in a high latitude. A very much lower degree of heat is required to produce vapor than might be supposed from the point of volatility of the substance whence it emanates, an instance in point being the familiar process of boiling water; but this is rather a *cloudy point* which would require the acumen of a certain celebrated jury to elucidate, and to their tender mercies it is perhaps the better part to consign it.

GENERAL REPORT UPON THE RESULTS AND EFFECTS OF THE "DRUG LAW," MADE TO THE SECRETARY OF THE TREASURY.

BY C. B. GUTHRIE, M. D.

The act of congress, approved 26th of june, 1848, entitled "an act to prevent the importation of spurious and adulterated drugs and medicines," having now been in existence and enforcement almost three years, the working of the law and its effects, immediate and remote, have become necessarily matters of fact, and are no longer left to conjecture and speculation.

At the time of the passage of this law by congress, no inconsiderable fears were entertained by its friends, and great hopes by its enemies, that it would be found impracticable to carry out its requisite provisions without great injury to that portion of our citizens engaged in the importation of this class of merchandize, in which event its repeal would, of course, have been urgently solicited.23

---

23 strong *prima facie* evidence of the popularity of this law may be found in this significant fact that not a petition for its repeal has ever been presented to congress.

In entering upon the duties of the commission, which i had the honor to recieve from the department, i was fully impressed with the importance of the information sought for, and the necessity of a candid, impartial and unbiassed examination of facts bearing upon the subject, and in making, to the department, this report, i have divided my results and facts into immediate and remote; the reasons for which, will appear in the detail. Under the general terms drugs and medicines, are embraced all articles intended for the treatment of the diseases of the human system, and though they admit of many subdivisions, these terms, included under the two heads of chemicals and compounds, and crude drugs, are all that is necessary for my purpose in speaking of the effects and applications of the law.

First, with regard to the effect upon chemicals and compound medicines.: previous to the passage of this law, no restriction was laid upon any class of medicines coming in under this head. If the importer paid the requisite duty, no questions were asked, no limit was fixed as to quality or condition. It needs no argument, but merely a mention of the fact, to show that any compound medicine or chemical preparation may be so made as to deceive the unsuspecting and uneducated, and even very often the druggist, apothecary, physician, and all, because they were not in the habit of analysing their articles, and were deceived by their external, often times very fine appearance. Under the combined influence of competition and avarice—two strong temptations, the manufacture of articles of this class had become systematised, and on purpose to supply the united states market.

The immediate and positive beneficial results of the law may be seen in the fact that now very few, if indeed any, spurious or sophisticated chemical preparations, for pharmaceutical purposes, are even offered at our ports, or by any possibility find their way into our markets. Manufacturing chemists and importers of this description of medicines, finding it impossible to get such goods through our custom houses, will, of course, not risk the loss of bringing them here, but in their stead will import such as are known to come up to our required standards. Under this general head of chemicals, may be included a large majority of the manufactured and compound medicines used in practice by the medical faculty, and all the most important usually purchased by others for domestic uses, more especially in the great west and south, where every man, almost, is obliged to learn the uses and doses of calomel, blue mass and quinine, &c. The certainty of purity in these articles alone, is a matter of no small moment to the community at large; of the probabilities of their home adulteration i shall also refer to elsewhere.

A few articles of this class may now and then, either through culpable negligence on the part of the inspector, or by being entered under a false name, be imported, but they must be few, and are daily growing less. An instance of this kind has occurred in new york, where a large lot of sulphate of lime was offered in market, under the name of precipitated chalk. The new york college of pharmacy, standing very properly as the guardians of the public health, and protectors of this act, for which they had petitioned and which they had agreed to support, by committee, reported the fact, and warned the holders of the consequences of continuing to sell the article as a medicinal preparation, upon which they very readily withdrew it. How it came into the city that committee have never been able to ascertain, whether imported under the head of plaster of paris, and thus escaping the eye of the inspector, or whether passed by him, or at some other port, without due test and examination, i am not able to say. That it was imported under a false name, is, to my mind, the most likely of all.

If our colleges of pharmacy in the different cities, as i have no doubt they will, continue to thus watch the articles offered them and the public, and act with the independence that has characterised them thus far, no deception of this kind will go long unexposed, and it will soon cease altogether.

No manufactured article, susceptible of adulteration, ought ever to be suffered to pass by the examiner of drugs without being *sampled* and tested by analysis, and no matter what its appearances, or what its label; neither the one or the other are guarantees of its purity, for both may alike be counterfeits. The more popular the maker, the higher his name and reputation, the more likely his name, label, bottle and article to be counterfeited, as has pelletier's name to the article quinine, others to iodide of potassium, &c. &c.

Secondly. The effects of the law upon crude drugs and medicines, such as leaves, barks, roots, gums, gum resins, &c. Upon these articles, the effect has been the same as upon chemicals and compound goods. Greater variations must of, course occur in their qualities, as many of them cannot be tested with accuracy; and of the rest, very imperfect standards are to be found in any of the works on pharmacy or materia medica now extant. This was heretofore left entirely in the hands of the examiner at each port, who has been obliged to fix his own standards when there were none laid down in the works referred to in the instructions of the department. Such has been the case with many of our most valuable and important articles of crude drugs, gums, and gum resins,—such as opium, scammony, &c. Such also has been the case with many of the roots and barks, as rhubarb and the cinchona and all its varieties. One may have fixed upon five per cent. Of morphine, and another upon eight, another ten, as the standard for opium. Again, the same might occur in admitting or rejecting scammony. One requiring sixty or seventy per cent. Of resin, another admitting or rejecting, merely from the physical appearance of the article.

So again with regard to barks, especially the cinchonas— one refusing to admit any except the true medicinal article; another admitting maricaibo and other false barks usually sold in market as pale bark, or used to adulterate that article.—but, upon the whole class of crude drugs, the effect has been highly beneficial. Greater care is taken in their selection and preparation for market, and a vast quantity of many kinds of barks and roots heretofore finding daily their way into market either in their simple worthlessness or mixed with purer and different articles, are now scarcely, if ever found; and if seen, they are about the last of their kind.—now and then, an article may get through our ports, by some adroit means of deception, or be slipped in at a port where there is no examiner, but this must be but seldom.—but recently, in new york, i saw several casks of gum guaic, the heads of which, for about six inches, were filled with a fair article, while the remaining portion of the cask was made up of the vilest trash imaginable. This is but a shallow trick that could not be often repeated, for though it might decieve the examiner (as it did not), it would meet detection in the hands of the jobber, who would not fail to claim damages from the importer at once. Another mode of evading the law, is by sending sample packages to the examining office, or such cases as are known to be all right, and getting the whole invoice passed by them. This can only be guarded against by the examiner being always upon the alert, and where there is the least doubt refusing to pass anything except what he sees and knows to be correct as to quality. The facility with which this fraud may be practised, led the convention of the colleges of pharmacy to recommend that every package should be examined; an opinion, i then and now fully concur in. Many similar instances, both in regard to chemicals, chemical preparations and all sorts of crude drugs, might be given, but they have no bearing upon the object of this report, only as they point to a necessity for the law's continuance.

Another immediate result of the law is the exclusion of damaged drugs. Heretofore no state of damage or decay, whether little or much, prevented an article, either manufactured or crude, being thrown into market and sold for whatever it purported to be, whether calomel half oxydyzed, iodide of potassium one-third deliquesced, rhubarb one-half rotten, senna in a similar or worse condition from being soaked with salt water—they each sold under their original names, and found their way into the bands of the buyers of *cheap goods*, either in that state or powdered or re-bottled, re-labelled, and done up good as new. The importer got his drawback of twenty-five, fifty, and seventy per cent. Of duty. The insurance company sold the goods and paid the difference; bargain getters purchased; the physician prescribed; the apothecary dealt out, and the patient, suffering under the pains and ills of lingering disease, swallowed; all but the last got their pay, while the poor man who bore the unrighteous accumulation of the whole, cursed his physician for not understanding his complaint, and perchance turned his face to the wall and died. This is no fancy sketch, but true, every word of it, and more than once acted out in the dream of every-day life.

Under the proper construction and administration of the law, all this will and is now mostly prevented. It must be evident that any article of medicine essentially damaged, is not fit to be given to the sick as a remedy. This is a very important point, and all examiners should be careful to enforce it strictly, regardless of the specious plea of interested insurance companies or individuals, for any other construction for their general or especial benefit or relief.

In few words then, may be summed up the immediate effects of this law: a purer and better class of chemicals and compound preparations, a material improvement in the quality of crude drugs imported, such as gums, barks, roots, leaves, and an almost entire exclusion of damaged and decayed drugs from our markets.

These results are, in themselves, sufficient to mark the law as one of great value, and to entitle it to a sure claim for perpetuity, and its provisions to a steady enforcement. But they are by no means all that it has accomplished. Its remote or secondary effects, which i propose to point out, are equally important, and they are found in the influence upon our home manufactures and trade.

It has often been claimed that the law was a tariff for protection to home adulteration, and while we shut out the evil in one way, we were equally exposed to it in the shape of home preparations; were this even true, it is no argument against the law for keeping out foreign adulteration, as it is very evident that if both are equally bad, no pure medicine can be had by those who require them, while if we are certain the foreign are pure, we have a choice between the pure and the sophisticated. But i am satisfied that the amount of home adulterations have been over estimated, and that under the effect of this law they are decreasing daily, and perhaps mainly because the demand is decreasing.

I have never believed, though it has been again and again asserted, that our medical gentleman to any great extent, who buy and use most largely of this class of goods, have desired to buy and use inferior medicines, because they were cheap, and my own direct intercourse and observation, as a druggist for five years, aside from a six years' experience in the profession, has satisfied me of the correctness of my views. I speak of the country at large. Wherever it has been the case, it has been the result of ignorance, as to the appearance and physical properties of drugs that has led them into this error, an error in which, from a like ignorance, they have been kept by their druggist, who has been imposed upon by the bland assurance of the importer or jobber, which led him to take all things of a like name as of the same quality. There are those who buy because cheap, and prescribe, and perchance hope for success in the use of such remedies, but they are not found among our medical gentlemen of education and character and entitled to the respect and confidence of the community at large. The flood of light thrown upon this subject of adulterations of medicines by the reports to congress; by the report of dr. Bailey, special examiner for the port of new york; reports to the american medical association, and by various other writers in our pharmaceutical and medical journals, through the newspapers of the day, and various other means to the people, has worked, and is working a revolution in the drug trade at large. By a desire and growing necessity for a proper education of pharmaceutists and druggists, a man is no longer considered competent to sell, dispose and deal out medicinal articles affecting the health, life and happiness of his fellow-beings, simply because he can calculate a per centage, or make a profit.

The reform in this department is, i know, but just beginning, though long needed, but it will progress, for public opinion demands, and will continue to demand it.

Physicians, professors of materia medica, and teachers of practical pharmacy and chemistry are feeling it, and the whole course of teaching upon this and kindred branches, has received more attention from both professor and pupil within the two past years, than ever before in the same length of time in the united states. From these combined sources will continue to flow a light that must shine upon and enlighten that ignorance which was permitting men to tamper with the life and health of the community. This has also had the effect to create a demand for pure medicines. Rhubarb is no longer rhubarb unless the quality is such as to commend it to the unfortunate consumer, and calling a thing by a good name is no longer sufficient to redeem it from its lack of curative properties and consequent worthlessness.

Again, the endeavor to come up to the law's standard for chemicals, the competition with the imported article, the increasing demand for good medicines, together with a commendable emulation among our chemists, has produced an improvement in this class of goods, sufficiently visible to refute all charges of home adulteration because protected from foreign competition; besides this, they are our fellow citizens, within reach of our complaints, with no intermediate dealer to shift the blame of impurity to the other side of the ocean, and thus wash his innocent hands at our cost. With this and the spirit of inquiry as to what we are selling, what we are buying, what we are administering, what we are swallowing with hopes of relief, that is abroad, no man can long escape detection, exposure and consequent loss of business, if engaged in the manufacture or sale of spurious goods.

These opinions are the result of the concurrent testimony of the different examiners, of various dealers in drugs throughout the country, from whom i had before and since my appointment to this commission been in receipt of information, and are fully borne out by my own extensive observation in almost every state in the union.

Without inquiring or pointing out the cause, the testimony to this effect, that the quality of drugs in general has improved much within the two past years, is almost universal; and a style of drugs and chemicals, and of medicinal preparations, may now be found on sale in our great commercial emporiums, of a quality and purity never before found, certainly not in the united states, and i question if any wherelse.

These are the results of my observations, both as to the remote and immediate, or special and general effects of the law. And i feel that the friends of the law have great reason to congratulate themselves and the community at large, upon the fullest realizations of their hopes as to the good accruing from this sanitary measure.

Those who were reaping an iniquitous harvest either through a desire to do evil for the purposes of gain (if any such there could have been), or through ignorance of the extent of such evil, must themselves feel that the law has worked no wrong to them even though it may have forced them into a different channel of trade. The only ones from whom we shall hear any complaints while the law is carefully and judiciously executed, or from whom we shall hear the plea for "unrestricted commerce," and the potency of the great laws of trade as in themselves sufficient for the protection of life and health, are those whose prototypes aforetime cried out "great is diana of the ephesians."

The value of their opinions may be measured by the sincerity of their professions, and the weight of their testimony calculated by the per centage of their gains.

I have pursued my enquiries among drug importers and jobbers, meeting both friends and enemies of the law, among retail apothecaries, professional men and their patients, and my conclusions are that no more popular act, stands upon our congressional record.

I have only to add my sincere wish, that it may long stand as a mark of the enlighted wisdom of the age and nation.

The above report is but the general report upon the working of the law.—it was, we understand, accompanied by a second private and detailed one, regarding the manner in which, at different localities, the law has been carried out.—editor.

ON THE MANUFACTURE OF NITRATE OF POTASH (SALTPETRE.)

Previous to the middle of the seventeenth century, the chief part of the saltpetre consumed in this country was obtained from refuse animal matters, as is evident from the following edict, issued by james i., for the regulation of the "mynes of salt peter."—"the king, taking into his consideration the most necessary and important use of gunpowder, as well for supply of his own royall navie, and the shipping of his lovinge subjects, as otherwise for the strength, safety, and defence of his people and kingdoms, and how greate a blessinge it is of almighty god to this realm, that it naturally yieldeth sufficient mynes of salt peter for making of gunpowder for defence of ittself, without anie necessitie to depend uppon the dangerous chargeable and casuall supply thereof from forraigne parts, hath sett downe certen orders and constitutions to be from henceforth inviolably kept and observed, for the better maynteyning of the breed and increase of salt peter, and the true making of gunpowder.

"noe person doe from henceforth pave with stone or bricke, or floare with boarde, anie dove-house or dove-cote, or laie the same with lyme, sand, gravel, or other thing, whereby the growthe and increase of the myne of salt peter maie be hindered or ympaired, but shall suffer the floure or grounde thereof to lye open with goode and mellowe earth, apt to breede increase of the myne and salt peter, and so contynue and keep the same.

"that no innkeepers, or others that keep stables for travellers and passengers, doe use anie deceiptful meanes or devices whereby to destroy or hinder the growthe of salt peter in those stables. And that no stables at all be pitched, paved, or gravelled where the horse feete used to stand, but planked only, nor be paved, pitched, or gravelled before the plankes next the mangers, but that both places be kept and maynteyned with goode and mellowe earth, fitt and apt to breede and increase the myne of salt peter, and laide with nothinge which may hurte the same.

"that all and every such person and persons as having had heretofore had anie dove-house, dove-cote, or stable (which were then good nurseries for the myne of salt peter) have sithence carried out the goode moulde from thence, and filled the place agayne with lyme, sand, gravel, rubbish, or other like stuff, or paved or floored the same, whereby the growthe of salt peter myne there hath been decayed and destroyed, shall and doe within three months next contryve to take up the pavements and boards agayne, and carrie out the said gravel, lyme, and offensive stuff from thence, and fill the place agayne with goode and mellowe earth fitt for the increase of salt peter, three foote deepe at the least, and so contynue and keepe the same for the breede of salt peter myne. No person, of anie degree whatsoever, was to denie or hinder the salt peter man workinge any earth; nor was anie constable to neglect or to forbeare to furnish him with convenient carriages necessarie for his worke; and every justice to whom the salt peter man should address himself for assistance was at his peril to fail to render it, that his majesties service might not suffer by his default. And no one was to give any gratuity or bribe to the salt peter man for forbearinge or sparinge of anie ground or place which may be digged or wrought for salt peter."

To lessen the annoyance to the owners of these dove-cotes and stable beds of saltpetre, and to promote the comfort of the pigeons, the saltpetre man was "to dig and carrie away the earth in such convenient time of the daie, and work it in suche manner as maie give least disturbance and hurte to the pigeons, and encrease of their breede, and in the chief tyme of breeding, that it be not done above two howers in anie one daie, and that about the middest of the daie, when the pigeons use to be abroade. And shall in like seasonable tyme carrie in the saide earth after it shall be wrought, and spreade itt there, and make flatt the floure of the dove-house, and leave itt well and orderlie."

In another proclamation, issued two years after this, it was ordered that whensoever anie ould building or house in london within three miles, is to be pulled down and removed, notice is to be given at the king's storehouse in southwark, that the deputy may first take as much of the earth and rubbish as in his judgement and experience is fitted for salt peter for the king's service."

Soon after, we find that this enactment which caused much complaint, was repealed. "the manufacture of salt peter," says the king, "had hitherto produced much trouble and grievance to the lieges, by occasioning the digging up the floors of their dove-cotes, dwelling-houses, and out-houses, and had also occasioned great charge to the salt peter men for removing their liquors, tubbes, and other instruments, and carrying them from place to place, but now, divers compounds of salt peter can be extracted by other methods, for which sir john brooke and thomas russell, esq., have received letters patent.

"to encourage so laudable a project, all our loving subjects," continues his majesty, "inhabiting within every city, town, or village, after notice given to them respectively, shall carefully and constantly keep and preserve in some convenient vessels or receptacles fit for that purpose, all the urine of man during the whole year, and all the stale of beasts which they can save and gather together whilst their beasts are in their stables and stalls, and that they be careful to use the best means of gathering together and preserving the urine and stale, without any mixture of water or other thing put therein. Which our commandment and royal pleasure being so easy to be observed, and so necessary for the public service of us and our people, that if any person be remiss thereof, we shall esteem all such persons contemptuous and ill affected both to our person and state, and are resolved to proceed to the punishment of that offender with that severity we may."

Sir john agreed to remove the liquid accumulations from the houses once in every twenty-four hours in summer time, and every forty-eight hours in winter time.

About the year 1670, the importation of saltpetre from the east indies (where it is obtained as a natural product, being disengaged by a kind of efflorescence from the surface of the soil) had so increased as to affect the home manufacture, which has since gradually declined and become extinct. The manufacture of saltpetre from sources of the kind above mentioned, is not followed in this country at the present day, and it will be unnecessary to indicate here the process employed in france, sweden, germany, and other countries for obtaining it by the decomposition of animal refuse, the more especially as full accounts are given in knapp's *technology*, ure's *dictionary of arts and manufactures*, and other standard chemical works; we shall therefore confine our attention to an account of the processes which have been proposed for obtaining nitrate of potash by the decomposition of nitrate of soda and other sources.

The first of these processes is that of adding nitrate of lime to a solution of sulphate of potash; sulphate of lime is precipitated, and nitrate of potash obtained in solution, which, on evaporation yields crystals of that salt.

Mr. Hill's method of manufacturing nitrate of potash is by decomposing nitrate of soda by means of muriate of potash. For this purpose the nitrate of soda is put into a suitable vessel, made of wrought or cast iron, and dissolved in as much water as is required, and then the equivalent quantity of muriate of potash is added; decomposition ensues, with the formation of nitrate of potash and muriate of soda; the greater portion of the latter is separated during evaporation, as it is equally soluble at all temperatures. The nitrate crystallizes on the cooling of the solution. Specimens of this nitre were shown at the great industrial exhibition.

Mr. Rotch's processes for converting nitrate of soda into nitrate of potash are as follows:—

First process with american potashes, (caustic).—in a suitable round-bottomed iron boiler, he dissolves 2000 LBS. Of the ashes in 1000 quarts of water, and then applies heat for three hours, at the end of which time the solution ought to be of a density of 45° baumè, (sp. Gr. 1.453). In a similar boiler he dissolves 1300 LBS. Of nitrate of soda in 1200 quarts of water, applying the heat as before, until the solution becomes of the density of 45° baumé. Both solutions are then allowed to stand for twelve hours to cool and settle. They should be heated to from 175° to 200° fah., and then both poured into a third vessel or crystallizing pan, when the double decomposition will take place, and the crystals of nitrate of potash be deposited, this first deposition giving from 700 to 900 LBS. Of good merchantable saltpetre.

Care must be taken not to let the heat fall below 85°, at which the crystals form; and the better and more regularly the heat is kept up, the speedier will be the deposition of the crystals. The mother-liquor should then be poured off, and the crystals collected and thrown into the centrifugal drying machines, where they may be washed with weak mother-liquors. The portion of nitrate of potash that is left in the mother-liquor may be obtained by crystallization as before.

Second process with carbonate of potash (pearlash).—the pearlash is dissolved in water, and the solution brought to a density of 40° baumé (sp. Gr. 1.384). This will cause whatever sulphate of potash may be contained in it to be deposited. The solution should then be left to stand for five or six days, after which it should be poured off, and diluted with water, until its density becomes 15° baumé (sp. Gr. 1,116). Caustic lime should then be added in the proportion of one-fourth of the weight of the original quantity of carbonate employed. It should then be poured off from the carbonate of lime formed, heated and mixed with the solution of nitrate of soda, as above described. The precise proportions that the caustic alkali should bear to the nitrate of soda, are forty-eight parts of the former to eighty-six parts of the latter. The materials to be used should be tested, so as to enable the just proportions to be arranged according to the formula just given. The patentee states that by this means a nitre is produced which is equal to the bengal saltpetre, after the latter has gone through the expensive process of refining.

A stockholm manufacturer says:—"on dissolving nitrate of soda in excess of caustic potash solution, and evaporating to 28° or 32° baumé (sp. Gr. 1.241 or 1.285), the chief part of the saltpetre crystallizes, contaminated by the magnesia which is precipitated, and a small quantity of carbonate of lime. In order to obtain the whole of the saltpetre, the solution must be concentrated to 45° or 50° baumé (sp. Gr. 1.453 or 1.530). Here however, a difficulty arises; the cast iron crystallizing vessels are not impermeable to the liquor, which, whatever the thickness of the vessels, oozes through them, thus occasioning great loss. The saltpetre which still remains in solution after crystallization in the caustic solution at 30° baumé (sp. Gr. 1.263), cannot be collected, and if it be employed in the manufacture of soap, this will be found to contain so large a proportion of saltpetre, that it deliquesces and falls to pieces in a few days."

"a method employed in the russian manufactories is first to dissolve the fine pearlash, and the nitrate of soda in the relative proportions of water required for their mutual decomposition, or rather with an excess of potash in such a quantity of water that the resulting product remains dissolved at 50° reaumur. The solution is then allowed to settle, whereby the carbonates of lime and magnesia are deposited, after which the liquor is run off into wooden crystallizing vessels. As soon as the temperature is lower than 50° reaumur, the principal part of the nitrate of potash crystallizes. The crystallization must now be very attentively watched, for as soon as the soda begins also to crystallize, the mother-liquors should be run off into other vessels, where a small quantity of nitrate of potash will crystallize, though the principal part will be soda. The nitrate of potash and the soda must then be purified by new crystallizations. The salts formed from the mother-liquors must be redissolved with the nitrate of potash or the soda, according to which of the two most predominates."

Messrs. Crane and jullion patented in 1848 the following method of manufacturing the nitrates of potash and soda:—the oxides of nitrogen evolved in the process of manufacturing oxalic acid, are mixed with oxygen gas or atmospheric air, and made to pass slowly through a chamber or other apparatus containing an alkali placed on trays (similar to the lime in a dry lime purifier), the mixed gases combine with the alkali, forming a nitrate of potash or soda, whichever alkali may have been employed.

De sussex's process for the manufacture of nitrate of potash is as follows:—a solution is made of 166 pounds of nitrate of lead, and another of 76 pounds of chloride of potassium. The two solutions are then mixed, when double decomposition takes place, chloride of lead being precipitated, and nitrate of potash obtained in solution. In order to avoid the presence of lead in the nitrate of potash, a small portion of caustic or carbonated lime or magnesia is added, by which means any portion of the chloride of lead remaining in solution is precipitated. The solution of nitrate of potash is then evaporated and crystallized.

Nitrate of soda is obtained in the same way, by substituting sixty-six pounds of chloride of sodium for the chloride of potassium above mentioned.—*pharmaceutical journal and transactions, july 1, 1852.*

ON TINCTURE OF OPIUM.

The pharmaceutical society of antwerp has employed a commission composed of its members to determine the best menstruum for the preparation of tincture of opium. It has arrived at the following results:—

1. Good opium gives, when treated with water, less extract than bad or adulterated.

2. By warm digestion, a stronger solution is obtained than by cold infusion.

3. Alcohol must be preferred to wine in the preparation of tincture of opium.

4. Narcotine, although alone insoluble in water, becomes partially extracted with the other ingredients of opium. When it is advisable to avoid the removal of narcotine, proceed as follows:—treat carefully prepared aqueous extract of opium with, boiling alcohol; this dissolves out the narcotine and morphine, from which solution, when cold, the narcotine separates.

After the precipitation, whatever ingredients are necessary to form the tincture are to be added to the alcoholic solution.

By this opportunity, the commission recommend another process by which morphine may be more readily separated from narcotine. One part of the opium is to be treated with four parts of alcohol. After the alcohol has been separated by filtration, the residue is again to be macerated with three parts of alcohol. The resulting tinctures, after being mixed, are to be set aside for twenty-four hours to allow the narcotine to separate; afterwards the morphine is to be precipitated with ammonia. To remove the last traces of morphine, the fluid, from which the precipitated morphine has been filtered, is to be kept in a warm place for two days, a little water having been previously added, when a fresh quantity of morphine will fall down. By this method, $\frac{1}{12}$ of the weight of the opium employed, can be obtained as morphine.—*annals of pharmacy and practical chemistry*.

PREPARATION OF PROPYLAMINE FROM ERGOTINE.

BY DR. F. L. WINCKLER.

The readers of the *new repertory for pharmacy*, part i., p. 22 already know that i have been for some time occupied with the investigation of ergot, and that i obtained, by the distillation of ergotine with potash, besides ammonia, a substance having a very unpleasant odor, which conducted itself as a volatile alkali, and possessed a narcotic and highly diuretic property. This confirmation of a result which i had obtained some years before, induced me to continue my experiments, and i have now arrived at the conviction that the volatile alkali which is extracted from ergotine by distillation with potash is propylamine $(n\ h_2\ c_6\ h_7$, or $n\ h_3\ c_6\ h_6)$ consequently the same which, according to the most recent experiments, is proved to be the product of decomposition of narcotine by potash, and the ingredient of herring-pickle. The smell itself made me imagine, long before i was acquainted with wertheim's experiments, that herring-pickle must likewise contain propylamine, and my experiments have fully confirmed this supposition, for in distilling herring-pickle with potash i obtained the same propylamine as that extracted from a concentrated aqueous solution of ergotine. The properties in which they agree are the following:—

1. Propylamine saturates acids completely, and thus forms salts soluble in water, and for the most part in spirit of wine, with the exception of sulphate of propylamine, which does not dissolve in the latter. Beautiful white crystals may, however, be produced from the concentrated aqueous solution by the admixture of alcohol of eighty per cent. Of strength. The salts of propylamine dissolved in water and treated with tannic acid produce a white (flocculent) precipitate; with chloride of mercury likewise, a white but pulverulent precipitate; with nitrate of silver a white (flocculent) precipitate; and with chloride of platinum a yellow precipitate (a crystalline powder). The salts of propylamine have a strong odor of fresh ergot,

much less of herring-pickle, and are easily decomposed by potash.

2. The concentrated aqueous solution being mixed with a fourth of its volume of tincture of iodine, a considerable dark yellowish-brown sediment is precipitated, and the supernatant fluid appears dark brownish-red. But in a very short time this sediment diminishes considerably, the fluid gradually changes color, so that in about twelve hours' time there will be left but very little orange-colored sediment, whilst the fluid itself will appear almost colorless. Immediately after the addition of iodine the very disagreeable odor of propylamine disappears, and the mixture acquires the odor of iodine.

3. When the neutral aqueous solution of sulphate of propylamine is evaporated in a water-bath it exhales a very disagreeable odor of herring, the solution becomes very acid, has only a weak odor of ergot, and all the re-actions cease. If this concentrated solution be digested with caustic lime in a still, there comes over, without the aid of artificial heat, almost pure propylamine, which has the odor of an ammoniacal liquid, and produces all the re-actions of pure propylamine.

Now the propylamine of ergot presents the very same results, and it is on this account that until lately, it has always been mistaken for ammonia. I am convinced that it constitutes the odorous principle of urine, perspiration, and in the blood, and is often the cause of the odor which we observe in the action of alkaline leys upon nitrogenous compounds. Propylamine belongs to the organic bases, and may be considered as the adjunct [*paarling*] of ammonia. I think i am justified in concluding, from the results of my experiments, that propylamine, *combined with an acid*, pre-exists in ergot as well as in herring-pickle, and is not produced by the potash, as is the case with narcotine. I have previously demonstrated the presence of formic acid in ergot, and it is with that acid that the propylamine seems to be united. I have not yet made any experiments with herring-pickle.

It will now be difficult to determine whether the medicinal activity of ergot depends on propylamine or not, for the neutral salts of propylamine dissolved in water are easily absorbed, and i hope to be able to induce physicians to make pharmacological and therapeutical experiments.

I have reasons to suppose that propylamine is likewise an ingredient of cod-liver oil, and being easily combined with iodine, it may soon be ascertained by practical application whether it ought not to be considered as the bearer (*träger*) of iodine. I propose to begin the necessary experiments in this respect as soon as my apparatus is entirely free from the odor of propylamine, in order to avoid all error.

Finally, i had the idea of trying an experiment with regard to propylamine upon my own urine, which i made after a supper consisting of roast veal, potato-salad, and a glass of water, and which was neither acid nor alkaline. I poured three ounces of the urine, fresh made and still quite warm, upon four ounces of burned lime, and submitted it to distillation. The distilled product had indeed the odor of pure propylamine, and re-acted strongly alkaline; but acted in a remarkable manner on tincture of iodine in the same way as liquid ammonia. After having neutralized it with sulphuric acid, the liquid showed when tested with tannic acid and nitrate of silver, an unmistakable proportion of propylamine. Might this be formed out of the urea? My experiment confirms, at all events, the opinion stated above; the beginning is made, and i may now pass from experiment to scientific deductions.

Remarks by dr. Buchner.—my friend, dr. Winckler, in communicating the above paper, very agreeably surprised me by transmitting at the same time specimens of his preparation of propylamine, and that too in quantities varying from one to two drachms, for which i hereby beg to express to him publicly my best thanks. I received from him, namely:—

1. The rough product of distillation of herring-pickle.

2. The aqueous solution of the sulphate produced from it.

3. The pure crystallized, and by spirit of wine, precipitated sulphate of propylamine.

4. The concentrated solution of pure propylamine.

5. The aqueous solution of the sulphate prepared with no. 4.

Hitherto i have only experimented with the preparations no. 2, 4 and 5, in order to verify and complete the statements of the above paper. All these solutions are quite colorless and clear, like water; they diffuse already at some distance a strong odor of herring; but the pure aqueous propylamine, when smelt at closely, has a pungent odor, very similar to that of liquid ammonia, which, however, at a distance, assumes, as it has been said, the smell of herring. This odor is so peculiarly characteristic, that i do not doubt, that even in water-closets, in consequence of fermentation, propylamine is developed, particularly as woollen clothes easily acquire there the odor of herring. All the conditions at least necessary for the formation of propylamine ammonia, and carbo-hydrogen, are to be found in water-closets. In a small close room its odor becomes insupportable, and affects strongly the head. Dr. Winckler, had therefore, good reasons to warn me against it. A young chemist, upon whose hand i dropped a very minute quantity of aqueous propylamine, for the purpose of ascertaining its taste, notwithstanding that he had been walking after that a considerable distance, and had been exposed to the air, smelt still, after some hours, so strongly of herring, that happening to to enter a company, he was spoken to about it by several persons. I mention this merely as a caution. The taste of pure aqueous propylamine is pungently alkaline, and hardly distinguishable from that of caustic ammonia.

The chemical re-actions of propylamine are well explained by winckler. Turmeric paper turns brown with it, but being exposed to the air, in which propylamine quickly evaporates, it resumes again its primitive yellow color.

Sulphate of propylamine (no. 3,) appears in small splendid white prisms, exposed to the air it evolves a distinct smell of herring, and has a pungent saline taste, like sulphate of ammonia; it is entirely neutral, and when moistened with water, it does not alter the color either of blue or red litmus-paper, or of turmeric-paper.

We have in solutions of silver and iodine, which are not precipitated by ammonia, very appropriate re-agents for distinguishing propylamine from ammonia. Propylamine, however, treated with sulphate of silver, gave me not a white, but a yellowish-brown precipitate; and this result suggested to me the idea, that formiate of propylamine might be present. This precipitate was easily and perfectly dissolved in caustic liquid ammonia. With an aqueous solution of iodine i acquired at one time, according to the quantitative proportion a brown, and at another time a beautiful yellow precipitate, which dissolved in an excess of iodide of potassium. I usually employ an aqueous solution of iodine in iodide of potassium instead of the tincture of iodine made with spirit of wine. The precipitate produced by iodide of potassium is, as i have just stated, either brown or yellow, provided that no excess of iodide of potassium be employed.—*buchner's neues repertorium*, bd. 1.

EDITORIAL.

We had intended once more to call the attention of our readers to the approaching meeting of the national convention, but have been anticipated by one of our colleagues in the communication which is subjoined, giving an account of both its origin and its objects. It is to be hoped that, as the convention will probably assume a permanent organization, its proceedings will take on a scientific character. Independent of the subjects which pharmacy, every where, presents, such a body would be a fit one to assist in ascertaining and developing the resources of our indigenous materia medica. Our country is rich in medicinal articles, but the properties of many of them are but imperfectly known, and comparatively little attention has been paid to their pharmaceutical preparation. Inquiries of this kind, carried on with the aid of physicians, particularly of those attached to hospitals, could not fail to produce important results, and they seem peculiarly adapted to the wants of the community and to the position of the convention.

THE NATIONAL PHARMACEUTICAL CONVENTION.

The second meeting of pharmaceutists, the first as a national convention, to which the convention of delegates from the several colleges of pharmacy, held in new york last october, may be considered the preliminary movement, will take place in philadelphia, on wednesday the 6th of october ensuing. The convention of last fall was held chiefly for the purpose of considering the important subject of standards of quality and purity which imported drugs ought to possess in order to regulate and render uniform the character required of them by the government inspectors, at the various ports of entry in the united states. Unofficially and officially the duty of affixing standards for imported drugs was, with propriety, assigned to the colleges of pharmacy. For this object they were called in convention for that time only, and permanent organization was not then anticipated. But on the meeting of the colleges, and their united action upon the one subject of such general importance, it was a natural consequence that a spontaneous and general feeling should arise in favor of the establishment of a national pharmaceutical organization, with an annual convention for the advancement of science and for the promotion of intercourse and good will among pharmaceutists generally. Accordingly the preamble and resolutions brought forward by the committee, subsequent to their report on the special business of that convention and its action upon it, were received with hearty favor. We think it would be well to recapitulate them:

"whereas, the advancement of the true interests of the great body of pharmacutical practitioners in all sections of our country is a subject worthy of earnest consideration; and whereas pharmaceutists, in their intercourse among themselves, with physicians and the public, should be governed by a code of ethics calculated to elevate the standard and improve the practice of their art; and whereas, the means of a regular pharmaceutical education should be offered to the rising pharmaceutists by the establishment of schools of pharmacy in suitable locations; and whereas, it is greatly to be desired that the united action of the profession should be directed to the accomplishment of these objects; therefore,

Resolved, that in the opinion of this convention, much good will result from a more extended intercourse between the pharmaceutists of the several sections of the union, by which their customs and practice may be assimilated; that pharmaceutists would promote their individual interests and advance their professional standing by forming associations for mutual protection, and the education of their assistants, when such associations have become sufficiently matured; and that, in view of these important ends, it is further

Resolved, that a convention be called, consisting of three delegates each from incorporated and unincorporated pharmaceutical societies, to meet at philadelphia, on the first wednesday in october, 1852, when all the importent questions bearing on the profession may be considered, and measures adopted for the organization of a national association, to meet every year.

In accordance with these resolutions, it was resolved that the president of the convention be requested to transmit an invitation to the authorized bodies, at least three months previous to the time of meeting, desiring such bodies to acquaint him with the names of the delegates they may appoint.

On motion, it was resolved that the new york delegation be appointed a committee to lay the proceedings of this convention before the secretary of the treasury of the united states, and afterwards have them published in pamphlet form.

Dr. Philbrick of boston, offered the following preamble and resolution, which were adopted:

Whereas, to secure the full benefits of the prohibition of sophisticated drugs and chemicals from abroad, it is necessary to prevent home adulteration; therefore,

Resolved, that this convention recommend to the several colleges to adopt such measures as in their respective states may be best calculated to secure that object.

On motion of mr Colould of boston, it was

Resolved, that a committee of three be appointed by this convention to act as a standing committee to collect and receive such information as may be valuable, and memorials and suggestions from any medical and pharmaceutical associations, to be presented at the next convention.

The president appointed g. D. Coggeshall of new york, s. M. Colcord of boston, and w. Procter, jr., of philadelphia, as the committee.

A vote of thanks to the officers was passed, and then the convention adjourned, to meet in philadelphia, on the first wednesday in october, 1852."

We hope that the considerations embraced in the preamble and resolutions of the committee will engage the thoughtful and earnest attention of every apothecary every where throughout the united states, who has a just sense of the proper dignity of his profession and an honest desire for its advancement, and that all will feel the importance of a general gathering at the approaching convention,—one that shall comprise a full representation of remote as well as adjacent districts of our extended country. In the words of the resolution, "three delegates, each, from incorporated and unincorporated pharmaceutical societies," are invited, but a feeling has been increasingly manifested since the last convention, to solicit representation from all districts, small as well as large, that in places where but few apothecaries are located—too few as they may think for efficient organization,—they should yet feel their individual responsibility, and be encouraged to depute one or more of their number to represent them. All, who come in the right spirit of regard for the cause, may be sure of being welcome.—a national pharmaceutical association will undoubtedly be organized on a similar plan to that of the medical profession, and in it individuals may be admitted to membership that are acceptable as worthy practioners of their art.

The convention will have many subjects of general interest to discuss and to arrange for future consideration Prominent amongst these will be, a code of ethics which should govern pharmaceutists in the performance of their duties, and in their intercourse with each other and with physicians; the importance of general conformity in practice with the united states pharmacopœia; the suppression of *home* as well as the exclusion of *foreign* adulteration; and the driving out of quackery into its own mean company. That all these ends can at once be attained is scarcely to be hoped for; but we trust the convention will be composed of men who appreciate the distinctness of the honorable practice of our profession from all malpractice and quackery, and who are fully disposed to mark the division clearly and broadly; so that persons governed by such opposite principles may take their separate places, and be esteemed accordingly.

We are authorized by dr. Guthrie, who, since the convention of 1851, has removed to memphis, tennessee, to request that the names of delegates may be reported to prof. William procter, philadelphia,—a convenient arrangement, as mr. Procter is one of the delegates to the next convention, residing in the city where it is to be held.

We would also invite the attention of pharmaceutists to the resolution introduced by mr. Colcord, of boston, and hope that any suggestions they may wish to offer, will be presented at an early day to one of the committee appointed, to rceive them.

POISONING BY ADULTERATED CIDER.

A number of cases of lead poisoning, two of which terminated fatally, have lately occurred at paris, which have been traced to the use of cider, clarified by a mixture of acetate of lead and carbonate of potassa. The history of this matter shows the efficacy of the french law regarding the use of poisonous substances, and the rigor with which it is enforced:—

Several manufacturers, were accused of having sold cider adulterated and containing substances injurious to health; others in addition to this, of having caused various internal injuries to different individuals, and one m. Henon, further of having thus caused the death of two individuals.

One of the witnesses testified, that he had purchased cider at the establishment of the defendant, that some days after drinking it he had been attacked with colic, and constant tremblings; by the advice of his physician, he sent a quantity of the suspected cider to the prefect of police for analysis. A number of other witnesses who had been poisoned, made statements to the same effect.

M. Chevallier deposed, that he had received a letter from the prefect of the police, enclosing one from the physician of the plaintiff, who stated that a number of his patients had been rendered ill by the use of this cider; that he had, in consequence of this, inspected the various establishments in which the manufacture of cider was carried on, and that he has ascertained the presence of lead in the cider obtained at establishments of the accused.

Several physicians testified, that the symptoms under which their patients (the witnesses) had labored, were due to lead poisoning.

M. Dubail, a *pharmacien*, testified that he had furnished m. Henon, (one of the accused), with a mixture of acetate of lead and carbonate of potassa, which m. H. Stated, that by the advice of one of his clerks, he intended to use in the clarification of cider. That he had cautioned m. H. Regarding its employment, and had furnished him with a re-agent for the purpose of detecting any lead which might not be precipitated in the cider thus clarified.

The trial was commenced on the 9th of may, continued upon the 11th, and judgment rendered on the 18th.

Henon, the use of whose cider had caused two deaths, was condemned to 18 months imprisonment and to pay a fine of 800 francs; a second, to 8 months imprisonment and a fine of 500 francs; a third, to 6 months imprisonment and 500 francs; while a fourth party, accused only of selling adulterated cider, but to the employment of which no injury had been traced, was imprisoned 3 months and fined 100 francs. M. Henon was condemned to pay 24,050 francs in addition as damages; another of the accused, the sum of 1500 francs.

Truly, if the prince president has been rather free in the employment of lead in the streets of paris, the government takes good care that its citizens shall not be poisoned by it with impunity.

ERRATUM.

—in the july no. Page 224, article announcing delegates to the convention for 1852, fourth line, for monday read *wednesday*.

UNITED STATES CUSTOMS.

NEW YORK, SEPTEMBER 25, 1852.

MR. GEORGE D. COGGESHALL.

Dear sir,—your kind and courteous favor of the 16th instant, on behalf of the publishing committee of the new york journal of pharmacy, asking "information respecting the character of imported drugs and medicines coming under my supervision; and also, information in reference to the general working and effect of the drug law of 1848," has been before me for several days, waiting such response, in the shape of a full and lengthy communication in detail, as it was my wish to furnish; but pressing and increasing official duties compel me, from want of time (not material), to forego that pleasure and confine myself to a brief statement of facts and data, which, together with some general observations, i am in hopes may, nevertheless, be found interesting to your readers.

As an evidence of the beneficial effects of the wise sanitary measure, in the success of which, we have all taken so much interest, i am pleased to say that the character and quality of the more important articles of drugs, medicines and chemical preparations, connected with medicine at present presented for entry from abroad, is greatly improved, and of a far higher standard of strength and purity than formerly; notwithstanding, as will be seen, i still have occasion to apply the "veto power"—a labor of love, which must, of necessity, be performed in order to arrest the unhallowed strides of deception and fraud which will ever be practised, to a greater or less extent, as long as we have those among us, engaged in any department of the drug trade, who, to put money in their purse, would endanger, if not sacrifice the lives of their fellow men. The law in question has now been in operation at this port something more than four years; and, with the exception of some eleven months, the duties and responsibilities of its administration have devolved upon me. On the 21st day of april, 1849, i made a report to the new york academy of medicine, on the practical operation of this law, and stated therein the more important articles of drugs and medicines, with the quantities annexed, rejected by me up to that date; but as that report is doubtless familiar to most of your readers, i have not deemed it necessary to repeat them here. The following are the more important articles, with the quantities annexed, that i have since rejected and condemned as not of the requisite strength and purity to be safely and properly used for medicinal purposes, viz:—

Senna,	31,838	Lbs.
Jalap root,	37,121	Lbs.
Rhubarb root,	5,782	Lbs.
Sarsaparilla,	65,374	Lbs.
Mezereon bark,	1,353	Lbs.
Opium,	3,164	Lbs.
Kino,	230	Lbs.
Scammony,	1,483	Lbs.
Aloes,	12,375	Lbs.
Squills,	1,626	Lbs.
Spurious peruvian bark,	304,135	Lbs.
Spanish saffron,	360	Lbs.
Ergot,	475	Lbs.
Chamomile flowers,	1,896	Lbs.
Assafœtida,	3,700	Lbs.
Worm seed,	230	Lbs.

Colchicum seed,	2,246	Lbs.
Valerian root,	650	Lbs.
Guaiacum,	9,300	Lbs.
Cream of tartar,	7,673	Lbs.
Magnesia (carb.),	2,867	Lbs.
Magnesia (calc'd.),	1,560	Lbs.
Althea root,	1,117	Lbs.
Liquorice root,	9,430	Lbs.
Bistort root,	140	Lbs.
Gentian root,	7,572	Lbs.
Gentian root, in powder,	430	Lbs.
Lavender flowers,	3,042	Lbs.
Poppy flowers,	190	Lbs.
Hellebore root (white),	460	Lbs.
Pareira brava root,	730	Lbs.
Cantharides,	1,276	Lbs.
Creosote,	140	Ozs.
Bromine,	430	Ozs.
Sulphate of quinine,	3,200	Ozs.
Iodine,	6,864	Ozs.
Hydriodate of potass,	3,720	Ozs.

Making altogether some five hundred and twenty thousand pounds, to say nothing of various articles in small quantities rejected from time to time, which i have not considered of sufficient importance to note down. This, together with the ninety thousand pounds previously rejected, as stated in an early report above alluded to, makes some six hundred and ten thousand pounds of various articles of drugs and medicines condemned by me as unfit for medicinal purposes since the law took effect at this port. What articles and in what quantities, were rejected during the eleven months that i was absent from the office, i am not advised, neither am i at this time able to say what has been done under the requirements of this act at the other ports of entry. I hope, however, that the special examiners can give a good account of their stewardship, and that they will not hesitate to do so, whenever the information is desirable as a means of pushing on the column of medical and pharmaceutical reform.

It will be seen by the above statement, that by far the largest quantity of any one article rejected, is that of spurious peruvian bark, or as it is generally known in commerce, carthagena and maracaibo bark; and that too, as a general thing of the poorest and most worthless quality. The best of this bark affords on analysis only an exceedingly small percentage of quinine, not unfrequently, but a mere trace; while, at the same time, it yields as high as two, and occasionally with choice samples, two and a half per cent of a *peculiar* alkaloid which has been named *quinidine*, in contra-distinction to quinine, cinchonine, and aricine, (the three alkaloids heretofore obtained from the different varieties of the cinchona tribe of plants,) from which it differs essentially in several respects.

What *is quinidine, medicinally understood?* How does *sulphate* of quinine *compare with sulphate of quinine* (from which it is very difficult to distinguish it by the naked eye,) medicinally, as a remedial agent in cases where the use of the latter salt is particularly indicated? These are important questions, and the subject is one very properly at the present time calling for prompt, patient, and persevering investigation by all those whose mission it is to prepare, dispense or prescribe the most efficient means wherewith to combat disease; the more so for the reason, that i have detected in most of the sulphate of quinine lately imported from abroad, more or less of this non-officinal, and (in my opinion) as compared with quinine, non-efficient substance yclept quinidine; a fact readily accounted for, when it is known that for the last year or two immense quantities of the bark in question, good, bad, and indifferent, have been exported from new grenada, (as well as much from this port that had been rejected) and purchased by foreign manufacturing chemists, for the purpose, as i have reason to believe, of mixing it with the *true* bark in the manufacture of sulphate of quinine; hence the hybrid salt now too frequently presented to entry; a practice that, if not speedily abandoned, will ruin as far as this country is concerned, the formerly well deserved reputation of more than one of the foreign manufacturers of sulphate of quinine i could name. The argument maintained by some of them that the article is used in their hospitals and found equal to pure quinine, will not answer on this side of the water; it smacks too much of the almighty dollar, even as i must believe (until further advised) at the expense of truth.

This comparatively inert substance, quinidine, is readily detected by using the method adopted by zimmer, and published in the march number of the pharmaceutical journal (london), and, as i was happy to see, transfered to the columns of the may number of your valuable journal. It is a test so perfect, so scientifically practical, and so simple withal, that any one possessing only a moderate share of chemical and analytical acumen can successfully apply it, even though perchance he may not be able to boast of wearing the mantle of the departed berzelins, or of having been a favorite pupil of liebig.

The law went into operation at this port on the 12th day of july, 1848, and it is worthy of remark, as a cause of gratulation, on the part of the early friends of the measure, that the importation of inferior and worthless qualities of many important drugs and medicines, has since gradually and greatly decreased in quantity. For instance, i rejected during the first seven months of the working of the law 19,989 pounds of rhubarb root; but i have since rejected only 5,782 pounds, being but a fraction over one third of the quantity. For the past eighteen months, i have not had occasion to reject a single pound. I rejected during the first nine months 3,347 pounds of opium; but have since, during a period of more than two years and a half of my administration of the law, as will be seen by the above statement, rejected only 3,164 pounds. For the past thirteen months i have rejected only nine hundred and fifty two pounds, while i have passed during that period not less than 70,000 pounds. During the first two months of the operation of the law, i rejected 1,414 pounds of gamboge, but have since met with that only which i was ready to pass without any hesitation. During the first nine months i rejected 2,977 pounds of gum myrrh, but all that has since been presented to entry at this port, i have found satisfactory. Thus might i continue, but time and space will not permit. Enough i opine, has been said and shown to satisfy even the most prejudiced and sceptical opponent of this wise measure, that if faithfully and judiciously administered, *and seconded with becoming zeal and honesty of purpose by the medical profession, the pharmaceutist and dispensing apothecary*, it is calculated and destined to effect most beneficial and lasting sanitary reforms throughout the length and breadth of our vast and glorious land. In a word, the law has operated thus far remarkably well considering the hasty manner in which it was framed and passed through congress. It is, in some respects imperfect, as must ever be the case with all new measures of legislation until their utility is tested by practical operation; but these imperfections were, some time since, brought to the attention of the secretary of the treasury, who, with his accustomed promptitude soon after instructed me to report to the department such manifestations and suggestions as my experience in the administration of the law should dictate as most desirable, practicable, and judicious; and, notwithstanding this important and responsible trust has necessarily been made the subject of the few occasional leisure moments i could from time to time command, apart from other official duties, it is nearly completed, and, in a manner too, as i have reason to believe, that will render the law, when amended as proposed, satisfactory to all honorable dealers, importers, owners, and consignees, and, at the same time do away with the not unreasonable objections entertained by our marine insurance companies; while its efficiency instead of being in any manner impaired by the amendments, will be more perfectly guarded and essentially strengthened. The particulars and details connected with this duty i must defer until another time; but i must be permitted before closing this communication to say, that to the present able and distinguished head of the treasury department, hon. Thomas corwin, is due a debt of gratitude, from all true friends of this important measure, not easily cancelled. Soon after he was called to take upon himself the responsibilities of one of the most important, and by far the most arduous offices under the general government, the downward and fatal tendency of a maladministration of the law was brought to his notice; when, rising *above all minor considerations*, he rescued it from impending danger, and placed it upon what he deemed a safe basis; and has since, on all occasions, lent a willing ear to every suggestion calculated to render it more perfect, to add to its efficiency, or perpetuate its usefulness. A noble example truly, and one well worthy of the man.

TO CONCLUDE, I BEG TO SAY, THAT ALTHOUGH I HAVE NOT THE HONOR OF BELONGING TO ANY PHARMACEUTICAL ASSOCIATION, I NEVERTHELESS TAKE GREAT INTEREST IN EVERYTHING CALCULATED TO ADVANCE THE GOOD CAUSE AND NOBLE CALLING IN which you have so long been engaged; and, i hope the day is not far distant, when every city and town of importance throughout this wide extended country, will be favored with an organization of the kind, radiating from a *national* pharmaceutical association as a common center. It would be of vast benefit to the community at large, as well as eminently useful to the medical profession; for as all must admit, it is of the most vital importance to the success of the physician, that his remedial agents are properly prepared by a well-bred and perfectly educated chemist and pharmaceutist; and, i may add my conviction, that medical and pharmaceutical chemistry, a part of medical education that has thus far been most unpardonably neglected, should be universally and efficiently taught in our schools of medicine.

I am, dear sir,

Very respectfully, your obd't. Serv't.,

M. J. Bailey, m. D.,

Special examiner of drugs, medicines, chemical medicinal preparations, &c.

ON THE USE OF COAL GAS AS A SOURCE OF HEAT FOR THE LABORATORY.

BY EDWARD N. KENT.

Having recently fitted up a new laboratory in which i have introduced coal gas as a source of heat, i have thought a description of the apparatus and manner of using it, would be interesting to chemists and pharmaceutists, as it has not been very generally applied to this purpose as yet in this country, although in england, where alcohol is dear, it has long been used as a substitute.

In the use of coal gas as a source of heat, the principal difficulty to be avoided, is its tendency to smoke; this i have accomplished in a variety of ways. The ordinary argand gas burner, fixed permanently upon a branch pipe passing up through the table, is one of the cheapest, and a convenient arrangement for many purposes, and to prevent smoke, a tall glass chimney, or a short sheet iron chimney, with every other hole in the burner plugged, so as to make separate and distinct jets for the air to pass through, is all that is necessary. A tripod or sheet iron cylinder, for supporting vessels over the flame, is an indispensable addition to this burner. There is one objection to this form of apparatus, which is, that it is *fixed*, and cannot be moved about like a lamp. To avoid this inconvenience, i have had a number of burners constructed in different ways, and connected with flexible tubes, so as to admit of a change of position, to any place within the length of the tube.

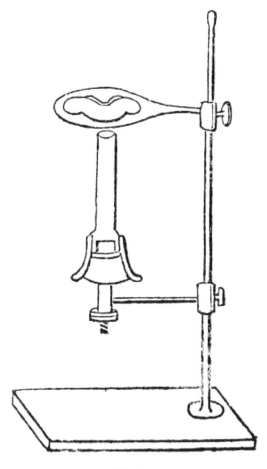

Fig. 1.

Figure 1, is a gas burner designed as a substitute for the rose lamp, and when connected to the gas pipe by means of a flexible tube, answers every purpose of that excellent lamp without being liable to the danger of catching fire, or to the necessity of replenishing during an operation, as is the case with most alcohol lamps. The above arrangement consists of an ordinary argand gas burner, with every other hole plugged, fixed to an arm with a socket and thumb screw, by means of which it can be raised to any height on the rod attached to a moveable wooden foot. The lower part of the burner is provided with a screw to which the flexible tube is attached, by means of a hare's gallows screw connector. The other end of the flexible tube should be provided with a stopcock, at its union with the fixed gas pipes for regulating the supply of the gas. Above the burner is a moveable ring, with socket and thumb screw, for supporting retorts, flasks, etc., at any desired height. A glass chimney is represented in the figure, but this may be replaced with a short sheet iron chimney, when part of the holes in the burner have been plugged as before mentioned. The above burner is well adapted for use with the wire gauze chimney, as the moveable ring with the addition of a wire tripod, answers as a support for a platina crucible. To insure a perfect combustion of the mixture of gas and air, i find that the sheet iron cylinder should be about ten inches high and two inches diameter. Over such a cylinder, with the upper end covered with wire gauze, it is an easy matter to fuse carbonate of soda, or other substance requiring a bright red heat. When the combustion is perfect with the above cylinder, the flame is of a pale blueish white color, like that of a solid flame from alcohol but much hotter. With the addition of a small conical chimney of sheet iron, placed over the mixed gas-burner, so as to bring the blue flame to a smaller compass, i find it a very convenient and powerful flame for bending glass tubes, by which tubes of any diameter, or the neck of a retort, may be easily softened and bent.

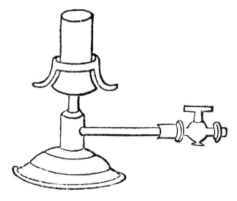

Fig. 2.

Figure 2, is an argand burner, with every other hole plugged, attached to a heavy brass foot, and with an arm and stopcock, to which a long flexible tube is attached, the other end of which is connected to a pendant above the table. This burner is well adapted for use on any part of the table, and may be used with an ordinary retort stand, or with a sheet iron cylinder, for supporting vessels over the flame. It has all the conveniences without the disadvantages of a berzelius' lamp, as it requires no wicks or replenishing, and cannot take fire; and the stopcock is not liable to get out of order, as is the case with the rack and pinion of the alcoholic lamp.

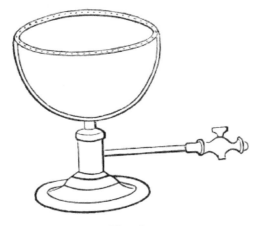

Fig. 3.

Figure 3, is a large burner, six inches in diameter, with the holes placed far enough apart to form distinct jets of the burning gas, by which means smoke is entirely prevented without the use of any chimney. This burner, like the preceding, is attached to a heavy brass foot, and with an arm and stopcock, to which a long flexible tube is attached, by means of which it can be moved to any part of the table.

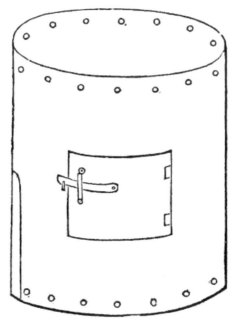

Fig. 4.

This burner is provided with a large sheet iron cylinder, (figure 4) with air holes at the top and bottom, a slit at the side, to go over the arm of the burner, and a door in front for convenience in lighting the gas, and thus forms a powerful and convenient gas furnace, by means of which a gallon of water can be easily boiled. With this arrangement the confined heat is so great, that it is necessary to protect the table from burning, by means of sheet iron, or other suitable material.

In point of economy, coal gas is cheaper than alcohol for fuel, even in america where the latter is so cheap, and the price of gas is comparatively high; and, it is to be hoped, that the price of the latter will be reduced, so that coal gas may yet be used with economy, as a source of heat for domestic as well as for chemical and pharmaceutical purposes. The present price should be no detriment to its free use, as it is, undoubtedly, the most cleanly and convenient fuel which can be used in the laboratory; and, as such, i would strongly recommend it to those, for whom the above description has been prepared.

NOTE UPON CICUTA (CONIUM MACULATUM) AND CONICINE.

Since stoerck, who first extolled the virtues of hemlock, this plant has undergone numerous alterations of credit and neglect which may be explained by the want of certainty, or rather by the irregularity, of its action.

An important work has just appeared on this subject, executed conjointly by a physician and pharmacien of lyons, mm. Devay and guillermond. This work, which developes and completes what has been said upon the medicinal virtues of hemlock, furnishes a new element which will fix, we believe, the therapeutic value of that substance. It is the substitution of the seed like fruits for the other parts of the plant. We will briefly explain the motive of that preference.

The principle to which cicuta owes both its toxicological and therapeutic powers has received the names of cicuta, coneine and conicine, the last of which is now generally adopted. It is a volatile alkaloid, of a sharp penetrating, disagreeable smell, somewhat like that of mice. It is of an oily consistence, and easily decomposed by heat. In these respects it resembles nicotine. But, a characteristic readily recognized and which distinguishes it from the latter, when shaken with water it again floats upon the surface, while nicotine is immediately dissolved by that liquid.

The volatility of conicine, the readiness with which it is decomposed by heat or time alone, are such that the lyonese experimenters do not hesitate to propose the abandonment both of the herb itself, and of all the pharmaceutic forms prepared by the aid of heat, or in which the conicine is susceptible of undergoing decomposition. We think this is going rather too far. The extracts of cicuta prepared with care, and particularly those prepared in vacuo, are of daily service. We have been able to verify by trituration with potassa, the presence of conicine in a hydro-alcoholic extract, a number of years old. But, notwithstanding recognising the fact that the preparations of cicuta of this kind are often inert, we agree with the experimenters that it is of consequence to escape from such a state of things.

The tincture of cicuta prepared with the fresh plant, is a very beautiful product, but made from parts of the plant containing but a small proportion of conicine, or at all events containing it in very variable proportions, may be inert or irregular in its action. What then is to be done? Employ conicine itself? But the preparation of the alkaloid is difficult; it is promptly decomposed by contact with the air and light, and the apportionment of its dose, offers serious inconveniences.

There is a organ of the plant in which its active principle is found in larger and more constant proportion, and under conditions in which it is better preserved than in any other; that organ is the fruit. It is at the moment of its most perfect development, when the plant commences to flower, that it contains the largest proportion of conicine, and that the principle is most perfectly elaborated. At a later period it disappears and is fixed in the fruit, in which it is concentrated in great quantity. It is in the fruit that we seek it when we wish to extract it. It is in the fruit we should seek it for medical use.

Pharmaceutical preparations. Formulæ.—"having shown by experiment as well as by reasoning, that the fruit of the cicuta (akène) should henceforth replace all the preparations of the plant employed in medicine: we have to make known the use we have made of this fact. It is important in the first place, that the fruit employed should be that of the great cicuta, and that it should not be mingled with seeds of the other umbelliferæ. They may be known by being almost globular with five crenelated sides.

When the fruit is divided, the sides fold in the form of a crescent. They do not possess like most of the other umbelliferæ, a peculiar aromatic odor. This appears to be covered by that of conicine. The fool's parsley, (æthusa cynapium,) the phellandrium aquaticum, the anise, bear fruits which, physically, have much resemblance to that of the cicuta; but, when the latter is pulverized, the characteristic odor which is developed is sufficient to enable us readily to recognize it. Another precaution to be taken is in relation to the time at which the fruit should be collected.

Those which were employed in our experiments and preparations had reached the perfection of their maturity. It is then it should be collected for medical use, because then it is isolated, so to speak, from the plant which produces it; the active principle exists then in them in a true state of concentration and permanence.

1st. Formulæ for internal use.—"the fruit of the cicuta does not need any complicated pharmaceutic preparation. It is active enough of itself to be employed in its natural condition. A very simple manipulation only seems necessary to facilitate its use. It is to reduce it to powder and to form it into pills, which, coated with sugar, may be preserved an indefinite time. We have thought best to give the pills two degrees of strength according to the following formulæ.

"pills of cicuta, no. 1.—take one gramme of the fruit of the cicuta recently pulverized; make with a sufficient quantity of sugar and of syrup a mass, to be divided into 100 pills. These are to be covered with sugar; each pill will weigh about 10 centigrammes. These are suited to persons who are not yet habituated to the use of the drug, and who are of a delicate constitution. We commence with two pills the first day, and the dose is augmented day by day to 10, 15, or 20. It is then most convenient to employ pills no. 2.

Pills no. 2.—take 5 grammes of the recently powdered fruit of the cicuta; incorporate them with a sufficient quantity of gum and sugar; divide as before into 100 pills, which are to be enveloped with sugar, each pill will weigh about 25 centigrammes.

"we will finish the series of internal medicines by the formula of a syrup of conicine, which will be of the greatest utility to practitioners.

"exhaust 10 grammes of the fruit of the cicuta, with alcohol at 28° c. (82 f.) So as to obtain 60 grammes, to which 3000 grammes of syrup, aromatised, *ad libitum*, are to be added.

"thirty grammes of this syrup represent 1 decigramme of the fruit or a milligramme of conicine. A teaspoonful being the equivalent of 30 grammes of syrup, the patient who takes one pill of no. 2. Will be able to take half a teaspoonful of the syrup.

Formula for external use.—*balm of conicine.*—the process which we employ to prepare the balm of conicine authorizes us to give it that name. It is in effect, a true solution in lard freed from the principles which retain it in combination, and as pure as the processes we have proposed for its extraction will permit. Thus, after having exhausted the fruit by alcohol, and after having separated as completely as possible the conicine by means of ether and caustic potash, confining ourselves to the precautions indicated below, we take: the ether of cicuta, obtained by the exhaustion of 100 grammes of the fruit, and 300 grammes of recently washed lard. We begin by evaporating the ether in the open air, that is, by pouring it little by little in a plate, and as soon as the greater part of it has been eliminated, and the conicine commences to appear upon the plate in the form of little yellow drops, separating themselves from the vehicle, the lard is to be incorporated with it by degrees, the whole being constantly stirred to facilitate the evaporation of the ether. A balm of conicine is thus obtained, exceedingly active and convenient for use.

The following is the mode of preparing the ether of cicuta: "the alcoholic tincture obtained by the complete exhaustion of 100 grammes of the fruit, is to be evaporated to the consistence of a syrup, and the alcohol is to be replaced by a small quantity of water. This leaves undissolved a thick green oil, entirely soluble in ether, and of which the quantity reaches the weight of 30 grammes. After having separated this green oil, we wash with ether the product of the alcoholic evaporation and obtain a yellowish resinous substance, which has no action on litmus paper and which has a strong odor, *sui generis*, different from that of conicine.

After having submitted the mother waters of the alcoholic extract to this preliminary treatment, we have introduced them into a flask having a capacity three times as great as their volume, and treated them successively with a concentrated solution of caustic potash and rectified sulphuric ether. Immediately after the addition of the potash, a well marked odor of conicine was manifest in the mixture, and the ether became strongly alkaline. We left the same ether, (about 20 grammes) upon the mixture for twelve hours, often agitating it. It was then decanted and replaced by fresh ether, and this was replaced until the ether became nearly insensible to litmus paper. We remarked that the first 20 grammes of ether took up nearly all the alkaloid. One hundred grammes of well rectified ether was sufficient to remove almost completely the alkaloid from the extractive and alkaline mixture derived from 100 grammes of the fruit of the cicuta.

SOLUTION OF CONICINE FOR INJECTIONS.

Tincture of the fruit,	100 grammes.
Lime water,	900 grammes.

Filter at the end of a few minutes.

"in this preparation we have thought best to employ lime water instead of simple water. We have remarked previously that the tincture of cicuta possessed no smell of conicine, but when lime water was added, the odor was instantly developed in a high dagree. The conicine is disengaged by the lime from its saline combination, and remains free, dissolved in the water."

Mm. Devay and guillermond, who, in their work, have been so just in their deductions, fail here, we think, in denominating syrup, injection, &c., of conicine, the various preparations of the fruits of the cicuta. It is only perhaps a matter of form, but it is important to avoid in materia medica a matter of form which may give rise to a false idea of things, which may in a word, induce error.

We have only occupied ourselves with the pharmacological part of the work of mm. Devay and guillermond. The bulletin de therapeutique will soon offer an appreciation of its therapeutical portion.—*dorvault.*— *bulletin de therapeutique.*

[the facts on which the preference of the seeds of conium to the preparations in ordinary use are founded, are by no means new. They have been long known and frequently commented on. From six lbs. Of the fresh and nine of the dried fruit, geiger obtained an ounce of conia, or, as the french chemists prefer to call it, conicine; while from 100 LBS. Of the fresh herb, he procured only a drachm. The fresh dried herb exhibited only traces of it. The extract prepared from the herb partakes necessarily of its uncertainty and inactivity. Most of what is found in the shop is entirely inert; while the best, that of tilden or of currie, which are superior to the best english extract we have seen, possess comparatively little power. If conium is to be retained in the materia media, it is evident that we should employ that part of the plant in which the active principle is contained in the greatest quantity, and in a condition least liable to alteration. We are as yet, however, very imperfectly acquainted with the properties, either medicinal or poisonous of conium; and, as the continuation of the memoir of mm. Devay and guillermond promises us a solution of the question, we await it with much interest.]—ed. New york journal of pharmacy.

ON THE MANUFACTURE OF WRITING INKS.

In the manufacture of good writing ink, more nicety is required in the choice of materials, as well as greater skill in manipulation, than is generally bestowed upon it.

The proportion of the various ingredients used is a matter of considerable importance, affecting in a great degree the durability of the ink.

Dr. Lewis's writing ink.—dr. Lewis, who instituted a series of very careful experiments on the manufacture of writing ink, found that equal parts of sulphate of iron and of galls gave an ink, which, although of a good color when first used, became yellowish-brown when the writing was kept for a moderate length of time, and that in proportion to the quantity of the sulphate, the inks were less durable in color, and that those in which the galls were in excess, were most durable.

He, therefore, recommended the following proportions as best suited for the manufacture of good writing ink:— powdered sulphate of iron, 1 OZ.; powdered logwood, 1 OZ.; powdered galls, 3 OZ.; gum arabic, 1 OZ.; white wine or vinegar, 1 quart.

Water will answer for common purposes, but white wine formed a blacker ink than water, and vinegar formed one still blacker than wine. The addition of spirit injured the color, and occasioned a precipitation of coloring matter—a decoction of logwood, instead of water, improved both the beauty and deepness of the black. The ingredients are to be put in a glass or other convenient vessel, not metallic, and the mixture shaken four or five times a day. In ten or twelve days it will be fit for use, and sooner if in a warm situation; but it continues for a long time to improve if left without decantation. When it is separated from the powdery residue, it will be kept in a good state with greater certainty, if some broken galls freed from the powder and some pieces of iron are put into it. Iron, however, is the only metal which it is safe to retain in contact with the ink.

Dr. Lewis gave the preference to distilled or rain water in the manufacture of ink, but it seems probable that a water containing a certain proportion of carbonate of lime is more suitable. In dyeing a black color by means of galls or sumach and copperas, hard spring water is preferred by some dyers. To produce in a liquid a given depth of color, distilled water requires more dyestuff than common spring water. This is illustrated in the following experiment, devised by mr. Phillips: into two glass jars of the same size, each half-filled with distilled water, introduce equal quantities of infusion or tincture of galls or sumach, and an equal number of drops (only three or four) of a solution of copperas; a faint purplish color will be developed in both jars, but if one is filled with spring water, the color in that rapidly becomes dark reddish-black, and one-half more water is required to reduce it to the same shade of color as the other. The water which is found by experience to be best adapted for dyeing with galls and sulphate of iron, differs from distilled water in containing sulphate of lime, carbonate of lime held in solution by free carbonic acid, and chloride of calcium. The beneficial ingredient seems to be the carbonate of lime, which possesses slight alkaline properties, for if the smallest quantity of ammonia or of bicarbonate of potash is added to the distilled water in the above experiments, the purple color is struck as rapidly and as deeply as in the spring water; chloride of calcium and sulphate of lime, on the contrary, produce no sensible change either in the depth of color or the tint. The effect is no doubt referable to the action of the alkali or lime on the proto-sulphate of iron, by which the sulphuric acid of the latter is withdrawn, and hydrated protoxide of iron set free, for protoxide of iron is much more easily peroxidized and acted upon by tannic and gallic acids (the dyeing principles of galls) when in the free and hydrated state, than when in combination with sulphuric acid. Neither the caustic fixed alkalies (potash and soda) nor their carbonates can be well introduced in the above experiments, as the slightest excess reacts on the purple color, converting it into a reddish-brown. Ammonia, lime-water, and the alkaline bicarbonates also produce a reddening, and if applied in considerable quantity a brownish tinge. It is very probable that the above-mentioned principle is applicable to the preparation of writing ink.

RIBANCOURT'S WRITING INK.—M. RIBANCOURT, WHO PAID MUCH ATTENTION TO THE PREPARATION OF INKS, STATED THAT NONE OF THE INGREDIENTS SHOULD BE IN EXCESS. "IF THERE BE A WANT OF THE MATTER OF GALLS, PART OF THE VITRIOL WILL NOT BE DECOMPOSED; IF, ON THE CONTRARY, THERE BE TOO MUCH, THE VITRIOL WILL TAKE AS MUCH AS IT CAN DECOMPOSE, AND THE REMAINDER WILL DE NEARLY IN THE STATE OF THE DECOCTION OF GALLS, SUBJECT TO CHANGE BY BECOMING MOULDY, OR TO UNDERGO AN

ALTERATION AFTER WRITING WHICH DESTROYS ITS LEGIBILITY MUCH MORE COMPLETELY THAN THE CHANGE UNDERGONE BY INK CONTAINING TOO SMALL A PORTION OF THE GALLS.

"it is doubtful whether the principles of the galls are well extracted by cold maceration, and it is certain that inks made in this way flow pale from the pen, and are not of so deep a black as those wherein strong boiling is recurred to."

From all the foregoing considertions, m. Ribancourt gives the following directions for the composition of good ink:—

"take 8 OZ. Of aleppo galls (in coarse powder); 4 OZ. Of logwood (in thin chips); 4 OZ. Of vitriol of iron; 3 OZ. Of gum arabic (in powder); 1 OZ. Of vitriol of copper; and 1 OZ. Of sugar-candy. Boil the galls and logwood together in 12 LB of water for one hour, or till half the liquid has evaporated. Strain the decoction through a hair sieve or linen cloth, and then add the other ingredients. Stir the mixture till the whole is dissolved (more especially the gum), after which leave it to subside for twenty-four hours. Then decant the ink, and preserve it in bottles of glass or stoneware well corked." The sulphate of copper must be omitted in the preparation of an ink required for steel pens.

Dr. Bostock's instructions for the manufacture of ink.—a few years since, dr. Bostock presented to the society of arts the following, valuable communication "on the properties of writing inks," which will be read with interest.

"when the sulphate of iron and the infusion of galls are added together, for the purpose of forming ink, we may presume that the metallic salt or oxide enters into combination with at least four proximate vegetable principles, viz: gallic acid, tan, mucilage, and extractive matter, all of which appear to enter into the composition of the soluble part of the gall-nut. It has been generally supposed that two of these the gallic acid and the tan, are more especially necessary to the constitution of ink; and hence it is considered, by our best systematic writers, to be essentially a tannogallate of iron. It has been also supposed that the peroxide of iron alone possesses the property of forming the black compound which constitutes ink, and that the substance of ink is rather mechanically suspended in the fluid than dissolved in it.

"ink, as it is usually prepared, is disposed to undergo certain changes, which considerably impair its value; of these, the three following are the most important:—its tendency to moulding; the liability of the black matter to separate from the fluid, the ink then becoming what is termed ropy; and loss of color, the black first changing to brown, and at length almost entirely disappearing.

"besides these, there are objects of minor importance to be attended to in the formation of ink. Its consistence should be such as to enable it to flow easily from the pen, without, on the one hand, its being so liquid as to blur the paper, or on the other, so adhesive as to clog the pen and be long in drying. The shade of color is not to be disregarded; a black approaching to blue is more agreeable to the eye than browner ink; and a degree of lustre or glossiness, if compatible with due consistence of the fluid, tends to render the characters more legible and beautiful.

"with respect to the chemical constitution of ink, i may remark that, although as usually prepared it is a combination of the metallic salt or oxide with all the four vegetable principles mentioned above, yet i am induced to believe that the last three of them, so far from being essential, are the principal cause of the difficulty that we meet with in the formation of a perfect and durable ink.

"i endeavored to prove this point by a series of experiments, of which the following is a brief extract.

"having prepared a cold infusion of galls, i allowed a portion of it to remain exposed to the atmosphere, in a shallow capsule, until it was covered with a thick stratum of mould, the mould was removed by filtration, and the proper proportion of sulphate of iron being added to the clear fluid, a compound was formed of a deep black color, which showed no further tendency to mould, and which remained for a long time without experiencing any further alteration. Another portion of the same infusion of galls had solution of isinglass added to it, until it no longer produced a precipitate; by employing the sulphate of iron, a black compound was produced, which, although paler than that formed from the entire fluid, appeared to be a perfect and durable ink.

"lastly, a portion of the infusion of galls, was kept for some time at the boiling temperature, by which means a part of its contents became insoluble; this was removed by filtration, when, by addition of sulphate of iron, a very perfect and durable ink was produced.

"in the above three processes, i conceive that a considerable part of the mucilage, of the tan, and the extract, were respectively removed from the infusion, whilst the greatest part of the gallic acid would be left in solution.

"the three causes of deterioration in ink, the moulding, the precipitation of black matter, and loss of color, as they are distinct operations, so we may presume that they depend on the operation of different proximate principles.

"it is probable that the moulding more particularly depends ©n the mucilage, and the precipitation on the extract, from the property, which extractive matter possesses of forming insoluble compounds with metallic oxides.

"as to the operation of the tan, from its affinity for metallic salt we may conjecture that, in the first instance, it forms a triple compound with the gallic acid and the iron, and that in consequence of the decomposition of the tan, this compound is afterwards destroyed. Owing to the difficulty, if not impossibility, of entirely depriving the infusion of galls of any one of its ingredients without in some degree affecting the others, i was not able to obtain any results which can be regarded as decisive; but the general result of my experiments favors the above opinion, and leads me to conclude that, in proportion as ink consists merely of the gallate of iron it is less liable to decomposition or to experience any kind of change. The experiments to which i have alluded above, consisted in forming a standard solution by macerating the powder of galls in five times its weight of water, and comparing this with other infusions, which had either been suffered to mould, from which the tan had been extracted by jelly, or which had been kept for some time at the boiling temperature, and by adding to each of these respectively both the recent solution of the sulphate of iron, and a solution which had been exposed for some time to the atmosphere.

"the nature of the black compound produced was examined, by putting portions of it into cylindrical jars and observing the changes which they experienced with respect either to the formation of mould, the deposition of their contents, or any change of color. The fluids were also compared by dropping portions of them upon white tissue paper, in which way both their color and their consistence might be minutely ascertained. A third method was to add together the respective infusions, and the solutions of the sulphate of iron, in a very diluted state, by which i was enabled to form a more correct comparison of the quantity and of the shade of the coloring matter, and of the degree of its solubility.

"the practical conclusions which i think myself warranted in drawing from these experiments are as follows:—in order to procure an ink which may be little disposed either to mould or to deposit its contents, and which at the same time may possess a deep black color not liable to fade, the galls should be macerated for some hours in hot water, and the fluid filtered; it should then be exposed for about fourteen days to a warm atmosphere, when any mould which may have been produced must be removed. A solution of sulphate of iron is to be employed which has been exposed for some time to the atmosphere, and which consequently contains a certain quantity of the red oxide diffused through it. I should recommend the infusion of galls to be made of considerably greater strength than is generally directed, and i believe that an ink formed in this manner will not necessarily require the addition of any mucilaginous substance to render it of a proper consistence.

"i have only farther to add, that one of the best substances for diluting ink, if it be in the first instance too thick for use, or afterwards become so by evaporation, is a strong decoction of coffee, which appears in no respect to promote the decomposition of the ink, while it improves its color and gives it an additional lustre."

Dr. Ure recommends the following formula for the manufacture of writing ink. To make twelve gallons take: 12lb of nutgalls; 5lb of green sulphate of iron; 5lb of gum senegal; 12 gallons of water. The bruised nutgalls are to be put into a cylindrical copper, of a depth equal to its diameter, and boiled during three hours, with three-fourths of the above quantity of water, taking care to add fresh water to replace what is lost by evaporation. The decoction is to be emptied into a tub, allowed to settle, and the clear liquor being drawn off, the lees are to be drained. The gum is to be dissolved in a small quantity of hot water, and the mucilage thus formed, being filtered, it is added to the clear decoction. The sulphate of iron must likewise be separately dissolved and well mixed with the above. The color darkens by degrees, in consequence of the peroxidizement of the iron, on exposing the ink to the action of the air.

But ink affords a more durable writing when used in the pale state, because its particles are then finer and penetrate the paper more intimately. When ink consists chiefly of tannate of peroxide of iron, however black, it is merely superficial, and is easily erased or effaced. Therefore, whenever the liquid made by the above prescription has acquired a moderately deep tint, it should be drawn off clear into bottles and well corked up. Some ink-makers allow it to mould a little in the casks before bottling, and suppose that it will thereby be not so liable to become mouldy in the bottles. A few bruised cloves or other aromatic perfume, added to ink, is said to prevent the formation of mouldiness, which is produced by the ova of infusoria animalcules.

The ink made by this prescription is much more rich and powerful than many of the inks commonly sold. To bring it to the common standard a half more water may safely be added. Even twenty gallons of tolerable ink may be made from the above weight of materials.

Scott's writing ink.—mr. Scott's method of manufacturing writing ink, as patented by him in 1840, is as follows:—take 48lb of logwood chips, and let them be saturated two days in soft water, then put the same into a close covered iron cauldron, and add 80 gallons of soft water; let these be boiled one hour and a half, when the wood must be taken out and the fluid left, to which add 48lb of the best picked aleppo galls in coarse powder; boil these half an hour longer, then draw off the fire, and let it remain in the cauldron twenty-four hours infusing, during which it is to be very frequently agitated; when the properties of the galls are sufficiently extracted, draw off the clear fluid into a vat, and add 40lb of pulverized sulphate of iron; let these ingredients remain a week (stirring daily), after which add four gallons of vinegar. Next take 7½LB of the best picked gum arabic, and dissolve it in sufficient water to form a good mucilage, which must be well strained, and then added to the fluid by degrees; let these stand a few days longer, when pour into the same 20 ounces of the concentrated nitrate of iron; let the whole stand by again until it has arrived at its height of blackness; next pour the clear fluid off from the sediment, and add to it the following substances, each prepared and ground separately:—

First, take half a pound of spanish indigo, which grind very fine between a muller and stone, adding by degrees portions of the ink until it is made into an easy soluble paste; next take well-washed and purified prussian blue five pounds, which prepare as the former, except grinding it in distilled water in lieu of the fluid, until it is formed into a soluble paste; also next take four ounces of gas black which results from the smoke of gas burners received on surfaces of glass, as is well known, which grind in one ounce of the nitrate of iron; when each is sufficiently fine, let them remain a few hours unmixed, when the whole may be incorporated with the fluid, and kept agitated daily for a week. The clear may then be poured off for use. The above will make eighty gallons of ink.

Dr. Normandy's black ink.—in order to supersede the use of nutgalls, dr. Normandy patented the following process for making black ink

Take either sumach, elm wood, elder, chestnut, beech, willow, oak, plum, sycamore, cherry, poplar wood, catechu, or any other wood or berry, or extract of vegetable substances, containing gallic acid and tannin, or either, and put this, previously reduced to powder, into a copper full of common water, and boil it until a sufficiently strong decoction be obtained.

The quantity of water must of course vary according to the sort of vegetable substance employed; catechu, for example, requiring less water than sumach, on account of the former being almost totally soluble. To this add a certain quantity of campeachy wood, of acetate and hydrate of deutoxide of copper, of sulphate of alumina and potash, of sulphate of protoxide of iron, in quantities which vary also according to the vegetable material first employed, and gum arabic, or the best sort of gum senegal, in the proportion of eighty pounds or thereabouts for 340 gallons of liquid; also a variable quantity of sulphate of indigo; the whole of these last ingredients, depending on the shade of the color intended to be produced, it is impossible to indicate absolutely the proportions in which they are to be used, as the taste and fancy of the operator must decide. Supposing, however, a blue black to be the color desired, and sumach, for example, the vegetable ingredient selected for the purpose, the proportions should be for 240 gallons: sumach, from 12 to 15 sacks, of four bushels each; campeachy logwood, 2 cwt. Or thereabouts, according as new or old chip is used; gum arabic, 80 LB. To 1 cwt.; sulphate of protoxide of iron, 1 cwt.; acetate and hydrate of deutoxide of copper, 4lb; sulphate of alumina and potash, 37lb; sulphate of indigo, 6lb, or even more, according to the intensity of the blue cast desired. If catechu were to be used instead of sumach, 1 cwt. Would be required, the proportions of the other materials remaining the same.

The variously colored precipitates which salts of iron form in the solutions of the above-cited vegetable astringent substances, all of which precipitates vary from the green to the brown (the decoction of nutgalls yeilding with salts of iron only a dark purple,) are the obstacles which have hitherto prevented the use of these vegetable substances, with a view to supersede nutgalls; but by means of the sulphate of indigo in various proportions, from the above-cited substances a liquid may be obtained, of different shades of color, from dark blue to most intense black, applicable to dyeing, staining, or writing, and which may be used with every description of pen.

Dr. Normandy's purple ink.—to produce a purple-colored ink called the "king of purples," dr. Normandy recommends the following proportions to be observed:—to twelve pounds of campeachy wood add as many gallons of boiling water; pour the solution through a funnel with a strainer made of coarse flannel, on one pound of hydrate or acetate of deutoxide of copper finely pulverized (at the bottom of the funnel a piece of sponge is placed), then add immediately 14lbs. Of sulphate of alumina and potash, and for every 340 gallons of liquid add eighty pounds of gum arabic or gum senegal. Let these remain for three or four days, and a beautiful purple color will be produced.

Dr. Normandy's blue ink.—dr. Normandy's blue ink is made by operating upon chinese blue or cyanoferruret of iron. The cyanoferruret of iron is to be ground in water with oxalic acid or bin-oxalate of potash, adding gum arabic in the following proportions: to seven ounces of water add three drachms of chinese blue, 1 drachm of bin-oxalate of potash, and 1 drachm of gum arabic; to these ingredients a solution of tin may be added.

Girond's substitute for galls.—the substitute for gallnuts, patented by m. Girond, of lyons, in 1825, is an extract from the shell of the chestnut, and also from the wood and sap of the chestnut-tree. The extract is denominated *damajavag*, and the mode of preparing it is by reducing the chestnut-shell into small pieces, and boiling them in water.

One hundred-weight of the shells of chestnuts broken into small pieces is to be immersed in about 180 or 200 quarts of water, in a vessel of copper or any other material, except iron, and after having been allowed to soak in this water for about 12 hours, the material is then to be boiled for about three hours, in order to obtain the extract. The wood of the chestnut tree may be cut into small pieces or shaved thin, and treated in the same way.

The extract is now to be drawn off from the boiler, and filtered through a fine sieve or cloth, after which the water must be evaporated from it until the extract is reduced to the consistence of paste.

It may now be cut into cakes of any convenient size, and dried in an oven of low temperature, and when hard, may be packed for sale, and used for any of the purposes in the arts to which gallnuts have been heretofore applied. The quantity of damajavag obtained from the above will be about 8 or 10 LBS.

In using this damajavag, it is only necessary to pound or otherwise reduce it to powder when it may be mixed with other ingredients as pulverized gall nuts.

The same chemical properties belong to the sap of the chestnut-tree, which may be extracted by tapping the trunk, and when so obtained, may be used for the same purpose as gallnuts.

Stephens' blue ink.—stephens' blue ink is prepared as follows:—take prussian blue, whether produced from a combination of prussiate of potash and salts of iron, or the prussian blue of commerce, as commonly manufactured, and put this into an earthen vessel, and pour over it a quantity of strong acid, sufficient to cover the prussian blue. Muriatic acid, sulphuric acid, or any other acid which has a sufficient action upon iron will do. If sulphuric acid is used it should be diluted a little, that is, with a quantity of water equal to about its bulk. The prussian blue is allowed to remain in the acid from twenty-four to forty-eight hours or longer, and then the mixture is diluted with a large quantity of water, stirring it up at the time, for the purpose of washing from it the salts of iron. When in this state of dilution, it is allowed to stand until the color has subsided, when the supernatant liquor is drawn off with a syphon and more water added to it. This process is repeated until the acid, with the iron, has been completely washed away, which is known by testing it with prussiate of potash, which will show if it yields any blue precipitate; if not, it is sufficiently washed. The product is then placed upon a filter, and suffered to remain until the liquid has all drained away.

The prussian blue, thus prepared, is reduced to a state containing less iron than the prussian blue of commerce, in which state it is more readily acted upon, and rendered soluble than in any other condition.

This prussian blue may then be placed in evaporating dishes, and gently dried. To form the prussian blue, so operated upon, into a solution, oxalic acid is added, and carefully mixed with it, after which cold water is added (cold distilled water is best) a little at a time, making it into a dense or dilute solution, according to the color required. The quantity of oxalic acid may vary according to the quantity of water used. It will be found that the prussian blue that has undergone the process of digestion, as described, requires but a small quantity of oxalic acid to dissolve it: about one part of oxalic acid will dissolve six parts of prussian blue, the weight taken before digesting in the acid. This will answer for a concentrated solution, but for a dilute solution more acid will be required.

(to be continued.)

VARIA—EDITORIAL.

QUINIDINE.

—sulphate of quinidine is advertised, "eo nomine," for sale in the london journals. What we get, as yet, occurs only as an adulteration of the sulphate of quinine. The same virtues, and to an equal extent, are ascribed by the advertisers to the new article, that are possessed by quinine. We do not know what authority there is for this statement, but it is exceedingly desirable that careful and well conducted experiments should be made to determine the properties and relative value of quinidine, quinoidine, and cinchonine. The great importance of quinine and its immense and constantly increasing consumption, long ago created a well founded anxiety lest the sources whence we obtain it should become exhausted or materially diminished. If the allied alkaloids will in any degree replace it, it is a fact of the highest value. Quinidine, in particular, is contained in some varieties of bark in which little or no quinine is found, and if the statements which have been made of the identity of its effects with quinine, probably without any better foundation than the closeness of resemblance of the two substances, should prove correct, the destruction of the cinchona calisaya which is going on, may be in some measure stayed.

EXTRACT OF BARK.

—a new article has appeared in our markets under the name of extract of bark. The specimen that came under our observation was a dark brown substance, homogenous, and about the consistence of dry opium. It was very little soluble in water, much more so in alcohol, and completely so in diluted sulphuric acid. From chemical examination it would appear to contain about 46 per cent of quinine, with perhaps traces of quinidine and cinchonine. At the price at which we hear it is offered it will be sought for by the manufacturers of sulphate of quinine.

SYRUP OF TURPENTINE.

—m. Trousseau often uses the syrup of turpentine in chronic catarrh of the bladder and the lungs, in old copious suppurations, etc., but as the standard works contain no formula, the preparation intended is not always obtained.

The following is the formula which has been published by m. Dorvault, according to the indications furnished by m. Trousseau, as being at once the most rational, and as furnishing a product preferable in all respects to that of the two formulæ given in the officine.

Turpentine,24	100 grammes.
Water,	375 grammes.

Digest during two days, taking care to agitate frequently; afterwards make a syrup after the manner of the balsam of tolu, by adding

White sugar,	750 grammes.

This syrup contains besides the resinous principles, the nature of which is not well ascertained, from 1-40 to 1-100 of its weight of the essence of turpentine.

It is limpid, of an aromatic odor—very sweet, and of an agreeable taste; it may be employed pure, or used to sweeten appropriate drinks.

Dose: from one to a number of tablespoonsful per day.—*bulletin de therap.*

24 the turpentine recommended by m. Dorvault is a variety of the strasburg turpentine, having an agreeable odor of lemon.

ALOINE.

—our readers will recollect that dr. Pereira has found aloine, the chrystalline neutral principle recently discovered in barbadoes aloes, by mr. Smith of edinburgh, in socotorine aloe juice, (new york journal of pharmacy, no. 6, p. 177.) Since then mr. Smith has succeeded in procuring it from socotorine aloes. It was much longer in crystallizing than when obtained from barbadoes aloes, but did so at last. When the impure product is recrystallized from rectified spirits it presents the same appearance as the purified crystal of barbadoes aloes (the crystals obtained by dr. Pereira which were spontaneously deposited from the juice, were much smaller) and seems identical with that substance. It has not yet been obtained from cape aloes, but undoubtedly exists in that substance, though probably from its inferior activity in much smaller quantity.

Aloine has been introduced into the practice of medicine in edinburgh, and the messrs. Smith have already (june) sold a quarter of a hundred weight of it. It is five times more active than good aloes—a single grain producing all the effect of a large aloetic pill; the edinburgh physicians describe it as acting "*tuto, cito, et jucunde,*" safely, speedily, and pleasantly. If this is meant altogether seriously, in the second of the characteristics it presents a marked contrast with the crude drug. From the convenience with which it may be exhibited, it bids fair to come into general and extensive use.

ACTION OF SULPHURIC ACID ON THE INSOLUBLE RESIDUE LEFT BY OPIUM, EXHAUSTED BY WATER. FORMATION OF A NEW ALKALOID,

BY M. STANISLAS MARTIN.

—the smallest object added to a kaleidoscope produces new shades and different images; so it is with vegetable chemistry; every practical man knows that a foreign body, an hours delay in executing a work already commenced, changes the nature of the products. Two experiments on the inert residue of opium, exhausted by water give another illustration of this truth.

The residue of opium submitted to fermentation, affords us a substance which has a great analogy to paramorphia; this substance has since been studied by m. A. Guergy. The account of the labor of that chemist has been reproduced in the review of the journal de pharmacie, 1849.

Our second operation consists in treating the residue of opium exhausted by water, with water acidulated with sulphuric acid. The result is the formation of an alkali which has many of the chemical properties of narcotine, but which differs from it completely by its insolubility in ether.

This alkali has no relation with codeine or narceine; besides we obtain an extractive matter, soluble in all proportions in water, to which it communicates the property of frothing like soap.

The following is the method of proceeding. The residue of opium, exhausted with water, is boiled in distilled water acidulated with sulphuric acid, after ten minutes ebullition it has the appearance of a thick magma; it is strained with strong expression; when the colature is cold it is filtered through paper.

The colature is highly colored; its odor is similar to that of opium, its taste is exceedingly bitter.

Ammonia is added until litmus paper is no longer altered; the liquid is filtered, the precipitate washed with distilled water, and permitted to dry; afterwards it is boiled with a sufficient quantity of rectified alcohol and again filtered. The alcoholic solution deposits on cooling, numerous needle like crystals, colored by a brownish bitter resin. It is purified in the ordinary manner.

What are the therapeutic properties of this alkaloid, of the extractive saponaceous matter, and of the brown bitter resin! Do they partake of the properties of opium? We know not; the physician alone can determine their value.— *bulletin de therapeutique.*

GELATINIZATION OF THE TINCTURE OF RHATANY.

—mr. Editor,—some years ago having occasion to prepare some saturated tincture of rhatany, about eighteen, ounces were put aside in a glass stoppered bottle. The tincture being examined but a short time since, was found to be gelatinized, as is generally the case with old tincture of kino. Having never seen such a change before, i sought information, and ascertained through the united states dispensatory that a french pharmaceutist in paris has remarked the same phenomenon, what is the cause of this remarkable change, attended as it is, with the loss of astringency? Is it not, perhaps, caused by the same action which produces peculiar exudation from the bark of certain trees possessed of tannin, retaining it for a while and afterwards, when cut up in logs, losing their tanning properties and exuding a species of ulmine? Is it not the same process which takes place in the decomposition of the kino and rhatany? But why is catechu exempt from such a decomposition? If you can enlighten me, and especially can explain how to prevent this change, you will much oblige myself and numerous readers.

LIST OF DELEGATES TO THE CONVENTION.

—on the sixth of this month the national convention will meet in philadelphia, and we see that our philadelphia friends, with a reference to the convenience of the delegates, have fixed upon 4 o'clock in the afternoon as the hour for assembling. The meeting will be held in the hall of the college of pharmacy, in zane street, above seventh, which has been placed at the disposal of the convention. As far as heard from, the following is a list of delegates:—

Philadelphia college of pharmacy,

Daniel b. Smith,

Charles ellis,

William procter, jr.,

Massachusetts college of pharmacy,

Joseph burnett,

Samuel colcord,

Samuel r. Philbrick,

Richmond pharmaceutical society,

Alexander duval,

John purcel,

Joseph laidley,

Maryland college of pharmacy,

George w. Andrews,

David stewart, m. D.

Cincinnatti college of pharmacy,

William b. Chapman,

Edward s. Wayne,

Charles a. Smith,

College of pharmacy of the city of new york,

George d. Coggeshall,

L. S. Haskell,

John meakim.

NEW YORK JOURNAL OF PHARMACY. NOVEMBER, 1852.

ACCIDENTAL SUBSTITUTION OF EX-TRACT OF BELLADONNA FOR EX-TRACT OF DANDELION. PROSECUTION OF THE MANUFACTURER.

In the Court of Appeals,

Samuel thomas, jr. And mary ann thomas, his wife,

Against hosea winchester.

Ruggles, *chief judge.*

This action was brought to recover damages from the defendant for negligently putting up, labelling and selling as and for the extract of *dandelion*, which is a simple and harmless medicine, a jar of the extract of *belladonna*, which is a deadly poison; by means of which the plaintiff, mary ann thomas, to whom, being sick, a dose of dandelion was prescribed by a physician, and a portion of the contents of the jar was administered as and for the extract of dandelion, was greatly injured, &c.

The facts proved were briefly these: mrs. Thomas being in ill health, her physician prescribed for her a dose of dandelion. Her husband purchased what was believed to be the medicine prescribed, at the store of dr. Foord, a physician and druggist in cazenovia, madison county, where the plaintiffs reside.

A small quantity of the medicine thus purchased, was administered to mrs. Thomas, on whom it produced very alarming effects; such as coldness of the surface and extremities, feebleness of circulation, spasms of the muscles, giddiness of the head, dilation of the pupils of the eyes, and derangement of mind. She recovered, however, after some time, from its effects, although, for a short time, her life was thought to be in great danger. The medicine administered was *belladonna*, and not dandelion.

The jar from which it was taken was labelled *"½LB. Dandelion, prepared by a. Gilbert, no. 108 john street, n. Y. Jar 8.02."* It was sold for, and delivered by dr. Foord, to be the extract of dandelion as labelled. Dr. Foord purchased the article as the extract of dandelion, from james s. Aspinwall, a druggist at new york. Aspinwall bought it of the defendant as extract of dandelion, believing it to be such.

The defendant was engaged at no. 108 john street, new york, in the manufacture and sale of certain vegetable extracts for medicinal purposes, and in the purchase and sale of others. The extracts manufactured by him were put up in jars for sale, and those which he purchased, were put up by him in like manner. The jars containing extracts manufactured by himself, and those containing extracts purchased by him from others, were labelled alike. Both were labelled like the jar in question, as "prepared by a. Gilbert." Gilbert was a person employed by the defendant, at a salary, as an assistant in his business. The jars were labelled in gilbert's name because he had been previously engaged in the same business, on his own account, at no. 108 john street, and probably because gilbert's labels rendered the articles more saleable. The extract contained in the jar sold to aspinwall, and by him to foord, was not manufactured by the defendant, but was purchased by him from another manufacturer or dealer. The extract of dandelion and the extract of belladonna resemble each other in color, consistence, smell and taste, but may, on careful examination, be distinguished, the one from the other, by those who are well acquainted with these articles. Gilbert's labels were paid for by winchester, and used in his business, with his knowledge and assent.

The defendant's counsel moved for a nonsuit on the following grounds:—

1. That the action could not be sustained, as the defendant was the remote vender of the article in question, and there was no connexion, transaction, or privity between him and the plaintiffs, or either of them.

2. That this action sought to charge the defendant with the consequences of the negligence of aspinwall and foord.

3. That the plaintiffs were liable to, and chargeable with the negligence of aspinwall and foord, and therefore could not maintain this action.

4. That according to the testimony foord was chargeable with negligence, and that the plaintiffs therefore could not sustain this suit against the defendant; if they could sustain a suit at all, it would be against foord only.

5. That this suit, being brought for the benefit of the wife, and alleging her as the meritorious cause of action, cannot be sustained.

6. That there was not sufficient evidence of negligence in the defendant to go to the jury.

The judge overruled the motion for a nonsuit, and the defendant's counsel excepted.

The judge, among other things, charged the jury that if they should find from the evidence that either aspinwall or foord were guilty of negligence in vending as and for dandelion the extract taken by mrs. Thomas, or that the plaintiff thomas, or those who administered it to mrs. Thomas, were chargeable with negligence in administering it, the plaintiffs were not entitled to recover; but if they were free from negligence, and if the defendant winchester was guilty of negligence in putting up and vending the extracts in question, the plaintiffs were entitled to recover, provided the extract administered to mrs. Thomas was the same which was put up by the defendant and sold by him to aspinwall, and by aspinwall to foord.

That if they should find the defendant liable, the plaintiffs in this action were entitled to recover damages only for the personal injury and suffering of the wife, and not for loss of service, medical treatment, or expense to the husband, and that the recovery should be confined to the actual damages suffered by the wife.

The action was properly brought in the name of the husband and wife, for the personal injury and suffering of the wife, and the case was left to the jury, with the proper directions on that point. *1 chitty on pleadings. 62 ed. Of 1828.*

The case depends on the first point taken by the defendant on his motion for a nonsuit; and the question is whether the defendant, being a remote vender of the medicine, and there being no privity or connexion between him and the plaintiffs, the action can be maintained.

If in labelling a poisonous drug with the name of a harmless medicine for public market, no duty was violated by the defendant, excepting that which he owed to aspinwall, his immediate vender, in virtue of his contract of sale, this action cannot be maintained. If a build a wagon and sell it to b, who sells it to c, and c hires it to d, who, in consequence of the gross negligence of a in building the wagon, is overturned and injured. D cannot recover damages against a, the builder.—a's obligation to build the wagon faithfully, arises solely out of his contract with b. The public have nothing to do with it. Misfortune to third persons, not parties to the contract, would not be a natural and necessary consequence of the builder's negligence; and such negligence is not an act immediately dangerous to human life.

So for the same reason, if a horse be defectively shod by a smith, and a person hiring the horse from the owner is thrown and injured in consequence of the smith's negligence in shoeing, the smith is not liable for the injury. The smith's duty in such case grows exclusively out of his contract with the owner of the horse; it was a duty which the smith owed him alone, and to no one else. And, although the injury to the rider may have happened in consequence of the negligence of the smith, the latter was not bound, either by his contract or by any considerations of public policy or safety, to respond for his breach of duty to any one except the person he contracted with.

This was the ground on which the case of *winterbotham vs. Wright. 10 mees and wellsby, 109*, was decided. A contracted with the post master general to provide a coach to convey the mail bags along a certain line of road, and b and others also contracted to horse the coach along the same line. B and his co-contractors hired c, who was the plaintiff, to drive the coach. The coach, in consequence of some latent defect, broke down; the plaintiff was thrown from his seat, and lamed. It was held that c could not maintain an action against a for the injury thus sustained. The reason of the decision is best stated by baron rolfe. A's duty to keep the coach in good condition was a duty to the post master general, with whom he made his contract, and not a duty to the driver employed by the owners of the horses.

But the case in hand stands on a different ground. The defendant was a dealer in poisonous drugs. Gilbert was his agent in preparing them for market; the death, or great bodily harm of some person was the natural and almost inevitable consequence of the sale of belladonna by means of the false label.—gilbert, the defendant's agent, would have been punishable for manslaughter if mrs. Thomas had died in consequence of taking the falsely labelled medicine. Every man who, by his culpable negligence, causes the death of another, although without intent to kill, is guilty of manslaughter. 2 *r. S.* 662. § 19. A chemist who negligently sells laudanum in a phial labelled as paregoric, and thereby causes the death of a person to whom it is administered, is guilty of manslaughter. *Tessymond's case, 1 lewins' crown cases, 169.* "so highly does the law value human life that it admits of no justification wherever life has been lost, and the carelessness or negligence of one person has contributed to the death of another." *Regina vs. Swindall, 2 car. And kir. 232–3.* And this rule applies not only where the death of one is occasioned by the negligent act of another, but where it is caused by the negligent omission of a duty of that other. *2 car. And kir. 368–371.* Although the defendant winchester may not be answerable, criminally, for the negligence of his agent, there can be no doubt of his liability in a civil action, in which the act of the agent is to be regarded as the act of the principal. In respect to the wrongful and criminal character of the negligence complained of, this case differs widely from those put by the defendant's counsel. No such imminent danger existed in those cases.

In the present case the sale of the poisonous article was made to a dealer in drugs, and not to a consumer. The injury, therefore, was not likely to fall on him, or on his vendee who was also a dealer; but much more likely to be visited on a remote purchaser, as actually happened. The defendant's negligence put human life in imminent danger. Can it be said that there was no duty on the part of the defendant to avoid the creation of that danger by the exercise of greater caution. Or, that the exercise of that caution was a duty only to his immediate vendee, whose life was not endangered? The defendant's duty arose out of the nature of his business, and the danger to others incident to its mismanagement. Nothing but mischief like that which actually happened could have been expected from sending the poison falsely labelled into the market; and the defendant is justly responsible for the propable consequences of the act.

The duty of exercising caution in this respect did not arise out of the defendant's contract of sale to aspinwall. The wrong done by the defendant was in putting the poison mislabelled into the hands of aspinwall, as an article of merchandize to be sold and afterwards used as the extract of *dandelion* by some person then unknown. The owner of a horse and cart, who leaves them unattended in the street, is liable for any damage which may result from his negligence. *Lynch vs. Mordon, 1 ad. And ellis, u. S. 29, 5 car. And payne 190. Illidge vs. Goodwin.* The owner of a loaded gun, who puts it into the hands of a child by whose indiscretion it is discharged, is liable for the damage occasioned by the discharge. *5 maule and sel. 198.* The defendant's contract of sale to aspinwall does not excuse the wrong done to plaintiffs. It was a part of the means by which the wrong was effected. The plaintiffs injury and their remedy would have stood on the same principle, if the defendant had given the *belladonna* to dr. Foord without price; or, if he had put it in his shop without his knowledge, under circumstances which would propably have led to its sale, on the faith of the label.

In *longmead vs. Holliday, 6 law and eq. Rep. 562*, the distinction is recognized between an act of negligence imminently dangerous to the lives of others, and one that is not so. In the former case, the party guilty of the negligence is liable to the party injured, whether there be a contract between them or not; in the latter, the negligent party is liable only to the party with whom he contracted, and on the ground that negligence is a breach of the contract.

The defendant on the trial insisted that aspinwall and foord were guilty of negligence in selling the article in question for what it was represented to be in the label; and that the suit if it could be sustained at all, should have been brought against foord. The judge charged the jury that if they or either of them were guilty of negligence in selling the *belladonna* for *dandelion*, the verdict must be for the defendant, and left the question of their negligence to the jury, who found on that point for the plaintiff. If the case really depended on the point thus raised, the question was properly left to the jury. But, i think it did not. The defendant by affixing the label to the jar represented its contents to be *dandelion*, and to have been "prepared" by his agent gilbert. The word "prepared" on the label must be understood to mean that the article was manufactured by him, or that it had passed through some process under his hand, which would give him personal knowledge of its true name and quality. Whether foord was justified in selling the article upon the faith of the defendant's label, would have been an open question in an action by the plaintiffs against him; and i wish to be understood as giving no opinion on that point. But it seems to me to be clear, that the defendant cannot in this case set up as a defence that foord sold the contents of the jar as and for what the defendant represented it to be. The label conveyed the idea distinctly to foord that the contents of the jar was the extract of *dandelion*, and that the defendant knew it to be such. So far as the defendant is concerned, foord was under no obligation to test the truth of the representation. The charge of the judge in submitting to the jury the question in relation to the negligence of foord and aspinwall, cannot be complained of by the defendant.

Judgment affirmed.

A COPY. H. R. Selden, *state reporter.*

Mem.—the original verdict against winchester was $800; the costs of appeal, &c. Swelled the amount to near $1,400, which was paid by winchester.

NOTES IN PHARMACY, NO. 5.

BY BENJAMIN CANAVAN.

SUCCI INSPISSATI PER AERE SICCO.

—i take occasion again to notice these preparations, for the reason, that i perceive from a note, by the editor of this journal, appended to an article on "cicuta," &c., in the last (september) number: that he considers the extracts of messrs. Tilden or currie, superior to the best english extracts he has seen. I think, however, that on reflection, he will agree with me that those prepared by means of a current of dried air—some of which so made have been imported and used here—must particularly, when there is anything volatile about them,—be superior to all others; indeed, so favorably am i inclined to regard this process, that i think the profession, medical and pharmaceutical, should *demand* its adoption by those engaged in the business of preparing extracts; until which is the case, i shall feel it incumbent upon me to use the imported article, as i have been in the habit of doing. Moreover, the relative virosity of the *narcotic plants* of the american and european continents are still in favor of the latter, although, if recent researches are to be depended upon, the difference is not so great as was supposed. Mr. Currie, i believe, prepares some at least, if not all his extracts with imported herbs, and in vacuo, and they are therefore the best made here; but these are the *dried* herbs, and cannot afford as good an extract, ceteris paribus, as when the fresh plant is used. The english extracts of indigenous plants are, strictly speaking, *inspissated juices*, according to the *london pharmacopœia*. The juice of a plant inspissated by air alone, and that quickly too, must be tantamount in its properties to the fresh plant whence obtained, so far as we are at present aware, or at least to the same, dried in the same equally safe manner; wherefore, i consider them preferable to all other preparations of the family of extracts.25

---

25 mr, Canavan mistakes—the assertion was that the extract of conium, prepared by tilden or by currie, was

superior to the best english extract of that article we have seen, and a comparison of the odor of the two articles, under the influence of a little liquor potassae, will readily convince the observer of its correctness. The question as to the other extracts is one of great interest, and we still believe it awaits a satisfactory solution.—[ed.]

SANGUINARINA.

—having been called upon to prepare some of this article, i undertook to do so by the process said to have been adopted by mr. Dana, viz.: displacing the root with dilute acetic acid; precipitating by ammonica; boiling with purified animal charcoal; treating with alcohol, and finally evaporating the alcoholic solution, by which i obtained from two ounces of the root, about twenty grains only, having the sensible properties of the article very strongly, and being of a reddish brown color, assuming, when finely pulverized, an ochreish hue. It has been described as a "white, pearly substance," which it might have become by more perfect discoloration, or the use of a different acid. The liquor from which it was precipitated, lost its peculiar taste, but not all its color, showing that the color of the root does not depend altogether on this principle, as was supposed. The article in question has been used by one practitioner, who stated it to have met his expectations, administered in doses of one sixth of a grain. The preparation in question is a very desirable one, as the objectionable taste of the ordinary preparations is a frequent bar to their use.

ALOINE.

—on this subject it may be well to mark the fact, that the officinal "ext. Aloe purificat," presents the active property of the aloes, freed from its griping quality, (though this is doubted; but the same doubt would seem to apply to aloine.) It is, however, about twice the strength of the crude extract, and is generally used when the "tuto cito et jucunde" effect is desired. The change which is supposed to take place in the aloine, from the heat used in the preparation of the purified extract, would only—

according to the messrs. Smith of edinburg—prevent its crystallization, and therefore the extract should be equally advantageous, except, perhaps, in regard of bulk, which is not a very *great* object.

ZIMMER TEST FOR QUINIDINE.

—in employing this test, some modification of the original directions is necessary, in order to success. The word *drop* is used, but it is doubtful whether *minim* may not be meant, and if not, the difference in density of the liquids used would prevent our getting, by dropping, the correct quantities. This i found to be the case, and to save future trouble i give the minutiæ of the experiment as i performed it, with success; no evidence of the presence of quinidine being shown, as was expected:

aquae gtt. Xxiij.

ACID. Sulph. C. P. Gtt. Vi.

AETHER sulph. *Concentr.* Gtt. Lx.

AQUAE ammonia f. F. F. Gtt. Xx.

Et agita bene.

In each instance, the drops were allowed to fall from the lip of an ordinary quart tincture bottle, except the sulphuric acid, which was contained in a small pint tincture bottle, and of which i used *three times the number of drops* directed; the drops being about one third the size of a drop of distilled water, which was shown to be correct, by the necessity for that quantity to effect a solution which took place without the aid of external heat. With regard to this matter of drops, it is a considerable eyesore. I would recommend to apothecaries, (perhaps it might be deemed worthy of the action of the convention), to agree upon some standard *size* for the drop,—say that of a drop of distilled water, under definite circumstances. It is true, we have a measure; but it is for minims not for drops, whilst in this way, by a little practice, the eye might be accustomed to the proper size of the drop, so that there would be little or no difficulty in obtaining an exact result, by increasing or diminishing the number of drops, according to the proportional size of its drop, to the standard one. Of course, when i speak of "keeping the drop in the eye," i do not mean to imply anything incompatible with the maine liquor law. I speak aquatically, not *spiritually*.

NATIONAL PHARMACEUTICAL CONVENTION.

According to the arrangement which had previously been announced, the national convention met in philadelphia, on wednesday the 6th of october, at 4 p. M. In the absence of dr. Guthrie, the president, the convention was organized by the appointment of mr. Coggeshall, of new york, as president *pro tempore*; mr. A. B. Taylor, of philadelphia, as acting secretary. A committee was then appointed by the chair, consisting of messrs. Ellis, of philadelphia, colcord, of boston, and laidley, of richmond, to examine the credentials of the delegates present; and to report a resolution in regard to the admission of such apothecaries as might be present, who, though not delegated by any incorporated institution, desired to attend the convention.

The committee reported that satisfactory credentials had been presented by the following gentlemen:—

From the massachusetts college of pharmacy—joseph burnett, samuel m. Colcord, dr. Samuel r. Philbrick.

From the college of pharmacy, of the city of new york—george d. Coggeshall, l. S. Haskell, john meakim.

From the richmond pharmaceutical society—alexander duvall, john purcell, joseph laidley.

From the cincinnatti college of pharmacy—william b. Chapman, charles augustus smith, edward s. Wayne.

From the philadelphia college of pharmacy--daniel b. Smith, charles ellis, william procter, jr.

From the maryland college of pharmacy—dr. David stewart, george w. Andrews.

Henry f. Fish, of waterbury, connecticut, as the representative of the apothecaries and druggists of hartford county, connecticut. The following resolution was also offered by the committee:—

Resolved, that those gentlemen whose interest in the object of the convention has induced them to meet with us on this occasion, be invited to take seats in the convention, and fully participate in its proceedings.

The report and resolutions were adopted, and the committee continued to act on claims of delegates, and others not yet arrived.

After the roll had been called, the following gentlemen were invited to seats in the convention, viz.:—

San francisco, california

Charles l. Bache,

New york

Eugene dupuy,

Philadelphia

Edward parrish and

Alfred b. Taylor.

A committee, consisting of one from each delegation, was then chosen to nominate officers for the convention, and on their nomination, the following gentlemen were duly elected:—

President

Daniel b. Smith, of philadelphia.

Vice presidents

George w. Andrews, of baltimore,

Samuel m. Colcord, of boston,

C. Augustus smith, of cincinnati.

Recording secretary

George d. Coggeshall, of new york.

Corresponding secretary

William procter, jr., of philadelphia.

After the officers had taken their seats, the following report was presented by the committee appointed at the convention, held the previous year at new york, "to act as a standing committee, to collect such information as maybe deemed valuable, together with memorials and suggestions from medical and pharmaceutical associations to be presented to the next convention."

"the undersigned, a committee appointed at the convention, held last year in new york, and instructed "to collect and receive such information as may be valuable, and memorials and suggestions from medical and pharmaceutical associations, to be presented to the next convention," respectfully report: that in the period that has elapsed since their appointment—notwithstanding the fact of their readiness to receive any communications, having been duly announced—they have received no contributions towards the end or object of their appointment, except those relating to the inspection of drugs. They have, however, not been unmindful of the duty imposed upon them, and now offer the following suggestions, as tending to aid the business of the convention, in so far as they exhibit some of the more prominent subjects, worthy of its serious deliberation and action.

1st, the number of pharmaceutists constituting the professional body in the united states is large, comprehends all grades of qualifications, and extends to every city and town in the country. The professed object of the present convention being to adopt measures calculated to benefit this large body of citizens, in a professional point of view, by showing that there exist many grounds of sympathy between them, notwithstanding the present want of united action; we believe, that the institution of a national association, whose members may come from all sections of the body, is calculated to enlist this feeling of brotherhood, and direct its power, as a reforming force, towards the elevation of the average standard of qualification now existing. In view of this, it is suggested, whether the passage of a resolution by this convention, resolving itself into a national association, should not properly engage its attention at its commencement, so that the important details of forming a constitution—explaining the nature of its organization, &c. &c., might receive the deliberate consideration they merit, before being adopted.

As the basis upon which the association will rest, will be the decision as to what shall constitute a member, we believe its ultimate usefulness will very much depend on the character of this decision, and we cannot refrain from presenting some reflections on the subject.

The inefficiency or inadequacy of the present basis, viz.:—delegates from incorporated and unincorporated societies is here demonstrated, by the small number who have been appointed in answer to the call; at least, this must be true, so long as the process of local organization is so dilatory. The aim should be, to enlist as much as possible of the talent now engaged in the pharmaceutical ranks.

We think, therefore, that membership in the proposed association should be of a representative character, to as full an extent as practicable. Colleges and societies of pharmacy should, of course, send delegates. Then, provision should be made for the apothecaries, in cities and towns where no society exists, whereby they may send representatives, to the extent of one for every ten apothecaries, in such places; each representative to bring with him a certificate from his constituents. Finally, to provide for the admission of isolated individuals, who may not have neighbors sufficient to entitle them to act as representatives, but who feel an interest in the association. Power should be given to the committee, on credentials, under certain restrictions.

The formation of the constitution, and the preparation of a code of ethics applicable to the present condition of the profession; sufficiently stringent to elevate the members above many things now too prevalent, and yet not so binding as to exclude a large number, who, though well disposed, are unable to free themselves from participation in acts contrary to the highest standard, without a sacrifice greater than could be expected of them, should engage the wisest action of the convention, to render them practicable in their working.

2nd, the subject of *pharmaceutical education* is, in the opinion of this committee, one of great importance, and deserving of the consideration of the committee, in several points of view. Indeed, the primary object of the convention being called, was in reference to the improvement of the standard practice throughout the country; and this cannot be effected without extending the present means of education, either by schools, or by an increase of facilities, offered by proprietors to their apprentices and assistants. In too many instances the proprietors are illy fitted to extend to those whom they have engaged to teach the business of a pharmaceutist the tuition that of right belongs to them. As schools of pharmacy are of gradual growth, and cannot be expected to exist, except in large cities, the convention would do well to consider what subsidiary means may be enlisted to reach those of our brethren who reside in small towns. One of the first of these collateral aids will be found in local organizations, embracing the proprietors in such towns where, by a union of their exertions and contributions they may encourage pharmaceutical literature, by forming libraries, and uphold among themselves correct practice,— the employment only of good drugs, and the receipt of fair prices.

In france, where but three pharmaceutical schools exist, there are such societies in all large towns, which have halls and libraries, where their young men and apprentices have opportunities for gaining knowledge; and laboratories wherein they occasionally perform operations not easily executed with the instruments and utensils most usually found in shop laboratories. If such associations can be formed by the proprietors, they will soon influence the apprentices, and thus effect the object aimed at, to a great extent.

The superior advantages of tuition in well conducted schools of pharmacy will not be doubted, especially when it is preceded by several years shop practice. Access to these, by young men at a distance, can always be had, when their circumstances enable them to attend, and thus finish their pharmaceutical education. The perfection of a school of pharmacy is attained by attaching to it a practical laboratory, wherein the advanced pupils can have an opportunity to become familiar with the more difficult manipulations of pharmaceutical chemistry, and of extemporaneous pharmacy. As yet, neither of the schools in this country have that addition, which arises from the fact, that the expense of conducting them, renders their support by the fees of the pupils almost impossible. We think the voice of the convention should be raised to encourage the formation of such schools, and also, to advocate the practice of preparing chemicals in the shop laboratory.

3rd, the apprenticeship system, which obtains, in many parts of the united states, is a subject worthy the consideration of the convention. The conditions, conducing to mutual advantage, between the employer and the employed, are not sufficiently attended to in general. Proprietors often do not consider the fitness of applicants, both as regards natural endowments and preliminary education, with that care and attention that a due regard to such applicants demands; and consequently, a large number of inefficient apothecaries are entailed upon the country— inefficient from lack of talent, or from disgust at a business for which they have no inclination. More attention to the claims of apprentices, on the *teaching* of their employers, should be advocated by the convention as due to the former, as advantageous to the latter, and eventually to the profession.

4th, the committee believe that the subject of *secret medicines*, or quackery, as applied to pharmacy, together with the course usually followed by quacks, in bringing their nostrums into notice, is becoming yearly more fraught with ill consequences, both to the consumers and the apothecaries, and merits the consideration of the convention, as to whether the reference of the subject to a committee to investigate, would not result in some advantage.

5th, the subject of the *inspection of imported drugs*, as regards the *actual* working of the law, is of deep interest to all. The possibility of bringing the influence of this convention to bear, in regard to the continuance in office of able men, solely on the ground of fitness, is worth consideration. The usefulness of this law rests absolutely on the ability and conscientiousness of the inspector, and if incumbents, perfectly satisfactory to those concerned, are removed on political grounds, and replaced by inexperienced and unqualified persons, it is apparent that the good results of the law will cease.

Whatever may be the efficiency of the law against the importation of inferior drugs, it will not reach those *at home*, who are disposed to resort to adulteration as a means of increasing their profits. The power of the general government ceases with the custom house. It will be necessary in order to reach this evil effectually, as far as it can be done by legislation; to induce our state legislatures and municipal authorities to authorize some form of inspection by which the delinquents can be reached; not the drug adulterator merely, but the medicine adulterator— the apothecary who scruples not to reduce the strength of standard medicines, that he may reduce his prices. Whatever may be the proper course of this convention, we believe that eventually the national association should urge, with all the force of its influence, the enactment of state laws tending to the reformation of these evils.

6th, the general adoption of our *national pharmacopœia* as a guide in the preparation of officinal medicines, is much to be desired. We believe that this convention should encourage its adoption, and should request the publishers of that work to issue a small sized cheap edition, so that every physician and apothecary shall have a copy. We also believe that a fruitful source of variation in the preparations of the shops, is the existence of a number of formulæ for the same preparation, as found in the british pharmacopœias parallel with that of our own code, in the commentaries in general use.

7th, the *indiscriminate sale of poisons* by druggists and apothecaries, as at present conducted, is a serious evil in the united states. Any views which may originate in the convention, tending to abate this evil, would no doubt have some influence, if circulated by its authority

8th, the separation of pharmacy from the practice of medicine, has long been effected on the continent of europe, by the direct interference of the government, each profession being in the hands of a distinct class of men. Inheriting, as we do, our medical institutions from great britain, the confusion of interests which has long prevailed there has in some measure descended to us; and many instances of medical practitioners conducting apothecary shops, like the so-called *apothecaries* of england, exist among us. The increase of this class in some localities has been marked of late years—a fact attributable to the "undue multiplication of graduates in medicine, who, finding the ranks of their profession so full as to render prospect of immediate success doubtful, turn their attention towards pharmacy, as a subsidiary means of support. As these mongrel apothecaries too frequently use their shops merely as stepping-stones to business, they tend directly to depreciate the standard of practice on the one hand, and tempt young apothecaries, who are struggling against the difficulties of an already excessive competition, to turn their attention to medical practice with or without a diploma, as may suit their circumstances or fancy, on the other, and thus complicate the confusion. As pharmacy never will advance as it should, whilst this amalgamation exists in cities and towns to any large extent, we earnestly recommend to this convention, that a voice may go forth at its present session, calling attention to this growing evil.

9th, believing, that if the pharmaceutists of the united states are true to themselves, the meetings of the association, of which the present may be considered the beginning, will annually increase in interest and importance, we would suggest—what must have occurred to many present—that they should be partially devoted to the advancement of pharmacy, as well as to the sciences on which it is based, by inviting contributions of original papers, and by committing subjects requiring investigation to suitable committees, who should report the results of their researches at the ensuing annual meeting, when, if they meet the approbation of the association, it might direct their publication. Participation in the proceedings of such a gathering of their brethren, would prove a powerful incentive to many pharmaceutists, whose tastes lead them into scientific paths, to cultivate their talents by the pursuit of investigations fraught with usefulness to their profession at home, and with honor to it abroad

And lastly, whatever may be the ultimate action of the convention, in relation to the subjects brought forward in this report, we would respectfully suggest that a full digest of its proceedings be directed to be published, and largely circulated among the pharmaceutists of the united states, as calculated to do much good.

(signed,)

Committee

William procter, jr.,

Samuel m. Colcord,

Geo. D. Coggeshall.

The second meeting of this association was mainly occupied in reading and discussing a draft of a constitution and code of ethics.

Third sitting, october 7th, 4 o'clock, p. M.

President in the chair.

On the roll being called, the delegates generally were present.

The minutes of the preceding sitting were read and adopted.

The president informed the convention, that the business committee not being ready to report, it was understood that dr. Stewart, examiner of drugs, &c., at the port of baltimore, had some statements to offer in regard to the working of the drug law at that port, and the convention assenting, requested him to proceed.

Dr. Stewart stated, that as there had been some difference of opinion among the drug examiners, as to the intention of the law in certain cases, he desired the opinion of the convention regarding the inferior class of cinchona barks that came from maracaibo, carthagena, &c., and other articles about which there is difference of opinion among druggists. In illustration of the difficulties of the subject, he remarked that one invoice of bark, that in a commercial point of view was not esteemed, and which came invoiced at ten cents per pound, had yielded, on analysis, two and a half per cent of cinchonine; whilst loxa bark, invoiced at thirty cents per pound, had afforded but a fraction of one per cent. He considered the admission of the barks in question as quite different from deteriorated or adulterated drugs, in as much as they possessed a range of power which, though inferior to the best peruvian barks, was yet useful, and capable of application in medicine.

He therefore offered the following resolution:

"resolved, that it is the opinion of this convention, that all varieties of drugs, that are good of their kind, should be admitted by the special examiners of drugs and medicines."

Pending the consideration of this resolution, mr. Coggeshall informed the convention that dr. Bailey, the special examiner of drugs for the port of new york, had furnished, at his request, a report on the character of imported drugs, coming under his supervision, and on the general working of the laws, which, by request, was read. (published in our last.)

A similar report from mr. Edward hamilton, late drug examiner at the port of boston, communicated to mr. S. M. Colcord, at his request, with a view to its being presented to this convention, was also read. (to be published in our next.)

Dr. Stewart then opened the debate on the subject, arguing that drugs, of whatever virtue or variety, so that they are good of their kind, should be admitted. In reference to barks he could say, that perhaps a larger amount of the varieties of that drug came to the port of baltimore than any other. That the merchants in that trade were so desirous of getting the best kinds, that it was quite usual for them to import specimens by way of the isthmus, and have them examined before ordering their invoices, to ascertain whether they would pass the custom-house, that he had, (as examiner at that port,) chemically examined a large number of samples of the barks, both peruvian and carthagena, and that the latter had invariably contained more or less of alkaloids, and were generally of good quality, of their kind.

He therefore considered the fact that a drug is, or may be used as an adulteration for other drugs, should not exclude it if it is used to any extent on its own merits. In illustration, dr. Stewart remarked that the examiner might go on a vessel and observe, side by side, two casks of oil, consigned to the same individual, one invoiced "cod liver oil," and the other "sperm oil." On examination he finds that they are what they purport to be; the suspicion would arise very naturally, that the latter was to be used for adulterating the former, yet, should sperm oil be excluded, because certain parties use it for an adulteration? He thought not, and on the same grounds he considered that the inferior barks and rhubarb should be admitted, although some persons may use them for adulteration.

At the request of the president, professor carson, of the university of pennsylvania, addressed the convention on the subject before it. He coincided generally with the views of dr. Stewart, as regarded the value of the drugs in question. He expressed the opinion that numerous varieties of the so-called carthagena and maracaibo barks, were possessed of decided medicinal virtue; that several kinds of european rhubarb were of much value in medicine, especially in times when the officinal varieties are scarce, and that these drugs should all be admitted, when not deteriorated or adulterated.

Mr. Haskell, of new york, advocated the same views, more especially, as related to english rhubarb, bringing forward the testimony of dr. Pereira, to the effect, that some specimens of banbury rhubarb were almost, if not fully equal to the chinese drug, and they were here even of rather higher price. He also stated, that a large demand existed in this country for the yellow carthagena barks, that the house, of which he was a member, sold large quantities in powder, and that the parties purchasing it did so, knowing its origin. He was not aware of the use to which it was put, but presumed that it was employed legitimately.

Mr. Fisk, of connecticut, stated, that through the part of new england that he represented, considerable quantities of the barks in question were used legitimately, as tonics; and that no instance of their being used as an adulteration of the peruvian barks had come to his knowledge.

Mr. Coggeshall on the other side of the question, called the attention of the convention to the item in dr. Bailey's report, showing that three hundred thousand pounds of these barks had been rejected at the port of new york, in about two years and a half. He argued that this bark was not consumed there; that it was not used in the manufacture of the alkaloids; that the allegation that it was used for making tooth powders would hardly account for the great consumption of it, and the question naturally arose for what purpose was it imported? He believed that it was used extensively to grind with the peruvian barks, as an adulteration, and to make an inferior extract, which could be done cheaply and profitably, and it was largely sold as an officinal preparation, that many of the persons who came to our cities to buy drugs, were not able to judge of their purity, and bought them without asking any questions, save, as regarded price,—and so convinced was he of the application of these false barks to these false purposes, that as a protective measure, in his opinion, they should be excluded. And also, in regard to english and other european rhubarb, that the argument of professor carson would not hold good while the markets were so well supplied with the russian and chinese varieties, to which the banbury, regarded as the best of the european, was so very inferior. It might be used as a dernier resort, but should only be so used. Entirely independent of this argument, however, mr. Coggeshall considered that european rhubarb should be excluded, because of its peculiar adaptation and general use as an adulteration, owing to its fine color, which enables the adulterator to improve the appearance of the inferior chinese variety, to mix it with the russian article in powder, without depreciating its appearance; or, as it is notoriously done, to a great extent, substitute it entirely for the true article.

Mr. Colcord, of boston, advocated the latter view, and hoped that the resolution would not pass.

Other members of the convention joined in the debate, after which, the question was taken on the resolution of dr. Stewart, and it was lost.

As the importance of the subject introduced by dr. Stewart, was fully appreciated by the convention, at the same time that no direct course of action seemed proper for it to pursue, the following resolution was offered by mr. Smith, of cincinnati, viz.:

"resolved, that the whole subject of the inspection of drugs shall be referred to a committee, who shall be instructed to confer with the examiners, and endeavor to arrive at some practicable means of fixing standards for imported drugs."

The resolution was unanimously adopted, and mr. Taylor, of philadelphia, mr. Meakim, of new york, and mr. Burnett, of boston, were appointed by the president, to carry it into effect.

On motion of mr. Procter, dr. Stewart, of baltimore, was added to the committee.

[this report is made up from the report of the executive committee, published in philadelphia. The conclusion of the proceedings will be given in our next.]

OBSERVATIONS UPON A GENERAL METHOD FOR DETECTING THE ORGANIC ALKALOIDS IN CASES OF POISONING.

BY PROFESSOR STAS, OF BRUSSELS.

Whatever certain authors may have said on the subject, it is possible to discover in a suspected liquid all the alkaloids, in whatever state they may be. I am quite convinced that every chemist who has kept up his knowledge as to analysis, will not only succeed in detecting their presence, but even in determining the nature of that which he has discovered, provided that the alkaloid in question is one of that class of bodies, the properties of which have been suitably studied. Thus he will be able to discover conia, nicotine, aniline, picoline, petinine, morphine, codeine, narcotine, strychnine, brucine, veratrine, colchicine, delphine, emetine, solanine, aconitine, atropine, hyoscyamine. I do not pretend to say that the chemical study of all these alkaloids has been sufficiently well made to enable the experimenter who detects one of them to know it immediately, and affirm that it is such an alkaloid, and not such another. Nevertheless, in those even which he cannot positively determine or specify, he may be able to say that it belongs to such a family of vegetables—the solanaceæ, for example. In a case of poisoning by such agents, even this will be of much importance. The method which i now propose for detecting the alkaloids in suspected matters, is nearly the same as that employed for extracting those bodies from the vegetables which contain them. The only difference consists in the manner of setting them free, and of presenting them to the action of solvents. We know that the alkaloids form acid salts, which are equally soluble in water and alcohol; we know also that a solution of these acid salts can be decomposed so that the base set at liberty remains either momentorily or permanently in solution in the liquid. *I have observed that all the solid and fixed alkaloids above enumerated, when maintained in a free state and in solution in a liquid, can be taken up by ether when this solvent is in sufficient quantity.* Thus, to extract an alkaloid from a suspected substance, the only problem to resolve consists in separating, by the aid of simple means, the foreign matters, and then to find a base which, in rendering the alkaloid free, retains it in solution, in order that the ether may extract it from the liquid. Successive treatment by water and alcohol of different degrees of concentration, suffices for separating the foreign matters, and obtaining in a small bulk a solution in which the alkaloid can be found. The bicarbonates of potash or soda, or these alkalies in a caustic state, are convenient bases for setting the alkaloids at liberty, at the same time keeping them wholly in solution, especially if the alkaloids have been combined with an excess of tartaric or of oxalic acid.

To separate foreign substances, animal or otherwise, from the suspected matters, recourse is commonly had to the tribasic acetate of lead, and precipitating the lead afterwards by a current of sulphuretted hydrogen. As i have several times witnessed, this procedure has many and very serious inconveniences. In the first place, the tribasic acetate of lead, even when used in large excess, comes far short of precipitating all the foreign matters; secondly, the sulphuretted hydrogen, which is used to precipitate the lead, remains in combination with certain organic matters which undergo great changes by the action of the air and of even a moderate heat; so that animal liquids which have been precipitated by the tribasic acetate of lead, and from which the lead has been separated afterwards by hydrosulphuric acid, color rapidly on exposure to the air, and exhale at the same time a putrid odor, which adheres firmly to the matters which we extract afterwards from these liquids. The use of a salt of lead presents another inconvenience, viz.: the introduction of foreign metals into the suspected matters, so that that portion of the suspected substance is rendered unfit for testing for mineral substances. The successive and combined use of water and alcohol at different states of concentration, permits us to search for mineral substances, whatever be their nature, so that in this way nothing is compromised, which is of immense advantage when the analyst does not know what poison he is to look for.

It is hardly necessary to say, that in medico-legal researches for the alkaloids, we ought never to use animal charcoal for decolorizing the liquids, because we may lose all the alkaloid in the suspected matters. It is generally known that animal charcoal absorbs these substances at the same time that it fixes the coloring and odoriferous matters.

[this is no doubt true; we must not use animal charcoal to decolorize, and then look for the alkaloid in the *liquid*, but we may use it, at least in the case of strychnia and some of the non-volatile alkaloids, to separate them, and then we look for them *in the charcoal*. See notice of graham and hofmann's process for detecting strychnia: *monthly journal*, aug., 1852, p. 140; *pharmaceutical journal*, vol. Xi., p. 504, may, 1852.]

The above observations do not proceed from speculative ideas only, but are the result of a pretty long series of experiments which i have several times employed for discovering these organic alkaloids. To put in practice the principles which i have thus explained, the following is the method in which i propose to set about such an analysis:— i suppose that we wish to look for an alkaloid in the contents of the stomach or intestines; we commence by adding to these matters twice their weight of pure and very strong alcohol;26 we add afterwards, according to the quantity and nature of the suspected matter, from ten to thirty grains of tartaric or oxalic acid—in preference tartaric; we introduce the mixture into a flask, and heat it to 160° or 170° fahrenheit. After it has completely cooled it is to be filtered, the insoluble residue washed with strong alcohol, and the filtered liquid evaporated in vacuo. If the operator has not an air-pump, the liquid is to be exposed to a strong current of air at a temperature of not more than 90° fahrenheit. If, after the volatilization of the alcohol, the residue contains fatty or other insoluble matters, the liquid is to be filtered a second time, and then the filtrate and washings of the filter evaporated in the air-pump till nearly dry. If we have no air pump, it is to be placed under a bell-jar over a vessel containing concentrated sulphuric acid. We are then to treat the residue with cold anhydrous alcohol, taking care to exhaust the substance thoroughly; we evaporate the alcohol in the open air at the ordinary temperature, or still better, in vacuo; we now dissolve the acid residue in the smallest possible quantity of water, and introduce the solution into a small test-tube, and add little by little pure powdered bicarbonate of soda or potash, till a fresh quantity produces no further effervescence of carbonic acid. We then agitate the whole with four or five times its bulk of pure ether, and leave it to settle. When the ether swimming on the top is perfectly clear, then decant some of it into a capsule, and leave it in *a very dry place* to spontaneous evaporation.

---

26 when we wish to look for an alkaloid in the tissue of an organ, as the liver, heart, or lungs, we must first divide the organ into very small fragments, moisten the mass with pure strong alcohol, then express strongly, and by further treatment with alcohol exhaust the tissue of everything soluble. The liquid so obtained, is to be treated in the same way as a mixture of suspected matter and alcohol.

Now, two orders of things may present themselves; either the alkaloid contained in the suspected matter is liquid and volatile, or solid and fixed. I shall now consider these two hypotheses.

EXAMINATION FOR A LIQUID AND VOLATILE ALKALI.

We suppose there exists a liquid and volatile alkaloid. In such a case, by the evaporation of the ether, there remains in the inside of the capsule some small liquid striæ which fall to the bottom of the vessel. In this case, under the influence of the heat of the hand, the contents of the capsule exhale an odor more or less disagreeable, which becomes, according to the nature of the alkaloid, more or less pungent, suffocating, irritant; it presents, in short, a smell like that of a volatile alkali masked by an animal odor. If we discover any traces of the presence of a volatile alkaloid, we add then to the contents of the vessel, from which we have decanted a small quantity of ether, one or two fluid drachms of a strong solution of caustic potash or soda, and agitate the mixture. After a sufficient time, we draw off the ether into a test-tube; we exhaust the mixture by two or three treatments with ether, and unite all the ethereal fluids. We pour afterwards into this ether, holding the alkaloid in solution, one or two drachms of water, acidulated with a fifth part of its weight of pure sulphuric acid, agitate it for some time, leave it to settle, pour off the ether swimming on the top, and wash the acid liquid at the bottom with a new quantity of ether. As the sulphates of ammonia, of nicotine, aniline, quinoleine, picoline, and petinine, are entirely insoluble in ether, the water acidulated with sulphuric acid contains the alkaloid in a small bulk, and in the state of a pure sulphate; but as the sulphate of conia is soluble in ether, the ether may contain a small quantity of this alkali, but the greater part remains in the acidulated watery solution. The ether, on the other hand, retains all the animal matters which it has taken from the alkaline solutions. If it on spontaneous evaporation leaves a small quantity of a feebly-colored yellowish residue, of a repulsive animal odor, mixed with a certain quantity of sulphate of conine, this alkaloid exists in the suspected matter under analysis. To extract the alkaloid from the solution of the acid sulphate, we add to the latter an aqueous and concentrated solution of potash or caustic soda, we agitate and exhaust the mixture with pure ether; the ether dissolves ammonia, and the alkaloid is now free. We expose the ethereal solution at the lowest possible temperature to spontaneous evaporation; almost all the ammonia volatilizes with the ether, whilst the alkaloid remains as residue. To eliminate the last traces of ammonia, we place for a few minutes the vessel containing the alkaloid in a vacuum over sulphuric acid, and obtain the organic alkaloid with the chemical and physical characters which belong to it, and which it is now the chemist's duty to determine positively.

I applied, on the 3d march, 1851, the process which i have described, to the detection of nicotine in the blood from the heart of a dog poisoned by two cubic centimetres [0.78 c.i.] of nicotine introduced into the œsophagus, and i was able in a most positive manner to determine the presence of nicotine in the blood. I was able to determine its physical characters, its odor, taste, and alkalinity. I succeeded in obtaining the chloroplatinate of the base perfectly crystallized in quadrilateral rhomboidal prisms of a rather dark yellow color, and to ascertain their insolubility in alcohol and ether.

I have applied the same process for the detection of conia in a very old tincture of hemlock, which my friend and colleague m. De hemptinne was so kind as to put at my disposal; and i was equally successful in extracting from the liquid colorless conia, presenting all the physical and chemical properties of this alkali. I was also able to prove that the ether which holds conia in solution, carries off a notable portion of this alkaloid when the solvent is exposed to spontaneous evaporation.

EXAMINATION FOR A SOLID AND FIXED ALKALOID.

Let us now suppose that the alkali is solid and fixed; in that case, according to the nature of the alkali, it may happen that the evaporation of the ether resulting from the treatment of the acid matter, to which we have added bicarbonate of soda, may leave or not a residue, containing an alkaloid. If it does, we add a solution of caustic potash or soda to the liquid, and agitate it briskly with ether. This dissolves the vegetable alkaloid, now free and remaining in the solution of potash or soda. In either case, we exhaust the matter with ether. Whatever be the agent which has set the alkaloid free, whether it be the bicarbonate of soda or potash, or caustic soda or potash, it remains, by the evaporation of the ether, on the side of the capsule as a solid body, but more commonly a colorless milky liquid, holding solid matters in suspension. The odor of the substance is animal, disagreeable, but not pungent. It turns litmus paper permanently blue.

When we thus discover a solid alkaloid, the first thing to do is to try and obtain it in a crystalline state, so as to be able to determine its form. Put some drops of alcohol in the capsule which contains the alkaloid, and leave the solution to spontaneous evaporation. It is, however, very rare that the alkaloid obtained by the above process is pure enough to crystallize. Almost always it is soiled by foreign matters. To isolate these substances, some drops of water, feebly acidulated with sulphuric acid, are poured into the capsule, and then moved over its surface, so as to bring it in contact with the matter in the capsule. Generally we observe that the acid water does not moisten the sides of the vessel. The matter which is contained in it separates into two parts, one formed of greasy matter, which remains adherent to the sides—the other alkaline, which dissolves and forms an acid sulphate. We cautiously decant the acid liquid, which ought to be limpid and colorless, if the process has been well executed; the capsule is well washed with some drops of acidulated water, added to the first liquid, and the whole is evaporated to three-fourths in vacuo, or under a bell-jar over sulphuric acid. We put into the residue a very concentrated solution of pure carbonate of potash, and treat the whole liquid with absolute alcohol. This dissolves the alkaloid, while it leaves untouched the sulphate of potash and excess of carbonate of potash. The evaporation of the alcoholic solution gives us the alkaloid in crystals.

It is now the chemist's business to determine its properties, to be able to prove its individuality. I have applied the principles which i have just expounded to the detection of morphine, iodine, strychnine, brucine, veratrine, emetine, colchicine, aconitine, atropine, hyoscyamine—and i have succeeded in isolating, without the least difficulty, these different alkalies, previously mixed with foreign matters.

I have thus been able to extract, by this process, morphine from opium, strychnine and brucine from nux vomica, veratrine from extract of veratram, emetine from extract of ipecacuanha, colchicine from tincture of colchicum, aconitine from an aqueous extract of aconite, hyoscyamine from a very old extract of henbane, and atropine from an equally old tincture of belladonna. Thus it is in all confidence that i submit this process to the consideration of chemists who undertake medico-legal researches.—*bulletin de l' académie royale de médecine de belgique*, tom. Vi., no. 2; *and edinburgh monthly journal of medical science.*

VARIA—EDITORIAL.

OINTMENT OF STAVESACRE IN ITCH.

—it has long been known that the itch is caused by the attack of a minute insect, the acarus scabiei, the male of which has only been lately detected, by the microscope. The ordinary sulphur ointment, though successful after repeated applications, in destroying the insect, often causes a good deal of irritation of the skin, and leaves the patient with an eruption as troublesome if not as permanent as the itch itself. M. Bourguignon, a french physician, finds that the infusion of the seeds of the stavesacre, (delphinium staphisagria) or a solution of the extract, not only speedily kills the insects and destroys their eggs, but that it has no irritating influence whatever upon the skin itself. He afterwards adopted an ointment, prepared by digesting over a vapor bath, for twenty-four hours, three parts of stavesacre seeds in five parts of lard, and straining the product while still liquid. He found that friction with this ointment cured the patient in four days, while seven days were required when sulphur ointment was used.

POISONOUS HONEY.

—the family of one of our most respectable wholesale druggists has lately suffered severely from symptoms of poisoning, caused by some honey which they had eaten. The family of one of his neighbors likewise, to whom, induced by its particularly fine appearance, he had sent some of the honey, were affected in a similar manner. The number of those who partook of the suspected article, all of whom were affected, though not to the same degree, renders it certain that the symptoms were not caused by any idiosyncracy, but were produced by some poisonous principle, probably derived from some narcotico-acrid plant on which the bees had fed.

On eating it there was an unpleasant sense of pricking and burning in the throat, nausea, and a burning sensation throughout the whole system, together with an immediate effect upon vision, approaching to blindness. Several of those who ate of the honey vomited violently and were in great distress. One was rendered entirely blind and insensible, and it was feared for some time might not recover. In the other cases the effect passed off in some ten or twelve hours. In one case a single drop of the honey, taken on the end of the finger from the box where it had leaked through a crevice, had such an effect on the sight that the person could not see to read a newspaper, but it passed off within an hour.

"we are not aware," continues our informant, "of any poisonous plants in the vicinity where the honey was made, except what is called kill-calf, (andromeda mariana) which is found in abundance on hempstead plains, at a distance of about a mile."

If, as is supposed, the poison was derived from some plant in which the bees had fed, it must have been elaborated or concentrated in the economy of the insect, or been the product of some reaction of the honey itself upon the poisonous principle, since no poisonous vegetable is known which would produce such effects, in such minute quantity.

NEW REMEDIES.

—dr. J. Y. Simpson, of edinburg, the discoverer of the anaesthetic properties of chloroform, has lately been experimenting on the physiological and therapeutical properties of a varitey of substances which have not previously been used in medicine. He finds that the alkaloid furfurine in poisonous doses, produces upon animals many of the symptoms of poisoning by quinine, and that in smaller doses on the human subject it acts as a tonic, if not an anti-periodic. He has likewise used nickel, generally in the form of sulphate, and finds that it is exceedingly analagous in its therapeutic effects to the salts of iron. In one instance, however, a case of severe periodic headache, it proved completely successful, after iron with quinine, and a great many other remedies had been tried in vain.

THE CONVENTION.

—the *event* for pharmaceutists in the past month, was the meeting of the convention at philadelphia. The number present was smaller than could have been wished, yet great as could reasonably have been anticipated. Eight states were represented, including mr. Bache, of san francisco, california, and there were delegates present from five colleges. We have devoted, perhaps, an undue portion of our space to a partial record of its proceedings. Though on particular points there were differences of opinion, yet on the whole the meetings were characterized by great unanimity of sentiment, as well as cordiality of feeling. Our great hope for the convention is, that it will form a bond of union among the scattered and divided members of the profession in the united states; that it will tend to bring them into one great body, united by common interests and common pursuits, that it will tend to soften commercial jealousies between individuals, as well as between states and cities; that it will enable the profession when united, to exercise its rightful and legitimate influence upon public opinion; that in the profession itself it will promote a more extended course of education, a higher standard of attainment and nobler principles of conduct. These are great aims and worthy of strenuous efforts, and it is to be hoped that no personal or sectional jealousies may be permitted to stand in the way of their attainment. The convention has made a good beginning, "esto perpetua."

COLLEGE OF PHARMACY OF THE CITY OF NEW YORK.

The regular winter course of lectures in this institution, will commence on monday, 1st instant, at 7 o'clock, p. M., and be continued four months, on monday, wednesday and friday evenings of each week, at the college rooms.

On materia medica and pharmacy, from 7 to 8 o'clock, by prof. B.w. mccready, m.d.

On chemistry, from 8 to 9 o'clock, by professor r. O. Doremus, m.d.

On botany, by professor i. F. Holton, of which further notice will be given.

The chemical lectures will comprise instruction in the science as extensively connected with many of the useful and ornamental arts, rendering them of great advantage to the community at large as well as to the apothecary.

In calling public attention to the present course, the trustees would more especially call upon the medical profession and druggists and apothecaries generally, to encourage them in carrying out, in the most effectual manner, the important design of providing, at a nominal expense, for a knowledge of chemistry, pharmacy, and the collateral sciences, to our future apothecaries, and to all others who will avail themselves of the facilities offered.

In urging these, the trustees have no selfish ends to attain beyond the gratification of ministering to the public good in the elevation of their profession; they desire to see their efforts appreciated and sustained by full classes, and would earnestly ask of their brethren to make sufficient sacrifice of time and convenience to enable their assistants and pupils to profit by the opportunity offered for their instruction. The advantages will recur directly to the employer in the improved capacity and usefulness of his assistants.

The trustees solicit the influence of the medical profession to aid them in cultivating a desire to improve this important auxilliary department of the profession, as the successful treatment of disease is greatly dependent on the integrity and intelligence of the apothecary.

Tickets for the course on chemistry, at $7, and on materia medica and pharmacy, at $7, may be procured from

Mr George d. Coggeshall, no. 809 broadway.

Mr. J. S. Aspinwall, no. 86 william street.

Dr. W. J. Olliffe, no. 6 bowery.

And at the college rooms, no. 511 broadway.

October, 1852.

Erratum.

—in the october no. On page 294, twentieth line from the top, for *manifestations*, read *modifications*.

NEW YORK JOURNAL OF PHARMACY. DECEMBER, 1852.

ON THE PRESERVATION OF IODIDE OF IRON.

BY HENRY WURTZ.

There can be no doubt that imperfections exist in many of the methods at present in use for the preservation of various articles of the materia medica. Wherever the fault may be in these cases, the evil is generally shared between the physicians and the patients, much the larger share of course, falling to the latter. The *iodide of iron* is one of these articles, and it will appear probable from the sequel that, in a multitude of cases, this remedy is administered to the patient in quantities which are inconstant and much too small to produce the effect contemplated by the physician in his prescription.

One method, extensively employed, of preserving iodide of iron, for use in medicine, is in the form of an aqueous solution in which a coil of iron wire is kept immersed. This method is given by pereira,27 as proposed by hemingway. Pereira also remarks in another place that "it is important to know, that by keeping a coil of iron wire in a solution of the protiodide, as suggested by mr. Squire, no free iodine or sesquiodide of iron is formed although the liquid may be fully exposed to air and light; sesquioxide of iron is formed, but if the solution be filtered it is found to contain protiodide only."

---

27 materia medica, 3rd am. Ed. 1, 745.

In a paper previously published in this journal, i have remarked with reference to this matter, that i should strongly suspect in this case a formation of a subiodide of iron and consequent abstraction of iodine from the solution.28 since that time i have been enabled to confirm this supposition by experiment. Pieces of iron wire placed in contact with a colorless solution of iodide of iron caused, in the course of a few hours, the deposition of a precipitate, which had a dark orange color quite distinct from the dark brown color of hydrated sesquioxide of iron precipitated from a solution of the protochloride of iron by metallic iron. This precipitate, being washed with distilled water until the washings gave no indication of the presence of *iron*, was still found to contain much iodine. No quantitative analysis of the precipitate, however, was attempted, for it was found that the washings which no longer contained a trace of iron still gave with nitric acid and starch, a strong iodine reaction, thus indicating that the subiodide of iron upon the filter, whatever its composition, was decomposed by the action of water and oxygen as soon as the neutral iodide of iron was washed out. This is probably the reason why previous observers have mistaken this precipitate for pure sesquioxide of iron, having continued washing the precipitate until the washing no longer gave an *iodine* reaction, instead of an *iron* reaction as in the plan adopted by me, and consequently until all the subiodide of iron was decomposed and nothing but sesquioxide of iron was actually left upon the filter.

The washings, however, after the removal of the iodide of iron, gave no iodine reaction with starch until after the addition of nitric acid; iodine, therefore, could only have been present in the form of hydriodic acid and the reaction by which the unknown subiodide of iron was decomposed may be represented as follows:—$2 fe i1X + 1Xh o + (3-1X)o = fe\ ^2o^3 + 1Xhi.$

Since the above experiments were made, i have found that i have, after all, merely been in a measure confirming an observation of the illustrious berzelius. *Gmelin's handbuch* under the head of *einfachiodeisen*, has the following, "nach berzelius ist das braune pulver welches sich beim aussetzen des wässrigen einfachiodeisens an die luft absetzt, nicht reines eisenoxyd, sondern ein basisches salz."[29]

It appears, therefore, that the method of preserving iodide of iron in solution, in contact with metallic iron is perfectly fallacious. This remedy, if preserved in solution at all, should be kept in bottles hermetically closed.

29 according to berzelius, the brown powder, which is deposited upon exposure of aqueous protiodide of iron to the air, is not pure sesquioxide of iron, but a basic salt.

OBSERVATIONS ON THE VOLA-TILITY AND SOLUBILITY OF CAN-THARDIN IN VIEW OF THE MOST ELEGIBLE PHARMACEUTICAL TREATMENT OF SPANISH FLIES.

BY WILLIAM ROCTER, JR.

Cantharides have been used in pharmacy since the days of hippocrates. It was not till 1810, however, that the principle giving them activity was isolated by robiquet (annal. De chimie lxxvi. 302,) and subsequently named *cantharidin* by dr. Thomas thompson. Since then various experimenters have been engaged in the chemical investigation of these flies, and in the more recent treatises they are stated to consist of *cantharidin, yellow fixed oil, green fixed oil, a yellow viscous substance, a black matter, ozmazome, uric acid, acetic acid, phosphoric acid*, and the *phosphate of lime and magnesia*. It is proverbial among apothecaries and physicians, that the pharmaceutical preparations designed to produce vesication, vary very much in their power as prepared by different individuals, and from different samples of cantharides by the same recipes. Is this variableness of power due to the inequality of strength of the commercial drug? Or, are we to attribute it to the treatment employed by the apothecary? The real importance of these queries demands an answer. To proceed properly, the investigator should examine cantharidin in a pure state, ascertain how far the statements of writers are correct, then by a series of analyses, quantitative as regards that principle, determine whether its proportion varies, and to what extent, in different specimens of cantharides of fair quality; and finally to test the preparations derived from the same samples and see how far they correspond with the inferences drawn from the ascertained properties and proportion of the active principle. I have at present undertaken to resolve but a part of these queries—yet by far the most important ones—as will be seen.

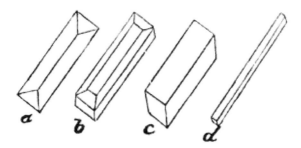

a   b   c   d

Cantharidin is a white, neutral substance, of which the formula according to regnault is $c_{10} h o_4$. Gmelin considers it of the nature of a solid volatile oil. As usually seen it has the form of minute flatted four-sided prisms (*c,*) much broken up, so as to appear like scales. When deposited from an ethereal solution of cantharides by slow evaporation, or from its solution in hot acetic acid by cooling, it assumes the form of flattened oblique four-sided prisms with dihedral summits, derived from the rectangular prism by the bevelment of its edges (see fig. *A* and *b* from *c.*) The crystals by slow sublimation are four-sided rectangular prisms of great brilliance and sometimes iridescent, *c* and *d*.

Solubility.—pure cantharidin is insoluble in water, hot or cold. It is slightly soluble in cold alcohol, readily so when hot. Ether dissolves it to a greater extent, yet much more easily hot than cold. Chloroform is its best solvent, cold or hot, as shown in a former essay (am. Jour. Pharm. Vol. Xxiii. 124,) and will remove it from the aqueous infusion of the flies. Acetic ether dissolves cantharidin, especially when hot, but does not retain much on cooling. When one part of cantharides is mixed with 20 parts of olive oil and heated to 250° fahr. It is completely dissolved. As the solution cools, the cantharidin rapidly separates in shining needles in such quantity as at first to give the oil a pulpy consistence. The clear cold oil retains sufficient to act as an efficient rubefacient but not as an epispastic. One part of cantharidin requires 70 parts of oil of turpentine to dissolve it at the boiling temperature, the greater part separating, as the solution cools, in long asbestos-like needles. A piece of paper saturated with the cold solution and applied to the skin under adhesive plaster did not vesicate. Acetone (from the distillation of acetate of lime) dissolves cantharidin with great readiness and ranks next to chloroform in this regard. The solution deposits the substance in crystals by evaporation. The commercial methylic alcohol or wood naphtha also dissolves cantharidin, but to a much less extent than acetone. When acetic acid SP. GR. 1.41 (U. S. P.,) is added to cantharidin, it but slightly acts on it in the cold; heat much increases its solvent power, which is lost on cooling and the substance deposited by standing, though not immediately. One part of cantharidin was mixed with 40 parts of *crystallizable* acetic acid and agitated together during five hours, but a small percentage was dissolved; but on applying heat the crystals were dissolved quickly. On standing, nearly all of the cantharidin was slowly deposited in regular crystals. To ascertain whether, as has been asserted,30 a combination was effected, and an *acetate* of cantharidin produced, an acetic solution of cantharidin was evaporated to dryness and the crystals mixed with strong sulphuric acid and heated till dissolved, while the nose was held near, without the slightest evidence of acetic odor; one twentieth of a grain of acetate of potassa was then added, which instantly evolved the well marked smell of acetic acid. Formic acid dissolves but a trace of cantharidin, cold or hot; and muriatic acid sp. Gr. 1.18 hardly can be said to act on it in the cold, but when boiling a minute portion is taken up. The same is true of phosphoric acid dissolved in five parts water. Sulphuric acid sp. Gr. 1.840, when heated readily dissolves pure cantharidin without being discolored, and deposits it in crystals unchanged by cooling. Hot nitric acid sp. Gr. 1.38, dissolves cantharidin readily, and deposits the greater part of it on cooling in brilliant crystals, unchanged. A concentrated solution of ammonia slowly dissolves cantharidin to a small extent, and yields it up on evaporation in crystals. Solutions of pottassa and of soda also dissolve this principle.

---

30 new york jour. Pharm. Vol. 1. P. 72.

Its volatility.—about ten grains of pure and perfectly dry cantharidin was spread on the pan of an oertling's balance, (sensitive to 1-150th of a grain,) and the equilibrium carefully adjusted with platina weights. After exposure for a week to the action of the air, a vessel of lime being present to keep the air dry, no change in the adjustment had occurred. To further test the volatility of cantharidin, a portion of it was put at the bottom of a dry test tube, through a paper funnel so as not to soil the sides, which was then fixed so as to dip half an inch in a mercurial bath having a thermometer suspended in it. It lost nothing appreciable after being kept at 212° f. For half an hour, no sublimate being visible with a lens. At 220° f. No visible effect was produced. Kept at 250° f. For twenty minutes, a very slow sublimation commenced. At 300° f. The vaporization was but slightly increased. The heat was then raised to 360° f., when the sublimation became more decided, yet still slow. Between 402° f. And 410° f. It fused, and rapidly sublimed at a few degrees higher. Cantharidin at this temperature volatilizes with great ease and condenses in beautiful well defined crystals like salicylic acid.

The specific gravity of cantharidin is considerable, as it sinks in nitric acid sp. Gr. 1.38; it is exceedingly acrid; its powder applied to the skin with a little oil, produces speedy vesication, and taken internally it is an irritant poison of the most virulent kind.

Such are some of the more prominent characters of this remarkable substance, which exhibits a permanence and want of affinity extraordinary in an animal principle. Let us now see how far experiments with cantharidin as it exists in the flies in substance, correspond with its behaviour in an isolated state.

1st. Is cantharidin, as it exists in spanish flies, volatile at common temperatures, or at the temperature usually employed in making the cerate; and if so to what extent?

A. Six hundred grains of powdered cantharides were put into a quart flask, a pint of water poured on, and macerated two hours. The flask was then adapted to a glass tubulated receiver by means of a long glass tube, the joints made tight, and the tube refrigerated throughout its length by a current of cool water, the receiver itself being surrounded by water. A sand-bath heat was then applied and the materials in the flask kept boiling during several hours, until half a pint liquid had distilled. The product in the receiver was opalescent with white particles floating through it, and had a strong odor of spanish flies. It was decanted into a bottle, and agitated repeatedly with half an ounce of chloroform, which dissolved the particles and removed the opalescence. The chloroform, when separated with a funnel, and evaporated spontaneously, yielded a colorless semi-crystalline residue, having a waxy consistence and a strong odor different from that of the flies. It fused at 120° fahr., was volatile *per se*, but was partially decomposed and condensed in drops which subsequently solidified. This substance is soluble in alcohol, ether and chloroform, is decomposed and dissolved by sulphuric acid, produces *no signs of vesication after forty-eight hours' contact with the skin* under adhesive plaster, and is most probably the same volatile principle that has been noticed by orfila.

The long glass tube was then examined for a sublimate, by rinsing it thoroughly with chloroform, which, on evaporation, afforded more of the same substance obtained from the distilled water, and like it did not produce vesication.

This experiment shows conclusively that cantharidin *does not volatilize to an appreciable extent with water evaporating from cantharides.*

B. More water was added to the residue in the flask, again boiled for fifteen minutes and thrown on a displacing filter, and water added to the solid residue, after the decoction had ceased to pass, until the absorbed liquid was displaced. The decoction was much less odorous than the distilled water, and had a deep reddish-brown color. Half of this was agitated repeatedly with chloroform. The latter decanted and evaporated yielded a crop of crystals intermixed with some coloring matter. A part of these heated in a tube over a lamp, gave immediately the brilliant crystaline sublimate of cantharidin well marked; another portion applied to the skin produced vesication in a few hours.

The other half of the decoction was evaporated to a soft extract by direct heat. This produced speedy and deep vesication, more effectual than that of pure cantharidin, as in the extract that principle was in a soluble state by virtue of the yellow matter of the flies.

C. The residual flies were then dried carefully and exhausted with ether, which assumed a deep green color. A green semi-fluid fatty oil was obtained by evaporation, from which a fluid yellow oil separated by standing, which produced a tardy vesication, not comparable with the aqueous extract.

D. One hundred grains of flies in powder were introduced into a test tube so as not to soil the sides. This was then kept at the temperature of 212° f. During six hours, by causing it to dip into a vessel of boiling water through a tin plate. The hygrometric water was removed as it condensed above. At the end of the experiment a minute deposit of microscopic crystals less than one thirtieth of a grain, was observed above the flies on the side of the tube.

E. Two hundred grains of flies were introduced into a two ounce retort, which they half filled, adapted to a two ounce receiver, and this again connected with a third vessel. The retort heated by a mercurial bath, was kept at 225° f., for two hours, without any product except a little odorous hygrometric water. The heat was then raised to 412° f., when a colorless oily matter flowed slowly into the receiver, mixed with water, whilst a crystalline matter mixed with oil collected in the neck. This crystalline matter mixed with the oil produced vesication when applied to the skin. The heat was now rapidly increased so as to produce brown vapors, from which was condensed a dark colored empyreumatic oil, abundant crystals of an ammonical salt collected in the tubes and on the sides of the receiver, whilst the aqueous liquor in the receiver was strongly ammonical. Neither the dark oil nor the crystals produced vesication, the high temperature having probably decomposed the cantharidin.

From these experiments it must be admitted that cantharidin is less volatile than has been asserted. The effect produced on the eye of the pupil of robiquet who was watching the crystallization of cantharidin during the evaporation of an ethereal solution, may be accounted for by the mechanical action of the dense ethereal vapor escaping near his eye, as he watched the process with a lens, carrying off some particles of cantharidin; and the readiness with which this principle may be brought mechanically in contact with the skin of the face, during a series of experiments, by want of care, will easily account for the occasional testimony of writers in favor of its volatility at low temperatures based on that kind of evidence. During the whole of the experiments detailed in this paper, the author has not experienced any inconvenience to his eyes or face except in two instances, once when decomposing cantharides by destructive distillation, during which some of the vapors escaped near his person, and again where a small capsule containing aqueous extract of cantharides was accidentally exposed to high temperature over a lamp so as to partially decompose it; he suffered slight pain for a few hours in the conjunctiva of both eyes.

It must also be admitted that the heat ordinarily employed in making the blistering cerate of the united states pharmacopœia, does not injure the preparation by volatilizing the cantharidin, and that the recommendation to digest the flies in the melted vehicle on a water bath is not only not injurious, but decidedly advantageous, as it increases, many fold, the solvent power of the fatty matter.

2d. Having ascertained the solvent powers of olive oil, oil of turpentine and acetic acid, on pure cantharidin, the following experiments were made with those menstrua, and with water, on the flies in substance:

A. One hundred grains of powdered cantharides were mixed with two hundred grains of olive oil in a large test tube, which was corked, and the mixture heated in a boiling water bath during four hours, with occasional agitation. The contents of the tube were then poured into a small glass displacement apparatus, surrounded with water kept hot by a lamp, and the saturated oil gradually displaced, without cooling, by the addition of fresh portions of oil. The oily liquid thus obtained had a deep green color, smelled strongly of the flies, and when applied to the skin produced full vesication in about twelve hours contact. After standing twenty-four hours shining needles of cantharidin gradually separated, but not in quantity.

B. One hundred grains of powdered flies were mixed with two hundred grains of pure oil of turpentine in a closed tube, heated in a boiling water bath four hours, and displaced while hot as in the preceding experiment. The terebinthinate solution had a dull yellow color, and was perfectly transparent as it passed, but in a short time numerous minute stellated crystals commenced forming, which increased in quantity by standing. The saturated cold solution, separated from the crystals after standing twenty-four hours, did not blister when applied to the skin.

C. One hundred grains of powdered flies were digested in a close vessel, at the temperature of boiling water, in three hundred grains of acetic acid sp. Gr. 1.041, for six hours, and then subjected to displacement in the hot filter above noticed. A dark reddish-brown transparent liquid passed, which had very little odor of flies, even when a portion was exposed until the acetic acid had nearly all evaporated. A portion of this liquid applied to the skin produced complete vesication in about ten hours. After standing a few hours, numerous minute granular crystals were deposited, which gradually increased in amount and size.

These three experiments prove that hot fatty matter is a good solvent for cantharidin as it exists in the flies, and that it retains more on cooling than either turpentine or acetic acid. That hot oil of turpentine is a good solvent for extracting cantharidin, although it does not retain much on cooling, and that officinal acetic acid at the temperature of 212° f. Will remove cantharidin readily from spanish flies, but retains but a part on cooling.

D. Five hundred grains of recently powdered flies, contained in a flask, were boiled in a pint of water, for an hour, and the clear decoction decanted, the residue again treated with half a pint of water, so as to remove all matter soluble in that liquid. The decoctions were mixed, filtered, and evaporated carefully to dryness. The extract was exhausted by repeated treatment with boiling alcohol, which left a dark colored pulpy matter, very soluble in water, from which it is precipitated by subacetate of lead. The alcoholic solution was now evaporated to a syrup, and on cooling yielded a yellow extract like mass, interspersed with numerous minute four-sided prisms. By washing a portion with water, the yellow matter was removed, leaving the crystals white and pure. The aqueous washings yielded by evaporation a residue of crystals, and does not vesicate. When the alcoholic extract was treated with chloroform the crystals were dissolved, and the yellow matter left. On evaporating the chloroform solution the crystals were re-obtained with all the characters of cantharidin. The matter left by chloroform was now treated with water, in which it dissolved, except a trace of dark substance, and was again evaporated carefully. It afforded a yellow honey-like residue, thickly interspersed with crystals and strongly acid to litmus, without vesicating power.

A portion of the yellow matter separated from the alcoholic extract by water was boiled with some cantharidin, filtered and evaporated. The residue treated with chloroform afforded no cantharidin; hence it would appear that although the yellow matter enables the cantharidin to dissolve in water and cold alcohol, when once separated its solvent power ceases.

Having now studied the effects of the ordinary solvents on cantharidin in a free state, and in the condition in which it exists in the insect, we are prepared to consider with some clearness, the pharmaceutical preparations of the spanish fly, and their action as vesicants.

A. If 1-30th of a grain of pure cantharidin, in fine powder, be placed on the skin of the arm and covered with a piece of warmed adhesive plaster, active vesication occurs in eight hours, with pain. If the same quantity of cantharidin be put on the other arm, a small piece of paper be laid over it, and then a piece of adhesive plaster with a circular hole in it be applied, so as to hold on the paper, no vesication occurs in sixteen hours, the powder remaining dry. If then a large piece of plaster be put over the whole, at the end of eight hours more no blistering action will have taken place. If now a trace of olive oil be applied to the back of the paper covering the cantharidin, and the plaster replaced, speedy vesication will occur. These experiments prove that cantharidin must be in solution to have its vesicating action, and that oily matter is a proper medium.

B. When powdered flies are stirred into the ordinary vehicle of resin, wax, and lard, so as to chill it almost immediately as was formerly directed, but little of the cantharidin is dissolved by the fatty matter, and when applied to the skin the process of vesication is retarded. If, however, the cerate be kept fluid for a length of time, say for half an hour, by a water-bath or other regular heat, no loss of cantharidin occurs by the heat, the active principle is in a great measure dissolved by the fat, and every part is impregnated and active. In the foregoing experiments it has been shown that twenty parts of olive oil will dissolve one of cantharidin when hot. If we admit with thierry that cantharides contain but four thousandths of their weight of cantharidin, the quantity contained in a pound of cerate is about *eight* grains, whilst the lard in the same weight of cerate is 1600 grains, or two hundred times the weight of that principle, not to speak of the influence of the wax and resin, which, in union, with the melted lard, act as solvents. Hence the whole of the cantharidin may be dissolved by the vehicle. Another advantage of employing a continued heat in digestion is the removal of the hygrometric water from the flies, which is the source of the mouldiness to which the cerate is prone in certain conditions.

In a former essay (amer. Journ. Pharm., vol. Xiii, p. 302,) i have advocated digestion in making this cerate, (a recommendation also made by mr. Donovan, of dublin, about the same time,) and also the use of a portion of the oil of turpentine to facilitate the solution of the cantharidin, but the foregoing experiments prove that fatty matter is quite as good, if not a better solvent alone than with turpentine.

C. It has been asserted long ago by beaupoil, robiquet and others, that water will perfectly extract the active matter from spanish flies, which these experiments corroborate. Hence it is easy to understand how the condensed perspiration may facilitate the action of a blister, especially when, as was formerly much the case, its surface is coated with the dust of the flies, and the skin moistened.

It is also clear why the unguentum cantharidis of the united states pharmacopœia is active although made with a decoction of flies, yet, in this preparation, care should be observed not to evaporate all the water, as on the existence of the aqueous extract in a soft state depends much of the efficiency of the preparation as an irritant dressing.

D. In the linimentum cantharidis, united states pharm., in which an ounce of flies is digested in eight fluid ounces of oil of turpentine, the cantharidin is to be the menstruum as 1 to 1500, a proportion probably quite sufficient to retain it in solution. The importance of the officinal direction to digest is evident. It is quite doubtful whether this liniment, as made by the process of dr. Joseph hartshorne, one part of flies to three parts of oil, will retain all the cantharidin after standing awhile.

E. The acetum cantharidis, (lond. Ph.) Made by macerating an ounce of flies in ten fluid ounces of acetic acid, 1.48, has been criticised by mr. Redwood, (pharm. Journal, oct. 1841,) who arrived at the conclusion that it owed its vesicating power almost solely to the acid, he not being able to discover cantharidin in it. The inefficiency of *cold* acetic acid as a solvent for *pure* cantharidin has been proven by the above experiments, and its efficiency when hot equally shown. There can be little doubt that the london preparation would be much improved by *digesting* the flies in the acid for an hour in a close glass vessel at the temperature of boiling water.

F. The *cantharidal collodion* of m. Ilisch has been considerably used as a vesicant in this country. Ether being a good solvent for cantharidin readily keeps that principle in solution. When applied to the skin, the escape of the ether leaves a coating of ethereal extract of cantharides, admixed with collodion. This preparation sometimes fails from a deficiency of cantharidin, at other times from want of a sufficient body in the collodion excipient, and it has been found more advantageous to treat the cantharides with ether till exhausted, distill off the ether, and add the oily residue to collodion of the proper consistence. The addition of a little olive oil, and of venice turpentine, as recommended by mr. Rand, will give more activity to the preparation, especially if a piece of oiled silk or adhesive plaster be applied over the part.

G. Besides these, many other epispastic preparations are made in france and other countries. The acetic alcoholic extract of cantharides of ferrari is made by digesting four parts of cantharides in sixteen parts of alcohol 36° b. Mixed with one part of acetic acid 10° b. In the opinion of the author, the acetic acid tends to prevent the crystallization of the cantharidin, a statement rendered doubtful by the above experiments, as that principle separates in crystals from an acetic solution of cantharides. The alcohol dissolves the green oil which gives to the extract a butyraceous consistence. This is undoubtedly an efficient preparation, and is used by spreading it on paper with a brush, and applying to the skin. Nearly all the french preparations direct digestion of from 2 to 6 hours, showing evidently that the experience of pharmaceutists is opposed to the opinion that cantharides is "a very volatile substance, even at common temperatures."

The vesicating tafeta of the codex, is that proposed by messrs. Henry & guibourt, and is made by fusing together one part of the ethereal extract of cantharides and two of wax, and spreading it on waxed paper or linen in the manner of adhesive plaster. This preparation is said to lose its efficiency by exposure to the air. How can this occur in view of the results which have been detailed above? Admitting the fact, it is not probable that the change lies in the strong tendency of the cantharidin to separate in crystals? A change easily observable in the ethereal extract. This is the chief objection to some otherwise excellent preparations of cantharides for vesication, and it is far more probably the true explanation, than, that volatility should be the cause.

The recently prepared and soft aqueous extract of cantharides has been shown to be a powerful epispastic. Will this extract of the consistence of honey, associated with sufficient acetic acid, alcohol, or acetone, to preserve it, keep without the gradual separation of the cantharidin? If so, it will undoubtedly prove one of the very best blistering agents, as by simply applying a covering of it over the surface of waxed paper, or adhesive plaster, with a camel's-hair brush, a perfect blistering plaster can be made quickly and neatly, and all tendency to change of aggregation by the action of the air on the menstruum avoided. This is a question now under trial, and should it result favorably, a formula will be published. The extraordinary tendency of cantharidin to crystallize, even under the most adverse circumstances, taken in connection with its insolubility, *per se*, has hardly received sufficient attention from pharmaceutists as a cause of the deterioration of cantharidal preparations, and the discovery of a menstruum, that will retain that principle in solution for an indefinite period, is a problem yet to be solved, and worthy the attention of pharmaceutical investigators.

Philadelphia, september, 1852.

ON GELSEMINUM SEMPERVIRENS OR YELLOW JASSAMIN.

BY WILLIAM PROCTER, JR.

Considerable attention has recently been turned to the yellow jassamin of our southern states, from the accidental discovery of certain remarkable effects produced by it when taken internally. A planter of mississippi having suffered much from a tedious attack of bilious fever, which resisted the usual medicines employed in such cases, requested one of his servants to obtain from the garden a certain root, from which he intended to prepare an infusion for drinking. By mistake, the person sent collected a different root, and administered the tea to his master, who, soon after taking it, was seized with a complete loss of muscular power, being, in fact, so completely prostrated as to be unable to move a limb or to raise the eyelids, yet he could hear, and could appreciate what was occurring around him. After some hours, during which his friends were watching him with much anxiety and little hope, he gradually recovered his muscular control, and was astonished to find that the fever had left him. Having ascertained from his servant what plant he had collected, he subsequently employed it successfully on his own plantation as well as among his neighbors. The history becoming known to a quackish physician, he prepared from it a nostrum called the "electrical febrifuge," in which, it was disguised by oil of winter-green, (*eclectic* dispensatory, page 186.)

The gelseminum is not noticed by dr. Griffith in his medical botany, nor in the recent edition of the united states dispensatory, and so far appears to have been used chiefly by the "eclectic" practitioners of cincinnati and other parts of the western states. The accompanying description of the plant is taken partly from a specimen sent from memphis, tennessee, where, in common with other parts of the south-western states, it is cultivated as an ornamental garden plant.

The gelseminum belongs to the natural order apocyneæ, so remarkable for the great activity of many of its genera, and the name of the genus, given by jussieu, is one of the ancient names of the jessamine, and that of the species arises from its evergreen foliage.

Gelseminum belongs to pentandria digynia of linnæus, and to the natural order apocyneæ of jussieu.

Generic characters.—regular, calyx five parted, (the sepals of this species being furnished with bract-like appendages) carolla funnel-form, border spreading, five lobed, nearly equal, capsule compressed, flat, two partible, two-celled, seeds flat and attached to the margins of the valves, (eaton.)

Specific characters.—the g. Sempervirens is known at the south under the names yellow jasmine, wild jasmine, and woodbine. In florida it flowers in march, and in mississippi and tennessee in may and june. Its stem is twining, smooth and glabrous; its leaves are opposite, perennial, lanceolate, entire, dark green above, paler beneath; with short petioles. The flowers, which are esteemed poisonous, are yellow, about an inch long and half an inch wide at the top, of a fine yellow color, and have an agreeable odor, which perfumes the air when they bloom. It grows luxuriantly, climbing from tree to tree, forming a delightful shade. According to eaton, from whose botany we glean part of the above botanical notice, there is a variety called inodorum which has scentless flowers.

The gelseminum is indigenous to the southern states, and its beauty has caused its introduction into the gardens.

Medical properties and uses.—the root is the part used, and the tincture is the preparation most usually employed, and, as made, must be a saturated tincture. The roots, in a green state, well bruised, are introduced into a suitable vessel, and covered with whiskey, or diluted alcohol. After standing two weeks, the tincture is separated by expression and filtered. It has a dark red color, and a pleasant bitter taste. The dose is from ten to fifty drops, The following account of its medical properties and effects is taken from a paper in the "eclectic medical journal," august, 1852, page 353, by f. D. Hill of cincinnati:

"gelseminum is stimulant, tonic, and anti-spasmodic. By its relaxing effect it produces gentle diaphoresis, and is said to be *narcotic*. Its effect in large doses, or doses too frequently repeated, is extreme relaxation, and general prostration of the whole muscular and nervous system. It will suspend and hold in check muscular irritability and nervous excitement with more force and power than any known remedy. It is of a pleasant bitter taste, and performs its wonder-working cures, in all febrile diseases, without exciting either nausea, vomiting, or purging. When enough has been given to produce its specific effect, the eye is dimmed, the vision clouded and double, the head light and dizzy. When these effects follow the administration of this remedy, no more should be given until the patient has entirely recovered from its influence. 'it maybe used in all species of fevers, nervous and bilious headache, colds, pneumonia, hemorrhages, leucorrhea, chorea, ague-cake, asthma, and many other diseases: but its efficacy has been most admired in all forms and grades of fevers.' it should always be used with great care and caution. The root is said to possess a resinous principle, which, when extracted by pure alcohol, will produce death in very small doses. But no such effect need be expected from the proper dose of the common tincture. There is danger of carrying it to such an extent as to suspend involuntary muscular action, and when this is the case, death must ensue. 'it is incompatible with no known substance, and may follow any *preceeding treatment with perfect safety.*' the dose is forty drops for an adult, and children in proportion to age and temperament. It is given either with or without quinine. It has been used alone for *chronic rheumatism*, in doses of forty drops, three times a day, with marked effects. Three or four doses, with a mild cathartic, will remove the redness and swelling attending inflamed sore eyes. Special attention should be directed to the general health and constitution of the patient before giving gelseminum. If the bowels be constipated they should be moved by a gentle aperient, and kept in a relaxed condition. It requires double the quantity to produce the effect on some that it does on others; and should the practitioner ever produce too great a degree of relaxation, he should lose no time in stimulating and toning up his patient."

The alleged effects of this plant on the human system, taken in connection with its medico-botanical relations, mark it out as being probably one of the most valuable of our indigenous remedial agents, and render it well worthy of the investigation of regular physicians.

ON THE MANUFACTURE OF WRITING INKS.
(*CONCLUDED FROM PAGE 316.*)

Prussian blue, that has not undergone digestion in acid in the way above pointed out, will require a much larger proportion of oxalic acid, from twice to three times its weight; and even then it will be greatly liable to precipitation after standing; but when treated in the way described, it is not liable to precipitate, but remains a permanent solution.

Stephens' red ink.—stephens' red ink is prepared as follows:—take a quantity of common soda, potash or carbonate of ammonia, to which is to be added, at intervals, twice its weight of crude argol in powder.

When the effervescence, arising from this combination, has ceased, pour off the solution, or filter it from the insoluble matter; to this, add by measure half the quantity of oxalate of alumina, or oxalo-phosphate of alumina, prepared by adding to precipitated alumina or phosphate of alumina, in a damp state, as much oxalic acid as will dissolve. Into this mixture, put, when cold, as much cochineal, first bruised or powdered, as will give it a fine red color, varying the quantity according to the shade of color required; and after letting it stand for the space of forty eight hours, strain it off for use.

Professor runge's writing fluid.—one of the least expensive formulas for the manufacture of a writing ink, is that given by professor runge, who says: "i have for some time endeavored to find a black fluid possessing the properties of forming no deposit, of adhering strongly to the paper, of being unaffected by acids, and lastly, what is of great importance, not acted upon by steel pens.

"after many experiments, i have succeeded in obtaining a composition of the kind required, very simple in its preparation, containing nothing but logwood, chromate of potash, and water, and free from vinegar, gum, copperas, blue vitriol, and even nutgalls. The low price of this writing fluid is also in its favor. It is prepared by simply adding one part of chromate of potash to 1000 parts of decoction of logwood, made by boiling twenty-two pounds of logwood in a sufficient quantity of water to give fourteen gallons of decoction; to this decoction, when cold, the chromic salt is gradually added, and the mixture well stirred. The addition of gum is injurious. In the preparation of this ink, it must be remembered that the yellow chromate and not the bi-carbonate of potash is employed, and great care is required to ensure due adjustment of the relative proportions of the ingredients used. The best way is to make a decoction of logwood, and *gradually* add to it, well stirring the mixture, as much solution of chromate as will give the shade required.

"it appears astonishing what a small quantity of the chrome salt is required to convert a large quantity of decoction of logwood into a black writing fluid; the fact is however certain, and care must be taken not to allow the proportion of chrome salt to exceed half a part for each 500 parts of decoction of logwood, as a larger quantity exercises a prejudicial effect in destroying the coloring matter of the liquid, whilst in the proportion above mentioned, a deep blue black writing ink is formed, which, unlike the ink made with tannogallate of iron, is perfectly fluid, forming no deposit. This writing fluid possesses another advantage; the paper which has been written upon with it may be washed with a sponge, or be left twenty-four hours under water, without the writing being effaced. Weak acids do not destroy the writing, nor do they even change the   shade, whilst that made with gallnuts is effaced, and the ink prepared with logwood and copperas is turned red.

"new steel pens are coated with a greasy substance, which prevents the ready flow of the ink; this should, therefore, be removed previous to use by moistening the pens with saliva, and then washing them in water. The application of an alkaline solution is still preferable to remove this greasy matter. The cleansing of the steel pens is absolutely essential in the case of using the ink above mentioned. I have used this ink upwards of two years, and my steel pens are not in the least degree affected. No rust is formed on the pens, so that after years of service the only wear experienced is that from constant use on the paper, thus rendering unnecessary the use of pens tipped with iridium and other hard substances."

ON THE GROWTH OF VARIOUS KINDS OF MOULD IN SYRUP.

Professor balfour, the professor of botany in the university of edinburgh, has read a valuable paper on this subject, at the botanical society in that city, in which he states that mould of various kinds, when placed in syrup, has a tendency to spread out and form a flat, gelatinous, and leathery expansion. This he shows by experiments, as follows:—mould that had grown upon an apple was put into syrup; and in the course of two months there was formed upon the syrup a cellular, flat, expanded mass, while the syrup was converted into vinegar.

Mould that had grown upon a pear was also put into syrup, and the same result was produced. He also experimented in the same manner with various moulds that were growing upon bread, tea, and some other vegetable substances; the effect produced, in most cases, was to cause a fermentation, resulting in the production of vinegar. In another experiment, a quantity of raw sugar, treacle, and water, were put into a jar, without any mould being introduced. When examined, after a lapse of four or five months, a growth like that of the vinegar plant was visible, and vinegar was formed. This plant was removed, and put into fresh syrup, which was followed again by the production of vinegar. It appears that, when purified white sugar only is used to make syrup, the plant, when placed in it, does not produce vinegar so speedily; the length of time required for the changes varying from four to six months. Dr. Balfour thinks this may possibly be owing, to the presence of some ingredient in the raw sugar and treacle, which may tend to promote the production of vinegar.

In connection with this subject, i may refer to the *vinegar plant*, which is considered by some eminent botanists to be an unnatural and peculiar form of some fungus. This plant, which has a tough gelatinous consistence, when put into a mixture of treacle, sugar and water, gives rise to an acetous fermentation. The vinegar, which is the result of this acetous fermentation, is of a syrupy nature; and when evaporated to dryness, a large quantity of saccharine matter is left. Various conjectures have been hazarded as to the origin of this vinegar plant; some stating that it came from south america, or other distant regions; and others that it is a spontaneous production. Dr. Lindley is of opinion that it is a peculiar form of *penicillum glaucum*, or common blue-mould. The general opinion appears to be, that it is in an anomalous state of mould, or of some fungus: and the peculiar form and consistence it assumes on different occasions, seems to depend upon the nature of the material in, or upon which, it makes its appearance.

CONSTITUTION OF THE AMERICAN PHARMACEUTICAL ASSOCIATION.

Whereas, the advancement of pharmaceutical knowledge and the elevation of the professional character of apothecaries and druggists throughout the united states are objects that are dear to us in common with all well disposed pharmaceutists; and, *whereas*, a large portion of those in whose hands the practice of pharmacy now exists, are not properly qualified for the responsible offices it involves, chiefly by reason of the many difficulties that impede the acquirement of a correct knowledge of their business;—

Therefore, we, the members of a convention now met at philadelphia, composed of apothecaries and druggists from different sections of the union, and from all the colleges and societies therein existing, with the object of deliberating on the condition of our profession, *do* hereby resolve and constitute ourselves into a permanent asociation, to meet annually at such times and places as may hereafter be determined, for more effectually accomplishing the objects for which we are now assembled; and do now adopt the following constitution:

SECTION 1.

This association shall be called "*the american pharmaceutical association.*"

SECTION 2.

Of the members.

Article i. All pharmaceutists and druggists who shall have attained the age of twenty-one years, whose character, morally and professionally, is fair, and who, after duly considering the obligations of the constitution and code of ethics of this association are willing to subscribe to them, shall be eligible for membership.

Article ii. The members shall consist of delegates from regularly constituted colleges of pharmacy, and pharmaceutical societies, who shall present properly authorized credentials, and of other reputable pharmaceutists feeling an interest in the objects of the association, who may not be so delegated, the latter being required to present a certificate signed by a majority of the delegates from the places whence they come. If no such delegates are present at the association, they may, on obtaining the certificates of any three members of the association, be admitted, provided they be introduced by the committee on credentials.

Article iii. All persons who become members of this association shall be considered as permanent members, but may be expelled for improper conduct by a vote of two thirds of the members present at any annual meeting.

Article iv. Every member in attendance at the annual meetings shall pay into the hands of the treasurer the sum of two dollars as his yearly contribution.

Article v. Every local pharmaceutical association shall be entitled to five delegates.

SECTION III.

of the officers.

The officers of this association shall be a president, three vice presidents, a recording secretary, a corresponding secretary, a treasurer, and an executive committee of three, which may include any of the members except the president, all of whom shall be elected annually.

Article i. The president shall preside at the meetings and preserve order. He shall nominate all committees, except a majority of the members present direct a resort to balloting or other means. He shall sign all certificates of membership, approve of all foreign correspondence, and countersign all orders on the treasurer drawn by the executive committee. And he shall, at least three months previously to the annual meeting publish a call in all the pharmaceutical and in such medical and other journals as he may select, stating therein the objects of the association, and the conditions of membership.

Article ii. In case of the temporary absence, or inability of the president, his duties shall devolve on one of the vice presidents.

Article iii. The recording secretary shall keep fair and correct minutes of the proceedings of the association. He shall keep a roll book of the members, and see that it is corrected annually, and he shall furnish to the executive committee a correct transcript of the minutes of the meeting for publication in the transactions of the association.

Article iv. The corresponding secretary shall attend to the official correspondence directed by the association with other bodies, or with its members, all of which correspondence shall be approved by the president.

Article v. The treasurer shall receive and take care of the funds of the association; shall pay its money only on the order of the executive committee, countersigned by the president; and shall present a statement of his accounts annually that they may be audited.

Article vi. The executive committee shall take charge of the publication of the proceedings of the association, including such papers on scientific subjects as it may direct to be published; attend to their distribution; pay the expenses incurred on behalf of the association at its meetings or in the interim, and report a statement of their transactions to the next meeting.

SECTION IV.

Of the meetings.

Article i. The meetings shall be held annually, at such time and place as shall be determined at the adjournment of the previous meeting, observing that no two meetings shall be held consecutively at the same place.

Article ii. The meetings shall be organized by the president of the previous year, or, in his absence, by either of the vice presidents in the order of their election, or, in their absence, by the recording secretary, who shall act *pro tempore* until the nomination and election of officers for the session.

Article iii. Immediately after the temporary organization of the association the roll shall be called, when a committee on credentials shall be appointed from the *members* present, to whom the certificates of delegates shall be submitted, and who shall examine the claims of all other applicants for membership before they are submitted to the association.

SECTION V.

This constitution may be altered or amended by a vote of three-fourths of the members present at any regular meeting, and notice to alter or amend the same shall be given at least one sitting before a vote thereupon.

CODE OF ETHICS OF THE AMERICAN PHARMACEUTICAL ASSOCIATION.

The american pharmaceutical association, composed of pharmaceutists and druggists throughout the united states, feeling a strong interest in the success and advancement of their profession in its practical and scientific relations, and also impressed with the belief that no amount of knowledge and skill will protect themselves and the public from the ill effects of an undue competition, and the temptations to gain at the expense of quality, unless they are upheld by high moral obligations in the path of duty, have subscribed to the following *code of ethics* for the government of their professional conduct.

Art. I. As the practice of pharmacy can only become uniform by an open and candid intercourse being kept up between apothecaries and druggists among themselves and each other, by the adoption of the national pharmacopœia as a guide in the preparation of officinal medicines, by the discontinuance of secret formulæ and the practices arising from a quackish spirit, and by an encouragement of that *esprit du corps* which will prevent a resort to those disreputable practices arising out of an injurious and wicked competition;—*therefore*, the members of this association agree to uphold the use of the pharmacopœia in their practice; to cultivate brotherly feeling among the members, and to discountenance quackery and dishonorable competition in their business.

Art. Ii. As labor should have its just reward, and as the skill, knowledge and responsibility required in the practice of pharmacy are great, the remuneration of the pharmaceutist's services should be proportioned to these, rather than to the market value of preparations vended. The rate of charges will necessarily vary with geographical position, municipal location, and other circumstances of a permanent character, but a resort to intentional and unnecessary reduction in the rate of charges among apothecaries, with a view to gaining at the expense of their brethren, is strongly discountenanced by this association as productive of evil results.

Art. Iii. The first duty of the apothecary, after duly preparing himself for his profession, being to procure good drugs and prepartions, (for without these his skill and knowledge are of small avail,) he frequently has to rely on the good faith of the druggists for their selection. Those druggists whose knowledge, skill and integrity enable them to conduct their business faithfully, should be encouraged, rather than those who base their claims to patronage on the cheapness of their articles solely. When accidentally or otherwise, a deteriorated, or adulterated drug or medicine is sent to the apothecary, he should invariably return it to the druggist, with a statement of its defects. What is too frequently considered as a mere error of trade on the part of the druggist becomes a *highly culpable* act when countenanced by the apothecary; hence, when repetitions of such frauds occur, they should be exposed for the benefit of the profession. A careful but firm pursuit of this course would render well-disposed druggists more careful, and deter the fraudulently inclined from a resort to their disreputable practices.

Art. Iv. As the practice of pharmacy is quite distinct from the practice of medicine, and has been found to flourish in proportion as its practitioners have confined their attention to its requirements; and as the conducting of the business of both professions by the same individual involves pecuniary temptations which are often not compatible with a conscientious discharge of duty; we consider that the members of this association should discountenance all such professional amalgamation; and in conducting business at the counter, should avoid prescribing for diseases when practicable, referring applicants for medical advice to the physician. We hold it as unprofessional and highly reprehensible for apothecaries to allow any per centage or commission to physicians on their prescriptions, as unjust to the public, and hurtful to the independence and self-respect of both parties concerned. We also consider that the practice of some physicians, (in places where good apothecaries are numerous) of obtaining medicines at low prices from the latter, and selling them to their patients, is not only unjust and unprofessional, but deserving the censure of all high-minded medical men.

Art. V. The important influence exerted on the practice of pharmacy by the large proportion of physicians who have resigned its duties and emoluments to the apothecary, are reasons why he should seek their favorable opinion and cultivate their friendship, by earnest endeavors to furnish their patients with pure and well-prepared medicines. As physicians are liable to commit errors in writing their prescriptions, involving serious consequences to health and reputation if permitted to leave the shop, the apothecary should always, when he deems an error has been made, consult the physician before proceeding; yet in the delay which must necessarily occur, it is his duty, when possible, to accomplish the interview without compromising the reputation of the physician. On the other hand, when apothecaries commit errors involving ill consequences, the physician, knowing the constant liability to error, should feel bound to screen them from undue censure, unless the result of a culpable negligence.

Art. Vi. As we owe a debt of gratitude to our predecessors for the researches and observations which have so far advanced our scientific art, we hold that every apothecary and druggist is bound to contribute his mite towards the same fund, by noting the new ideas and phenomena which may occur in the course of his business, and publishing them, when of sufficient consequence, for the benefit of the profession.

VARIA—EDITORIAL.

THE JOURNAL.

—with the present number, the first volume of the journal is completed. In a pecuniary point of view its success has fully equalled the expectations of its originators; it is no longer an experiment, but is established on a firm basis, and will be continued with increased energy and a larger experience in the art of journalism. We have tried to keep faithfully in view the objects with which the journal was commenced; while we have endeavored to present to our readers whatever of general interest or importance has been published abroad, we have the gratification to believe that some contributions to the general stock have first appeared in our pages which would otherwise never have seen the light. But those who confine the benefit of a journal solely to the information it imparts have but a limited view of its usefulness; an account of what is done abroad excites but little emulation compared with far humbler efforts made by our own friends, and in our own neighborhood, and the encouragement and promotion of such efforts is a large good, quite independent of the results that may be attained. The mere attempt to write on a subject like scientific pharmacy leads to a close scanning of the foundation of our opinions, to renewed experiments to ascertain their justness, to more enlightened views of the connection and bearing of our science. In this way we hope to see the good done by the journal greatly increased. The contributors to its pages have hitherto been but few in number, but its columns are open to all. They are controlled by no clique, are subservient to no views of merely personal advancement, and we will gladly, welcome communications from all quarters, judging of them only by their merit and usefulness.

THE DRUG INSPECTION LAW.

We had intended to have made some remarks on the debate which took place in the convention regarding the admission of certain articles, under the law for the inspection of imported drugs, which, though possessing medicinal properties are, we believe, merely used for the purpose of adulterating other and better articles, but willingly give place to the subjoined communication from dr. Guthrie, which, on the whole, advocates views similar to our own. With regard to the carthagena barks, as they are termed, we confess to a desire for further information. Those barks vary very much from each other. Though not rich in quinia, some of them contain a large per centage of alkaloids, which are closely allied to it. We hope that the committee to whom the subject was referred by the convention will not only cause proper analyses to be made of the commercial varieties of these barks, but will have experiments instituted regarding their comparative therapeutic value. The hospitals of our country afford abundant cases of malarious disease, and, we have no doubt, the physicians attached to them would be ready to institute trials which would afford a satisfactory solution to this important question.

Geo. D. Goggeshall,

My dear sir,—the proceedings of the national pharmaceutical convention have just come to hand, and been perused by me, with no ordinary degree of interest.

You have known somewhat of my anxiety concerning these preliminary and forming stages of an association of this character, and will readily believe that i have awaited the results of the late convention, from which, most unfortunately for myself, i was compelled to be absent, with great solicitude. That solicitude has been relieved, and in its stead i have the assurance that a good foundation to a national structure has been laid, towards which hope points and expectation looks with joyous anticipations of future good.

I may be permitted to congratulate you upon the successful labors of the convention, and more especially upon the fact that you have avoided any untenable false ground both in the convention and organization of the association.

That old stumbling block of "all drugs good of their kind," in reference to our drug law, i see made its appearance again, but this time from a quarter i little expected. But it had, notwithstanding its new paternity and eminent godfathership, only, so far as i can see, the same lame, diffuse and weak conclusions to back it.

I was the more surprised at seeing the resolution in the form offered as coming from my friend dr. Stewart, of baltimore, because i had considered him as one who held entirely opposite opinions, and from this fact, that in a communication made to me in january last, as special agent of the treasury department, charged with the examination of the practical workings of the drug law, he says, "i have inspected several hundred thousand dollars worth of one drug which requires some particular notice, as i understand your views and mine correspond with regard to it, and you have succeeded in arranging a uniform system of examination at the different ports.

The prominent principles upon which its value is based vary from about one to four per cent. The commercial article of the best varieties is graduated by the quantity of valuable element above referred to, but with regard to the inferior kinds this is not the case, as i have found upon repeated analyses that what are called bastard varieties (which are not used for extracting the valuable principles above referred to) *sell at* higher prices in proportion to their resemblance to the *officinal kinds*. Even in cases where they contain no valuable medicinal constituents they are invoiced at 3 to 4 times the price of the other varieties on board the same vessel containing 3 per cent. Now if our object in this law is to discourage the introduction of those articles that are used for the purpose of adulterating medicines, it is manifest that the true interest of all will be served by admitting those only of the bastard varieties that are *equal* to the inferior officinal varieties, particularly as they happen to be at a lower cost and are very abundant." This is dr. Stewart, jan. 9, 1852. The whole of his report to me, a very interesting and able document, i intend publishing, and have delayed it for the purpose of accompanying it with some other matter of the same nature, not yet in hand.

If i understand him correctly, he took entirely opposite ground in the convention, and i certainly shall look with no ordinary interest for some explanation of a change so entire, in one whose position and well earned reputation give him importance and great influence in the final settlement of this matter. What new light has shone upon his path? What new facts has he to offer? I say *final* settlement, because i see by the appointment of a committee to whom the matter was referred, that the whole subject is but laid over. Although the convention negatived the resolution, as it did a *similar* one a year ago in new york, they seem disposed to endow the question with as many lives as are fabled of the cat.

Notwithstanding all the reasoning of the author of the resolution, backed by the eminent professor, and aided by other reasons, thick no doubt as blackberries, you practical men who buy and sell these articles, were not convinced and never will be. They may cry out for "tooth powder," until the demand for dentrifice shall quadruple, and tell us of the legitimate use of carthagena or maracaibo barks; (what is its legitimate use?) All in vain, for it is too well known that the main use of the article is to adulterate the genuine barks. Why does the drug examiner at baltimore, dr. Stewart, say that the "bastard varieties *sell at higher* prices in proportion to their *resemblance to the officinal kinds*?" Why this demand for such as resemble the genuine, but to supply it to the buyers of peruvian bark for the genuine and officinal. There can be no other conclusion. If more proof is wanting i take the remark of the gentleman from new-york, that the "house he was connected with sold large quantities in powder, and the parties purchasing did so knowing its origin." No one could doubt this statement, at least as to the quantity annually purchased, who will go through half-a-dozen drug stores in any of the country villages or small towns any where in our country from maine to louisiana.

He will have offered prime, best quality cinchona bark for 40 to 100 cents almost any where, and in one half the cases the venders believe they are selling what they offer, for they bought it for that. Is this not so, or is it all bought for "tooth powder?" One half the druggists who go to our large cities, buy "pale yellow" and red bark, and never think to enquire for the inferior barks, and once drive these last from our seaboard cities, and we shall have done with them.

You are aware that i have had some opportunity of becoming acquainted with the drug trade of our country, and i assure you that throughout its length and breadth there is more worthless peruvian bark sold and consumed by far than of the genuine, mostly, i hope through ignorance, but many times knowingly on the part of the dealer.

The same that has been said of these false barks, may be said of english rhubarb; when it is not sold for and in the place of turkey, it is used to make powdered turkey out of. But the resolution does not stop short at these two articles, as the discussion seemed to. There is "false jalap" undoubtedly good of its kind, but unfortunately for the buyer the kind is good for nothing, although it makes extract of jalap, that in looks cannot be told from the genuine.

There is also egyptian opium, and a false sarsaparilla and many other important drugs, that should have received the attention of the friends of this resolution, all of which, i beg to assure them, are undoubtedly good of their kind.

But i have written more than i designed by far, as the subject grows upon my hands, though i regard it a very important one, and vitally so to the drug law which lies at the very foundation of all beneficial results to grow out of this association, and the position of the association as to the whole subject is equally important, for if we unfortunately commit ourselves to a wrong principle in the start, and especially upon this standard of purity as applicable to our drug examiners, which is now regarded as a test question by the community at large, we lose all hold upon their confidence, and with it all hope of effecting any good either to ourselves as a profession or to the community in general.

My chief object in addressing you this communication (intended for the new york journal of pharmacy, if you choose so to use it) is to record my experience as differing in toto from those of dr. Stewart and prof. Carson, and to elicit a full discussion of the whole matter. Let us have light! Light! Light enough to settle this question, especially about the barks, for they are the source of this whole contention after all. There must be data enough to be had, upon which to form an opinion, and a correct one as to the medicinal virtues of maracaibo, and carthagena barks, as well as of english rhubarb, false jalap, egyptian opium etc., etc.

I shall be perfectly satisfied if the labors of this committee result in fixing a definite standard of strength, or amount of alkaloids required to be found in barks before consumed for medicine, and therefore admissible under the act, but satisfied at nothing short of this, for till that is done there will never be any uniformity in the action of the law. I had designed to make some remarks upon the requirements of the law and its needed emendation which i must defer to more leisure.

Yours, ETC., c. B. Guthrie.

Memphis, tenn., november 2, 1852.

Introductory lectures are generally very common-place affairs. Custom has prescribed that every year the different medical schools shall be opened with them; and custom, too, has prescribed for them a certain limited range of topics. Year after year, in a hundred places, the same round is gone over, and the same good advice is listened to, and neglected. Dr. Bartlett has broken through all this. He has chosen for the subject of his discourse the character and writings of the father of medicine, and he has illustrated them well and thoroughly. This is not the place for a detailed notice of the lecture. Yet we cannot but call attention to the playful humour, the kindly and genial spirit which set off and enliven its details, and which breathing from the whole air and features of the man, render him one of the most agreeable lecturers to whom we have ever listened.

EXCHANGES.

—hitherto the exchanges of this journal have not been conducted with proper regularity. It has neither been transmitted punctually to other journals, nor have they been received regularly in return. For the future this will be corrected; the journal will be forwarded immediately on its publication; and we hope our contemporaries will observe a like regularity with us.

Lightning Source UK Ltd.
Milton Keynes UK
UKHW010943281222
414514UK00004B/241